Problem Oriented Approaches in Interventional Cardiology

Problem Oriented Approaches in Interventional Cardiology

Edited by

ANTONIO COLOMBO MD
EMO Centro Cuore Columbus, San Raffaele Hospital, Milan, Italy

GORAN STANKOVIC MD
Clinical Center of Serbia, Belgrade, Serbia

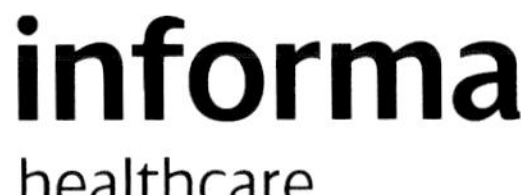

First published in the United Kingdom in 2007 by Informa Healthcare, 4 Park Square, Milton Park, Abingdon, Oxon OX14 4RN. Informa Healthcare is a trading division of Informa UK Ltd. Registered Office: 37/41 Mortimer Street, London W1T 3JH. Registered in England and Wales number 1072954.

Tel: +44 (0)20 7017 6000
Fax: +44 (0)20 7017 6699
Email: info.medicine@tandf.co.uk
Website: www.informahealthcare.com

A CIP record for this book is available from the British Library.
Data available on application

ISBN-10 1 84184 631 7
ISBN-13 978 1 84184 631 6

Distributed in North and South America by
Taylor & Francis
6000 Broken Sound Parkway, NW, (Suite 300)
Boca Raton, FL 33487, USA

Within Continental USA
Tel: 1 (800) 272 7737; Fax: 1 (800) 374 3401
Outside Continental USA
Tel: (561) 994 0555; Fax: (561) 361 6018
Email: orders@crcpress.com

Distributed in the rest of the world by
Thomson Publishing Services
Cheriton House
North Way
Andover, Hampshire SP10 5BE, UK
Tel: +44 (0)1264 332424
Email: tps.tandfsalesorder@thomson.com

Composition by Egerton + Techset

Printed and bound in Spain by Grafos SA Arte Sobre Papel

Contents

Contributors

Flavio Airoldi
Interventional Cardiology Unit
San Raffaele Hospital and EMO Centro Cuore Columbus
Milan
Italy

Babak Azarbal
UCLA School of Medicine
Division of Cardiology
Los Angeles, California
USA

Rade Babic
Institute for Cardiovascular Disease Dedinje
Belgrade
Serbia

Lutz Buellesfeld
HELIOS Heart Center Siegburg
Siegburg
Germany

Qi-Ling Cao
The Congenital Heart Center
Departments of Pediatrics and Medicine
University of Chicago Hospitals
Pritzker School of Medicine
Chicago, Illinois
USA

Alaide Chieffo
Interventional Cardiology Unit
San Raffaele Hospital
Milan
Italy

Antonio Colombo
EMO Centro Cuore Columbus
San Raffaele Hospital
Milan
Italy

Simon Corbett
EMO Centro Cuore Columbus
Milan
Italy

John Cosgrave
EMO Centro Cuore Columbus
Milan
Italy

George Dangas
Centre for Interventional Vascular Therapy
Columbia University Medical Center
New York-Presbyterian Hospital
Cardiovascular Research Foundation
New York, New York
USA

Carlo Di Mario
Department of Clinical Cardiology
Royal Brompton Hospital
National Heart and Lung Institute
Imperial College School of Medicine
London
UK

Konstantinos Dimopoulos
Department of Clinical Cardiology
Royal Brompton Hospital
National Heart and Lung Institute
Imperial College School of Medicine
London
UK

Eric Eeckhout
Centre Hospitalier Universitaire Vaudois
Lausanne
Switzerland

Ted Feldman
Evanston Hospital
Cardiology Division
Evanston, Illinois
USA

Westby G. Fisher
Evanston Hospital
Cardiology Division
Evanston, Illinois
USA

Francisco Garay
The Congenital Heart Center
Departments of Pediatrics and Medicine
University of Chicago Hospitals
Pritzker School of Medicine
Chicago, Illinois
USA

Mohamed Abdel Ghany
Cardiology Department
Mirano Public Hospital
Mirano
Italy

Liviu Ghilencea
Department of Clinical Cardiology
Royal Brompton Hospital
London
UK
Clinic of Cardiology and Internal Medicine
Bucharest Emergency Hospital
Bucharest
Romania

Grégoire Girod
Centre Hospitalier Universitaire Vaudois
Lausanne
Switzerland

Neil Goyal
Department of Medicine, Division of Cardiology
Center for Interventional and Vascular Therapy
Columbia University College of Physicians and Surgeons
New York, New York
USA

Raghava R. Gollapudi
Scripps Clinic Green Hosptial
La Jolla, California
USA

Eberhard Grube
HELIOS Heart Center Siegburg
Siegburg
Germany

Ziyad M. Hijazi
Sections of Pediatrics and Cardiology
University of Chicago Hospitals
Pritzker School of Medicine
Chicago, Illinois
USA

Barry T. Katzen
Baptist Cardiac and Vascular Institute
Miami, Florida
USA

Susheel Kodali
Columbia University Medical Center and the Cardiovascular Research Foundation
New York, New York
USA

Alessio La Manna
Department of Clinical Cardiology
Royal Brompton Hospital
London
UK
Department of Cardiology
Ferrarotto University Hospital
Catania
Italy

Thierry Lefèvre
Institut Cardiovasculaire Paris Sud
Massy
France

Amir Lerman
Division of Cardiovascular Diseases
Mayo College of Medicine
Rochester, Minnesota
USA

Yves Louvard
Institut Cardiovasculaire Paris Sud
Massy
France

Alexandra A. MacLean
Division of Vascular Surgery
The Johns Hopkins Hospital
Baltimore, Maryland
USA

Roxana Mehran
Columbia University Medical Center and the Cardiovascular Research Foundation
New York, New York
USA

Gary S. Mintz
Cardiovascular Research Foundation
Washington, DC
USA

Jeffrey W. Moses
Center for Interventional Vascular Therapy
Columbia University Medical Center
New York, New York
USA

Issam D. Moussa
Department of Medicine, Division of Cardiology
Center for Interventional and Vascular Therapy
Columbia University College of Physicians and Surgeons
New York, New York
USA

Dimitris Nikas
Cardiology Department
Mirano Public Hospital
Mirano
Italy

Eugenia Nikolsky
Rambam Medical Center
Division of Invasive Cardiology
Haifa
Israel

Matthew J. Price
Scripps Clinic Green Hosptial
La Jolla, California
USA

Bernhard Reimers
Cardiology Department
Mirano Hospital
Mirano
Italy

Frank Renders
Centre Hospitalier Universitaire Vaudois
Lausanne
Switzerland

Christan Roguelov
Centre Hospitalier Universitaire Vaudois
Lausanne
Switzerland

Asu Rustemli
Columbia University Medical Center and the Cardiovascular Research Foundation
Department of Medicine
Division of Cardiology
New York, New York
USA

Horst Sievert
Cardiovascular Center Frankfurt
Sankt Katharinen Hospital
Frankfurt
Germany

Gregg W. Stone
Columbia University Medical Center and the Cardiovascular Research Foundation
New York, New York
USA

Jennifer Sugita
Cardiovascular Center Frankfurt
Sankt Katharinen Hospital
Frankfurt
Germany

Paul S. Teirstein
Scripps Clinic Green Hosptial
La Jolla, California
USA

Swee Guan Teo
HELIOS Heart Center Siegburg
Siegburg
Germany

Jonathan Tobis
UCLA School of Medicine
Division of Cardiology
Los Angeles, California
USA

Giora Weisz
Center for Interventional Vascular Therapy
Columbia University Medical Center
New York, New York
USA

Steven D. Wolff
Columbia University Medical Center and the Cardiovascular Research Foundation
Department of Medicine
Division of Cardiology
New York, New York
USA

Preface

We think we have outlined in this book a mature technical description for the usage of drug-eluting stents. Despite all the worrisome information about drug-eluting stents, I remain convinced that these devices represent a major advance in the treatment of coronary artery disease. Even though the principles of evidence-based medicine must remain second to providing hard data, drug-eluting stents are saving lives!

Perhaps the problem is that these devices are such powerful tools that we are often so enthused by the lovely angiographic result that we do not give sufficient attention to proper patient selection or to optimal stent implantation. We are now performing procedures with drug-eluting stents that we never dreamed of doing a few years ago. The low late loss is sometimes used as justification for accepting sub-optimal results, and this may be one of the problems.

Instead of defining how drug-eluting stents should be implanted, in this book we are trying to give some direction. I write this preface when the book is nearly in print and already I would like to add new information and make additional changes. If I can but highlight two important points this book hopes to make, I would stress the value of optimal stent deployment and the value of intravascular ultrasound. Maybe it is now time to begin another book about optimal drug-eluting stent implantation with intravascular ultrasound guidance. I can already imagine how excited Goran Stankovic will be about this new task, only a few weeks after having completed the current book.

More importantly I would like to express my thanks to all the contributors who worked so hard and productively to deliver all the chapters in time. We all know how easy is to say yes when a colleague asks about writing a chapter in a new book and how demanding it is to realize that the deadline is looming and so much work still needs to be done. All the co-authors have been able to meet the deadline and to deliver enjoyable and useful write-ups.

I am hopeful everybody will find the time spent reading this book a useful experience and I hope many patients will benefit from the efforts all the contributors have put into this work.

Antonio Colombo

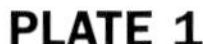

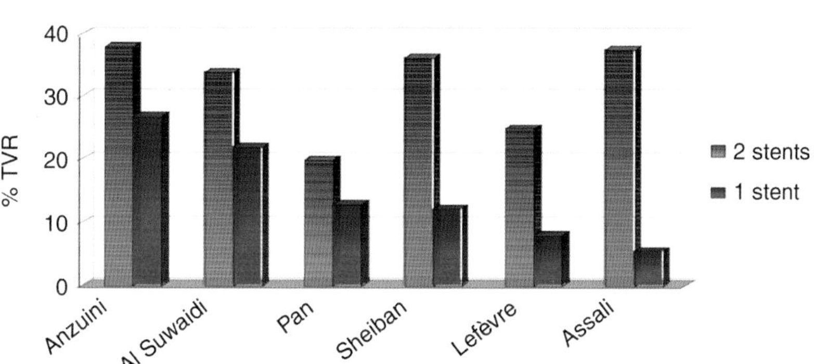

Figure 4-14 Target vessel revascularization rates in studies comparing two stent strategy vs. single stent strategy with bare metal stents. *Abbreviation*: TVR, target vessel revascularization.

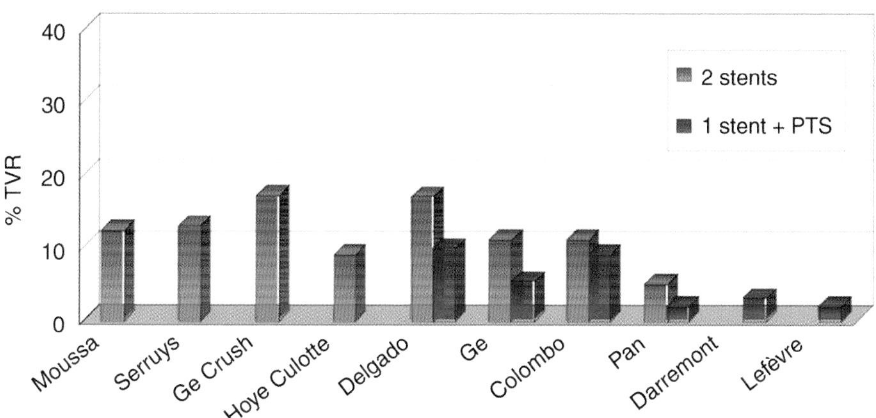

Figure 4-15 Target vessel revascularization rates in studies comparing two stent strategy versus single stent strategy with drug-eluting stents. *Abbreviations:* PTS, provisional T stenting; TVR, target vessel revascularization.

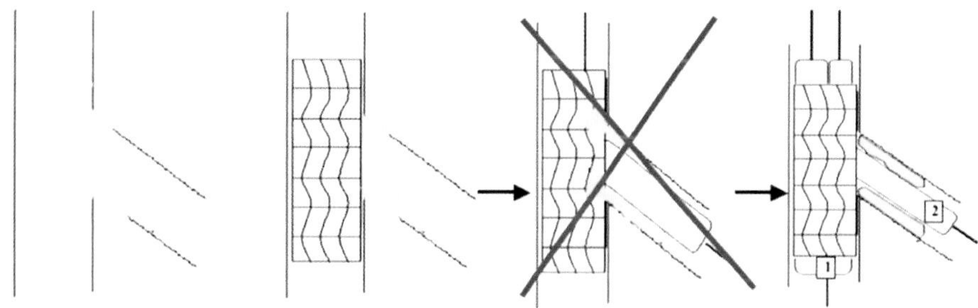

Figure 4-18 Plaque shifting toward the main branch following side branch balloon inflation.

PLATE 2

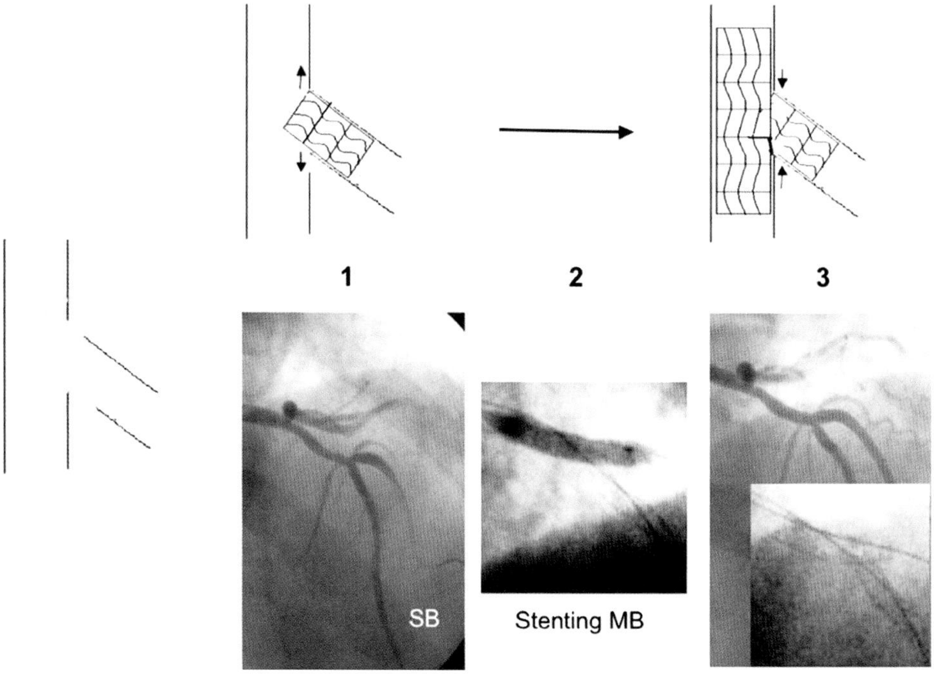

Figure 4-19 Plaque shifting toward the main branch following initial stent deployment in the side branch.

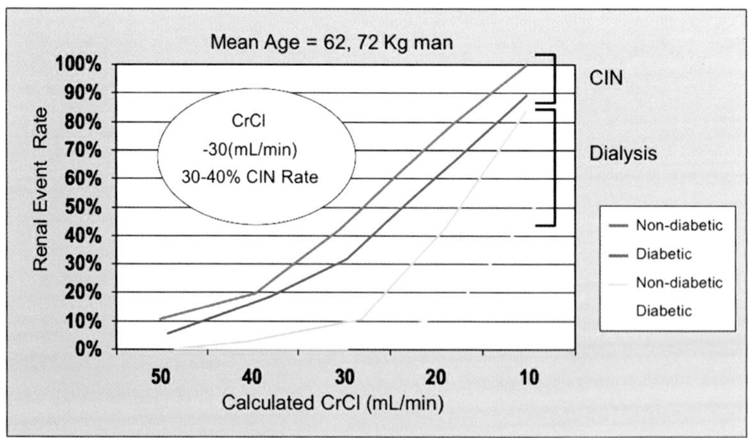

Figure 12-1 Validated risk of acute renal failure requiring dialysis after diagnostic angiography and/or angioplasty. A mean contrast dose of 250 mL and a mean age of 65 years is assumed. *Abbreviations*: CrCl, creatinine clearance; CIN, contrast induced nephropathy. *Source*: From Ref. 23.

PLATE 3

(A)

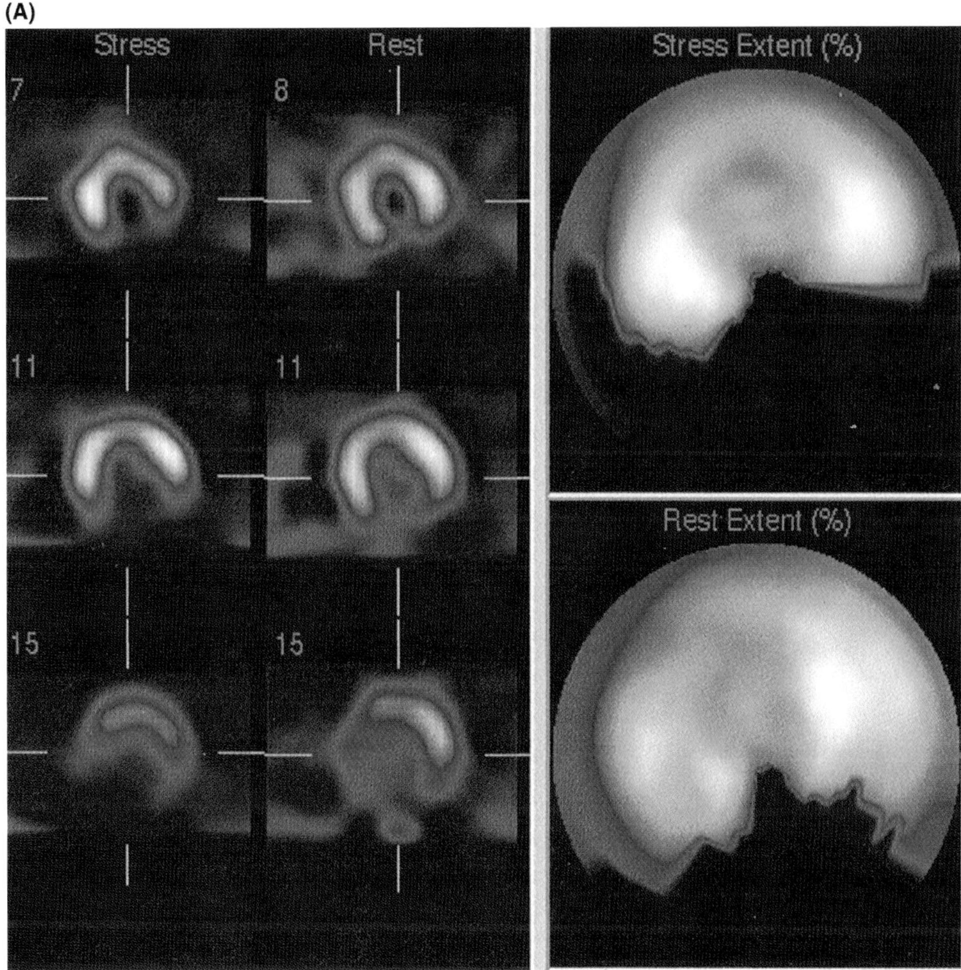

Figure 15-4 (**A**) A SPECT stress perfusion study showing an inferior infarct with mild peri-infarct ischemia.

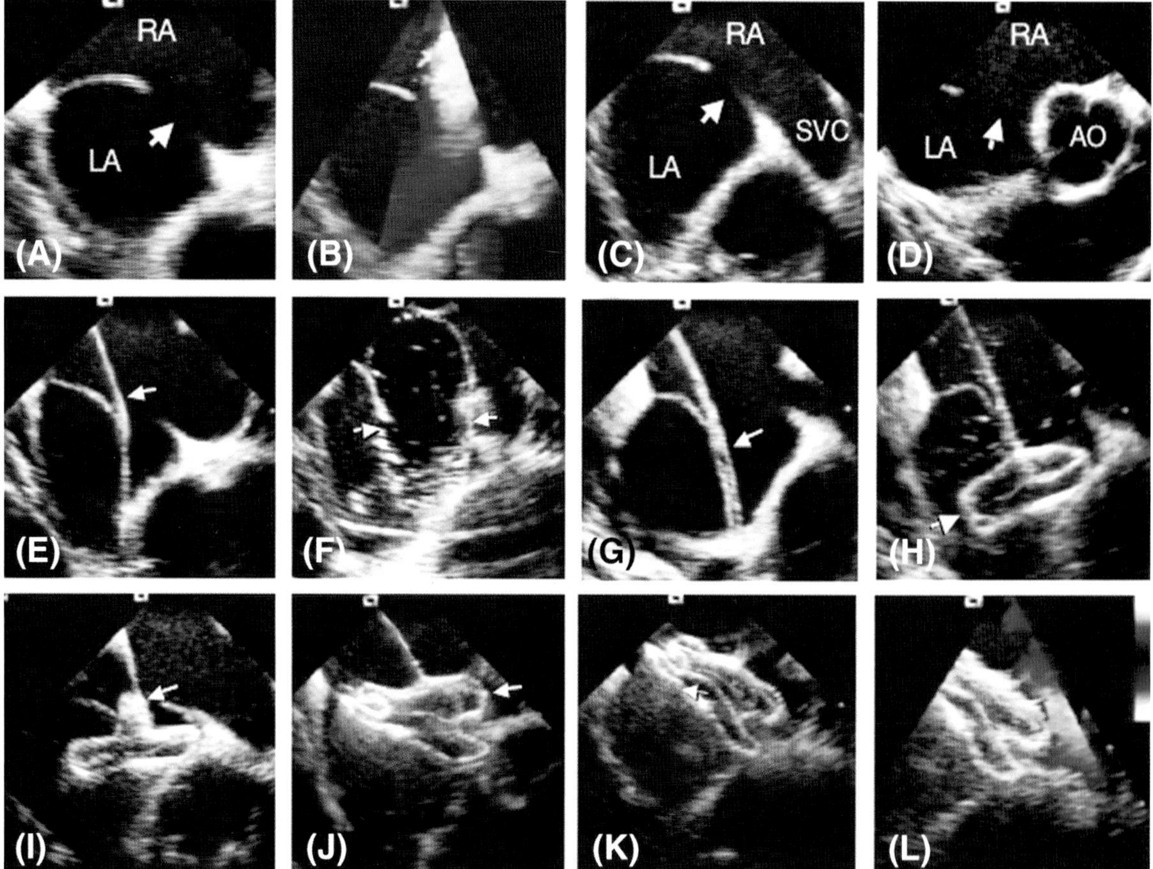

Figure 19-2 Intracardiac echocardiographic (ICE) images in a 42-year-old female patient with a 24 mm secundum atrial septal defect (ASD) as measured by ICE. (**A,B**) Septal view without and with color Doppler demonstrating the ASD (*arrow*) and left to right shunt. (**C**) Bicaval long axis view demonstrating the superior and inferior rims and the defect (*arrow*). (**D**) Short axis view demonstrating the absence of anterior rim, good posterior rim, and the ASD (*arrow*). (**E**) Passage of the guide wire (*arrow*) through the ASD to the left atrium to the left upper pulmonary vein. (**F**) The sizing balloon when left to right shunt ceased indicating the "stop-flow" diameter (*arrows*) of the defect. (**G**) Passage of the delivery sheath (*arrow*) through the defect to the left upper pulmonary vein. (**H**) Deployment of the left atrial disk (*arrow*) of a 30-mm Amplatzer® septal occluder in the left atrium. (**I**) Deployment of the connecting waist (*arrow*) in the defect. (**J**) Deployment of the right atrial disk (*arrow*) in the right atrium. (**K**) After the device has been released indicating good device position. (**L**) Bicaval view after the device has been released indicating good device position and no shunt. *Abbreviations*: LA, left atrium; RA, right atrium; SVC, superior vena cava; AO, aortic valve.

1

Prevention and treatment of procedural complications

Eric Eeckhout, Amir Lerman, Christan Roguelov, Grégoire Girod, and Frank Renders

- **Step 1: Know your patient • Step 2: Assess the indication for percutaneous coronary intervention**
- **Step 3: Judge the intrinsic risk of the intervention • Step 4: Predefine your strategy**
- **Step 5: Inform and obtain a written/documented consent from your patient • Step 6: Secure vascular access • Step 7: Work according to the predefined strategy; try to keep it simple; remain calm, patient, and alert • Step 8: Communicate with and observe your patient throughout the procedure**
- **Step 9: Know how to treat and anticipate the most common complications**
- **Step 10: Look for the hidden complication • Step 11: Stop in "peace" • Conclusion**

In the field of interventional cardiology, safety and long-term efficacy are at present the two most important goals when performing percutaneous coronary intervention (PCI). Technology has come a long way to improve the long-term outcomes of patients, although complications are mostly due to human errors and seldom because of technology failure. Operator's expertise is a key element in the prevention of complications. Therefore, education and training of future professionals are essential. The objective of this chapter is to propose a stepwise checklist-based safety approach to PCI, to discuss the most common complications occurring during PCI, and to provide recommendations in anticipating and handling them in a philosophical rather than dogmatic perspective.

STEP 1: KNOW YOUR PATIENT

He who intervenes should know his patient very well.

A careful study of the patient's records, including medical history, pertinent laboratory tests, and indication for diagnostic angiography, cannot be omitted before scrubbing in. Classically, five baseline questions always come back: (*i*) Does the patient have a history of contrast reactions and, if so, has it been adequately addressed? (*ii*) Can hemostasis be assured (once the introducer is in place)? (*iii*) What is the renal function level and have potential problems been anticipated (e.g., stopping nephrotoxic drugs, fluid administration)? (*iv*) Has the diabetic patient been prepared according to standard practice (i.e., stopping metformin)? (*v*) Has the vascular access been defined and prepared accordingly (e.g., Allen test for radial approach, vascular examination for femoral approach)? These items seem trivial and very easy to accomplish; unfortunately, however daily practice teaches us that they are often neglected.

Step 1: Know your patient

- Carefully review the patient's records.
- Check and anticipate:
  - Potential contrast reaction
  - Hemostasis
  - Renal dysfunction
  - Potential problems with diabetics
  - Patency of vascular access route

STEP 2: ASSESS THE INDICATION FOR PERCUTANEOUS CORONARY INTERVENTION

The only objective of PCI is clinical benefit for the patient.

The European Society of Cardiology and the American Heart Association–American College of Cardiology (AHA/ACC) have edited and updated the guidelines for PCI in 2004 and 2005, respectively. In view of the many possible reasons one might have to perform PCI in a given patient, it is important to remember that PCI is intended to improve symptoms and potentially also prognosis. Indirect evidence or objective proof of ischemia and/or myocardial viability is an essential prerequisite for PCI. In the era of ad hoc interventions and in busy programs, one might be seduced to overlook this and be victimized by the oculo-stenotic reflex. Except in cases of primary PCI for acute myocardial infarction, our interventions mostly palliate patients, which of course, if lasting, is already a great achievement. Today, the balance between surgery and PCI for complex and multivessel coronary artery disease is shifting in favor of the latter, at least in terms of volume. The cardiologist is the gatekeeper to intervention, and the large majority of patients prefer PCI as a first intervention for obvious reasons. Still, it is at present unclear if sequential drug-eluting stent placement improves survival in these patients to the same extent as surgery, especially in diabetics.

The decision to propose PCI or surgery to a given patient should be guided by the estimated risk and success rate of the selected strategy. This important decision should be made before informing the patient. If the indication is clear, if the interventional risk low or acceptable given the clinical condition, and if the strategy paved to success, the operator should proceed with informing the patient.

Step 2: Assess the PCI Indication

- Clinical benefit is the primary objective of PCI.

STEP 3: JUDGE THE INTRINSIC RISK OF THE INTERVENTION

Basic clinical, hemodynamic, and angiographic features should be used for risk assessment.

In the surgical field, precise risk scores (Euroscore, Parsonnet) have been developed to estimate the early mortality hazard related to the intervention. Identical risk models have been published in interventional cardiology. They take into account clinical, hemodynamic, and angiographic features and can therefore be calculated from a careful review of the patient's records and cine-images. Classical clinical and hemodynamic features include: age, diabetes, degree of emergency, peripheral vascular disease, and left ventricular dysfunction with shock in particular.

The 1990 updated AHA/ACC lesion classification included 11 angiographic variables to predict procedural success and risk up to a certain extent. More accurate and recent classifications have been provided by other authors and by the Society for Cardiac Angiography and Interventions. Actual angiographic determinants for increased complications are saphenous vein graft and left main lesions, inability to protect side branches, bifurcation lesions, large thrombus burden, important calcifications, and angulations >45°.

Interventional risk scores such as the model can be used to make a global risk assessment that can be compared to a surgical score. Particularly, patients with anatomy at risk require a clear predefined strategy to anticipate and minimize complications.

Step 3: Judge the interventional risk

- Parameters for risk models:
  - Clinical
  - Hemodynamic
  - Angiographic
- Integrate your risk assessment in your predefined strategy.

STEP 4: PREDEFINE YOUR STRATEGY

An optimal strategy helps you through half the procedure.

1. Guiding catheters are the "back-bone" of interventional cardiologists. First they transport wires, balloons, stents, and potentially frenzy devices to the coronary circulation. Second, they allow invasive arterial pressure measurement and consequently hemodynamic monitoring. Third, they regulate the quality of contrast injections.

   At the start of the procedure, the operator has to balance the advantages and disadvantages of a larger sized guiding catheter. All of the above are easier to accomplish with a larger guiding catheter but it comes with a higher bleeding risk. Still, getting stuck in a 0.068-in. 6 French guiding catheter, although unlikely with low profile balloons and stents, in a complex bifurcation lesion with loss of wire access can turn into a nightmare. Another crucial function of guiding catheters is support. As a rule, increased support equals more aggression and increased risk for guiding catheter-induced coronary dissections. Personal experience as well as reviews indicate that, besides perforations of any kind, this is the most reported complication. Again, the operators need to balance their decision at the level of support. Proper alignment of the extra backup guiding catheter is crucial to diminish the risk for dissection. A slight LAO cranial view (e.g., 10°–10°) is optimal for the right coronary artery, and alignment can mostly be achieved by further clockwise rotation after initial intubation of the ostium. For the left system, alignment depends on the size, orientation, and length of the left main artery and can be judged in most classical incidences. Opposite to more or less "passive" support stands "active" support—deep intubation with softer and thinner guiding catheters. The choice depends on the trainer's and operator's preferences. Proper alignment, particularly for active support is a major safety issue to ensure smooth transition from catheter to vessel wall.
2. The guidewire is the extention of the guiding catheter beyond the level of the lesion. Therefore, support besides torque control, steerability, flexibility, and crossibility are major considerations in guidewire choice. There is an excellent variety of wires available depending on the difficulty of access or the indication for PCI (e.g., the whole spectrum of wires for chronic total occlusion). Besides a classical workhorse wire, a modern catheterization facility should have a variety of wires on hand for particular indications.
3. The predefined strategy should optimally be decided up to the level of the balloon and stent. The issue of direct stenting is beyond the scope of this chapter. Briefly, a careful angiographic study allows proper selection of candidates for direct stenting.
4. The interventional strategy should consider the need for intra-aortic balloon counter pulsation or cardiac assist devices right from the start and not when hemodynamic collapse occurs.
5. Routine surgical backup in current PCI practice is questionable. Still, depending on the myocardium at risk and the anticipated difficulty of the procedure, "true surgical-back" with a fully available and informed surgical team is essential.
6. Finally, the strategy should include pharmacotherapy including monitoring of anticoagulation, and the need for inotrope support and for platelet glycoprotein IIb/IIIa receptor antagonists.

We equate this predefined strategy to a "flight plan prior to take-off." In the era of ad hoc PCI,

Step 4: Predefine your strategy

- Ad-hoc PCI-staged or deferred?
- Interventional strategy:
  - Guiding catheter: size and curve?
  - Guidewire(s)?
  - Direct stenting?
  - IABP-assist device?
  - Need for surgical back-up?
  - Which pharmacotherapy?
- Know your own boundaries!

where information and consent forms have been made available to the patient prior to diagnostic catheterization, both strategic evaluation and risk assessment allow selection of the best candidates for immediate PCI. Other patients will need a more profound discussion prior to PCI. Finally, it may be judged wise to stage procedures in patients with multivessel disease.

STEP 5: INFORM AND OBTAIN A WRITTEN/DOCUMENTED CONSENT FROM YOUR PATIENT

Do not decide for but with your patient.

At present, it is unconscionable to start a PCI procedure without clear and objective information to the patient (or family, and/or responsible physician). This should include a description of the potential risks, complications, and also benefits of the procedure. The therapeutic alternatives (in particular, surgical and/or medical therapy) should be stated and compared to PCI. It is also of utmost importance to inform them about the expected long-term outcome. Finally, a written/signed informed consent must be available from the patient (or the patient representative) as proof of adequate transmission of information.

Step 5: Informed consent

- Inform about risk, complications, and benefit.
- Describe the therapeutic alternatives.
- Inform about the expected long-term outcome.
- Obtain a written/signed informed consent.

STEP 6: SECURE VASCULAR ACCESS

Puncture and puncture well.

It is now obvious that major bleeding complications at puncture sites impair prognosis in patients undergoing PCI. Therefore, the quality of vascular access cannot be neglected.

The common femoral artery is the most frequent access site for PCI. Review of adequate puncture techniques is beyond the scope of this chapter, still a few points need to be stressed: (*i*) Avoid aggressive, repetitive, and transvascular punctures. (*ii*) ensure hemostasis between failed attempts, and seek help from a colleague when necessary. (*iii*) In case of complications (retrograde dissections) consider, particularly in elective interventions, stopping the procedure. (*iv*) Do not continue your procedure unless you have hemostasis, even with an introducer in place. (*v*) Be extremely careful and consider a radial approach in certain patients at risk, i.e., those with diffuse disease of the aortic wall or history of previous cholesterol embolism or severe peripheral vascular disease. (*vi*) Finally, the optimal entry site into the common femoral artery is located at the level of the head of the femoral bone (easily visible on fluoroscopy). Again, all this information is basic but often neglected.

The radial approach is an elegant alternative to femoral access. Excellent miniaturized puncture kits are now available, largely facilitating the technique, which is particularly indicated in those patients at risk for bleeding or other complications at the femoral site; e.g., severe obesity, excessive or cumulative use of antiplatelet agents, anticoagulation, fibrinolysis, hypertension, low body weight, peripheral vascular disease, and extreme tortuosity of the femoral and ileac axes. Nevertheless, procedural times and radiation hazard tend to be slightly higher. Complications at the radial site are potentially more dangerous and training is again crucial to minimize this. Hands-on transradial training is available and we strongly recommended such a training course before embarking in this technology. At minimum at least one operator in the team should be familiar with the radial access.

Step 6: Secure vascular access

- Hit the artery from the first stick.
- Obtain hemostasis between failed attempts and/or seek help.
- Do not continue the procedure in case of bleeding, even with the introducer in place.
- At least one operator on the team should be familar with the radial approach.

STEP 7: WORK ACCORDING TO THE PREDEFINED STRATEGY; TRY TO KEEP IT SIMPLE; REMAIN CALM, PATIENT, AND ALERT

Work out your strategy, step by step.

In the "executive" phase, the operator will develop the intended strategy. This is the moment of truth, as the predefined strategy will be challenged for its appropriateness. In general, "routine PCI" cases mostly work out fine. Actually, they still apply for the vast majority of interventions. One may consider performing the more difficult cases with two operators who can interact and adapt if the strategy fails. In an attempt to overcome failure, work from simple to complex and try to stay calm and patient. Again, this can be achieved more easily by two operators, shifting hands throughout the procedure. As mentioned previously, a careful study of angiographic images sets the tone for the difficulty of a particular intervention. Failure should not lead to heroic attempts or use of techniques the operator is not comfortable with. The operator and the team should know their own limitations and ask for help or refrain from further attempts. Many complications occur at this later stage where a tired and less alert team applies a more aggressive and often less well-known strategy.

To be alert, the interventionalist needs to be fit and "in good shape." In view of the overall activity of many interventional cardiologists, this may become an issue of concern for the future. A classical primary PCI program in an average-sized hospital (with less than four or five operators) plus daily lab activity and social and/or family events on the weekend (to compensate) may lead to chronic fatigue. At least in civil aviation this situation is considered unacceptable.

Step 7: Work according to strategy

- Apply your intended strategy.
- Consider working with two operators depending on the anticipated difficulty.
- Work from simple to more complex.
- Remain calm and patient.
- To be alert you need to be fit!

STEP 8: COMMUNICATE WITH AND OBSERVE YOUR PATIENT THROUGHOUT THE PROCEDURE

The patient's overall well being is based on empathy and confidence.

Most patients are barely sedated during intervention and some may be particularly sensitive to any conversation occurring in the lab. With few exceptions, an anesthesiologist is not present during the procedure. For this reason, the operator, the technicians, and the nursing staff should regularly communicate with patients for any concerns they may have. These may be technical questions in relation to the intervention but mostly and particularly during long procedures, patients may complain of fatigue, fear, and/or back pain. It is essential to foresee and manage these issues: (*i*) risk for vagal reactions, which are not all benign (e.g., in the hemodynamically unstable patient) and (*ii*) a suffering patient stresses most operators and puts their alertness at risk.

Step 8: Communicate and observe

- Regularly communicate and observe the patient.
- Avoid unrelated conversations in the lab during the intervention.
- Anticipate and/or promptly treat any discomfort.

STEP 9: KNOW HOW TO TREAT AND ANTICIPATE THE MOST COMMON COMPLICATIONS

Don't repeat the old ones and learn from the new ones.

The most commonly reported complications are related to vascular access problems, guiding catheter or wireinduced aorto-coronary and coronary dissections, critical wire loss across a lesion, perforation, and foreign body loss. All of these complications are mostly related to human error.

The vascular access issue has been discussed previously.

Aorto-coronary or near ostial coronary dissections induced by catheters are a classical complication and are quite often associated with loss of wire access to the true lumen. The right coronary artery mostly behaves differently from the left with risk for potential collapse of the true lumen. In case of ostial right coronary artery occlusion, it is advised to use a conventional right Judkins guiding catheter in order to stay slightly out of the ostium versus trying to find the true lumen with a soft floppy wire. Occasionally, a wire can be hooked into a small atrial branch to stabilize the guiding catheter. It is still unclear and a case-to-case decision must be made for surgery if PCI persistently fails. If a stent has been placed previously in a more distal segment of the artery and the dissection occurred proximally to the stent, the false lumen definitely stops at the stent entry site, leaving a limited time for the operator to try and regain the true lumen from the ostium and beyond the stent.

Collapse of the left main artery is less frequent and often a more or less complex stenting strategy can solve the problem. Again, loss of wire access following guiding catheter-induced dissections might be considered a professional mistake, but experience indicates that this occurs quite frequently. On occasion, the wire keeps the true lumen partially open and collapse of the neglected dissection occurs after pulling it out. The only solution is rewiring of the true lumen with soft wires and stenting of the dissection entry site. Intravascular ultrasound can be extremely helpful in cases where the angiogram does not provide sufficient information. Surgery should be considered for persistent failure, depending on the extent of ongoing transmural ischemia.

Dissections extending into the aortic wall have a dramatic angiographic appearance. Often, they can be treated by conventional or covered stent implantation to be expanded at low pressure. Surgery is rarely needed and is characterized by high mortality rates. Transesophageal echocardiography (and if needed computed tomography) enables judgment of the extent of the dissection and the need for surgery. Tamponade can further complicate the clinical picture and should be addressed promptly by either percutaneous or surgical means.

Vascular perforation is a chapter on its own and far beyond the scope of this chapter. Briefly, not all perforations are evident at first sight. Frequently overlooked are the greyish spots occurring during primary PCI at the tip of a hydrophilic wire while on a cocktail of full anticoagulation and platelet glycoprotein IIb/IIIa receptor antagonists. This may lead to delayed tamponade a few hours after the patient has returned to the ward. Prompt recognition and counterbalance of the therapeutic effect of these drugs is recommended. On the other hand, it is also important to realize that not all perforations require a covered stent. One should classify and quantify the perforation, continuously monitor hemodynamics, and identify the exit and destination of the perforation. Frank rupture into the pericardial cavity with immediate hemodynamic collapse fundamentally differs from a perforation into the right ventricle or a perimyocardial hematoma. The first will require prompt balloon angioplasty to seal the exit, pericardial drainage, and potential covered stent implantation. The latter may be treated either by heparin reversal and/or prolonged balloon inflation or no specific therapy at all.

Progress in crimping technology explains why stent loss has become relatively rare. Stents slipping of the balloon in the coronary circulation (especially if lost distally with a wire across) can probably best be left in situ and gradually expanded from low profile to normal ballooning. Capturing by a variety of wiring or snaring techniques can be considered for those stents lost more proximally, bearing in mind the risk of damage to the proximal vessel wall. Stents pulled out from the coronary artery on the wire (e.g., captured by an inflated small balloon) should be taken down to the iliac level and retrieved by a homo- or contralateral snaring technique.

Unfortunately, trial and error goes hand-in-hand with expertise. It is often said that if one has not had a particular complication, it will occur with time and more experience. The hospital morbidity–mortality conferences, local staff meetings, and case review sessions on a local or international level are of educational value, demonstrating a palette of these complications and their management.

Step 9: Know how to treat common complications
• Vascular access injury • Guiding catheter or wire induced dissections at the aorto-coronary or coronary level • Perforation • Foreign body loss • Critical wire loss accross a lesion

STEP 10: LOOK FOR THE HIDDEN COMPLICATION

Look and think twice and, if needed, seek advice.

During intervention, the clinical status of the patient may deteriorate without any clear explanation. Potential causes may include aortic dissection, contrast reactions, retroperitoneal bleeding, and others. It is imperative to take adequate diagnostic and therapeutic measures before proceeding further with the intervention. It is strongly advocated to seek advice from another or a more experienced operator. A fresh look into the whole clinical picture by a third person can be lifesaving.

Step 10: Look for the hidden complication
• The patient is always right—look and think twice for the clue. • Ask advice from a third person for a new and fresh look.

STEP 11: STOP IN "PEACE"

Take a last look at the global picture.

It is again trivial to mention that at least two orthogonal views with high quality images are required to make a final judgment of the angiographic result. Especially in this era of drug-eluting stents, we believe that proper postdilation (with short noncompliant balloons) is part of good clinical practice. Intrastent haziness should be clarified, diagnosed, and may need a control angiography. Important in- or outflow dissections cannot be left untreated. Intravascular ultrasound is particularly helpful in this situation.

A variety of femoral vascular closure devices are available. In experienced hands, they are excellent tools that increase the patient's comfort. They should only be used by well-trained operators in patients without any contraindication for their use.

Most patients leave the hospital the day following the intervention. This is the ideal occasion to check the secondary prevention program. Furthermore, the importance of antiplatelet therapy should be clearly explained to the patient (and eventually to the referring physician), as premature discontinuation has now clearly been associated with an increased mortality. It is imperative that the patient has fully realise the crucial role of these drugs and lifestyle recommendations.

Step 11: Stop in "peace"
• Obtain excellent angiographic images for a final judgment. • Do not leave angiographic uncertainties unsolved. • Ensure a secondary prevention program. • Stress the crucial role of the dual antiplatelet therapy.

CONCLUSION

To avoid and manage complications during PCI, risk assessment and a predefined stepwise strategy are crucial. The operator and the team should be aware of their boundaries and stay alert and calm throughout the procedure. They should be able to treat the most common complications with the necessary equipment and backup. During complex procedures especially, the whole team should not be focusing on the angiographic images alone. Procedural success in itself is a great achievement, but the final objective is to combine this with a well-considered secondary cardiovascular prevention.

2

Coronary guidewires

Antonio Colombo, Rade Babic, and Simon Corbett

The history and development of guidewires closely follows that of coronary angioplasty. The original Gruentzig balloon was equipped with a rudimentary fixed wire for better direction and alignment, but it did not provide real steerability (1). The subsequent development of the independent, removable guidewire system (2) and the steerable guidewire (3) were vital determinants of interventional success and improvement in safety.

Coronary guidewires are designed with the following functions in mind: to track through the vessel, to access the lesion, to cross it atraumatically, to steer into or away from side branches, and to provide device delivery support and unhindered device movement. Thus, optimal wire selection may make the difference between procedural success and failure. With this in mind, we feel confident to further extend the remark of Cournand in his Nobel lecture (4): "the cardiac catheter was ... the key in the lock" to "nowadays, the coronary guidewire is the master key to all locks."

In this chapter we discuss our approach to wire selection and describe our experience with what we consider to be the major categories of contemporary wires. We do not imply that what follows is an exhaustive description of all the currently available wires, as even a brief perusal of equipment catalogs reveals a potentially bewildering array of wires. However, on closer inspection, it can be relatively easily appreciated that there is a much smaller number of categories of wires designed for particular tasks and lesion subsets than the vast majority of wires fall into, and we hope to provide a comprehensive discussion of these. Finally, we must also acknowledge that for many operators, ourselves included, day-to-day choice of wires is often influenced by other factors such as previous experience and familiarity with particular wires and manufacturers, not to mention what equipment is actually stocked on the shelves in the catheter lab. If we, therefore, appear to give undue prominence to particular products, then that is because this chapter intentionally reflects our actual practice and experience rather than any underlying conflict of interest.

Finally, we have deliberately avoided discussing rarely used wires (such as neurological wires) or specific "tricks" where guidewires play another role, such as anchoring the guiding catheter, use in "focused force angioplasty"(5), as well as temporary pacing (6–8) and intracoronary echocardiography (ECG) recording (6), since we consider these to be beyond the scope of this chapter.

BASIC GUIDEWIRE STRUCTURE

Knowledge of the basic structure and construction details of guidewires is important to enable better comprehension of their characteristics and performance, allowing their full potential to be realized.

There are three main components of guidewire design: central core, outer covering, and flexible distal tip. The wire tip may be further subdivided into spring coil and short distal tip weld. On the top of these structural components, all guidewires have a specific surface coating applied (Fig. 1).

The central core is the longest portion of the guidewire. It is the stiff part of the wire and tapers distally to a variable extent in different wires. In two-piece core wires, the distal part of the core does not reach the distal tip of the wire, and is supplemented by the shaping (or forming) ribbon, which extends to the distal tip. In one-piece core wires the tapered core itself reaches the distal tip weld. The two-piece design provides easy shaping and durable shape memory, while the one-piece wires provide better force transmission to the tip and greater "tactile response" for the operator.

Guidewire central cores have traditionally been manufactured from stainless steel, but nitinol or similar proprietary elastic nickel titanium alloys are increasingly being used. Stainless steel provides superior torque characteristics, can deliver more push, and provides good shapeability of the tip in core-to-tip design wires. However, stainless steel guidewires are more susceptible to kinking. A proprietary modification of stainless steel called Durasteel® is employed as the core material of certain wires (e.g., Whisper®, Abbott Vascular/Guidant, Santa Clara, CA, and PT²®, Boston Scientific, Natick, MA) and is said to offer better tip shape retention and durability. With its greater elastic properties, nitinol is pliable yet remains supportive, albeit with less torquability than stainless steel. In addition, nitinol guidewires are generally considered kink resistant and have a tendency to return to their original shape, making them potentially less susceptible to deformation during prolonged use.

Some guidewires have a composite core design, employing stainless steel for the longer proximal part within the wire shaft, and a more elastic alloy at the tapered distal part within the wire tip, such as nitinol Runthrough® NS (Terumo Medical Corp., Somerset, NJ) or Elastinite® (BMW Universal, Abbott Vascular/ Guidant, Santa Clara, CA).

The outer covering on the central core is designed to keep the overall diameter consistent (typically 0.014 in. or 0.36 mm), complementing the core's physical properties and also providing a smooth and noninteractive surface. Guidewires may be categorized into two types according to the material used for the covering: polymer sleeve or metal coil. The majority of wires have metal coils, while a minority have full polymer cover to the tip such as the Whisper wire, PT² wires, and the Shinobi® wires (Cordis, Johnson & Johnson, Miami, FL). The smooth nature of polymer sleeves means that they provide less tactile feedback to the operator as compared to metal coil wires. In addition, all polymer sleeve guidewires are hydrophilic, a property that carries both advantages and disadvantages, as will be discussed later. Metal coils, in addition to providing better tactile feedback, also tend to provide better radio-opacity.

The distal tip is a flexible, radio-opaque part of the wire, often considered as its "business

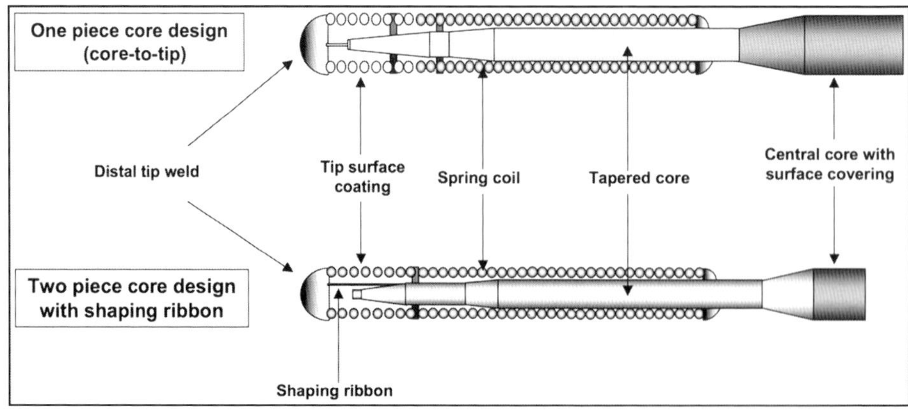

Figure 1 Components of guidewire construction.

end." It usually consists of spring coil extending from the distal untapered part of the central core toward the distal tip weld. It integrates the tapered core barrel, as well as the shaping ribbon in two-piece wire designs. This spring coil may be of variable length from 1 to 25 cm, with the radio-opaque section located at its terminal end. The distal tip weld is a short (up to 2 mm) compact cap forming the true distal end of the wire and is designed to minimize trauma while the wire is traversing the vessel.

Radio-opacity is an integral feature of guidewire design, being important for adequate visualization of the wire tip in the vessel. The length of the radio-opaque section varies from wire to wire, although the distal tip portion is always radio-opaque (usually of the order of 2–3 cm, and up to 30 cm at maximum). Some wires have additional radio-opaque reference markers, which allow the operator to measure longitudinal distances within the vessel of interest.

All guidewires are manufactured with a surface coating, which reduces friction and facilitates trackability, as well as reducing interaction with platelets and thrombogenicity. This surface covering must be chemically stable, biocompatible, thermo-resistant, and durable during sterilization. The most commonly used surface coating materials are: PTFE (Teflon®), fluororesin, medical-grade silicone, and proprietary hydrophilic coating. Most wires are coated by PTFE or fluororesin over the proximal shaft and by silicone or hydrophilic coating at the distal tip segment. Hydrophilic wires require hydration by submersion in water. The coating thereby absorbs moisture, becoming very lubricious and slippery. Medical-grade silicone coating is less lubricious, while PTFE offers the lowest degree of lubricity. Fluororesin is commonly used for covering wire shafts, and provides low friction, with good durability and biocompatibility.

Since the advent of monorail technology, most wires are now 185 to 190 cm long, but 300 cm wires are available if over-the-wire equipment is to be used. Most manufacturers also provide detachable extensions, which lengthen 185 to 190 cm wires for over-the-wire use, if necessary. Besides extending a standard length wire that is already positioned across a lesion, other ways to exchange an over-the-wire balloon without sacrificing its position include: "flying exchange" (9) by applying contrast/saline injection from the inflation device at high pressure (14 bar) through the central lumen of the balloon, use of exchange devices such as the Magnet® (Boston Scientific, Natick, MA), using the back end of a regular coronary wire (10), or cutting the balloon shaft during its removal, with two cuts usually being sufficient (11).

GUIDEWIRE CHARACTERISTICS

While each individual proprietary wire has its own characteristics dependent on its construction and composition, all wires can be considered as having or providing each of the following fundamental properties: flexibility/stiffness, supportability, torquability, lubricity, shapeability, and shaping memory.

It should be noted that with specific in-vitro laboratory testing, it is possible to derive reproducible quantitative measures for most of these guidewire properties. These data are occasionally used for benchmark testing and comparison of different wire brands and modes, particularly for marketing purposes. Nevertheless, in day-to-day practice we think that subjective assessment of these properties is often of greater value in informing one's personal experience and approach to wire selection.

Flexibility/stiffness

Flexibility/stiffness is the key determinant of tip strength. Flexible wires are soft and generally considered atraumatic. As stiffness increases, they become less flexible and potentially more traumatic. This property is directly related to the design and construction of the distal portion of the central core and the distal tip. It is also the basis of commercial labeling of guidewires as extra-floppy/light, floppy/soft, medium/standard and stiff. Besides determining their interaction with the lesion and the wall surface, higher guidewire flexibility commonly imposes higher tendency of tip prolapsing. However, tip prolapsing may show useful in specific situations when purposely utilized [such as for quick access down the vessel avoiding side branch or stent struts entrapment, or for the pop-up engagement of side branch at steep angle by pulling back the wire] (Fig. 2) (12). At the opposite pole, tip stiffness becomes an essential characteristic required for some types of lesions such as chronic total occlusions.

In benchmark testing, please note that Asahi Intecc (Aichi, Japan) measures tip flexibility/stiffness via tip deflection on pushing downwards (axial stiffness), whereas other manufacturers measure this property by deflection caused when a load is applied laterally (lateral stiffness).

Guidewire support

Guidewire support refers to the longitudinal rigidity of the guidewire shaft, proximal to the very distal portion that determines stiffness. It is the key determinant of the support that the wire will provide for device delivery. This supportive portion of the guidewire needs to be positioned across the lesion in order to allow equipment delivery. When using wires with greater support, vessels tend to become straightened. This may facilitate device delivery through tortuous or heavily calcified vessels (Fig. 3), but it increases device and wire contact with the wall, increasing not only resistance to device advancement but also the likelihood of vessel wall injury. Occasionally, high support wires act as a "cheese cutter" when the wire is so straight and stiff that it cuts through the vessel curvature, requiring exchange to a less supportive one. Less supportive wires conform more to the normal vessel anatomy, and cause less trauma, but require more trackable devices. We therefore recommend that one should aim to use a wire that provides the minimal level of support necessary for procedural success. As for stiffness and torquability, it is the design and construction of the central core, which largely determines the amount of support provided.

Torquability

Torquability refers to the degree of transmission of the operator's torque of the wire outside the guiding catheter to the tip inside the coronary artery. It is therefore a key determinant of the operator's ability to precisely steer and direct the wire through the vessel and lesion, as well as toward or away from side branches. Differences in core design, core composition, tip stiffness, and the surface coating all alter the torquability. In an ideal world, all wires would provide 1:1 torque, but in reality only a minority of wires are close to achieving this. An additional guidewire

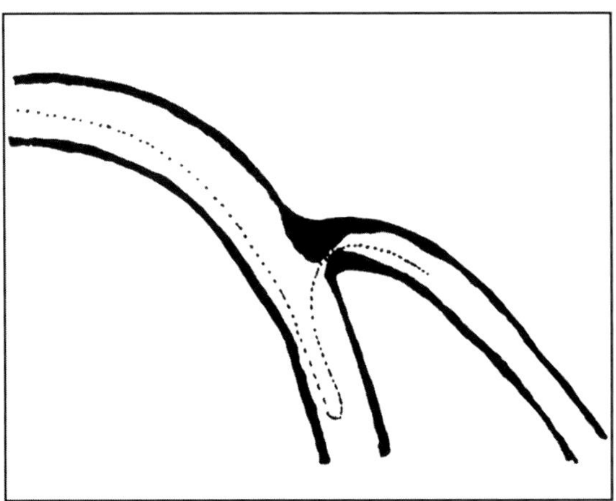

Figure 2 Wire prolapsing: Pulling the wire back to advance it into the angulated side branch. *Source*: Adapted from Ref. 12.

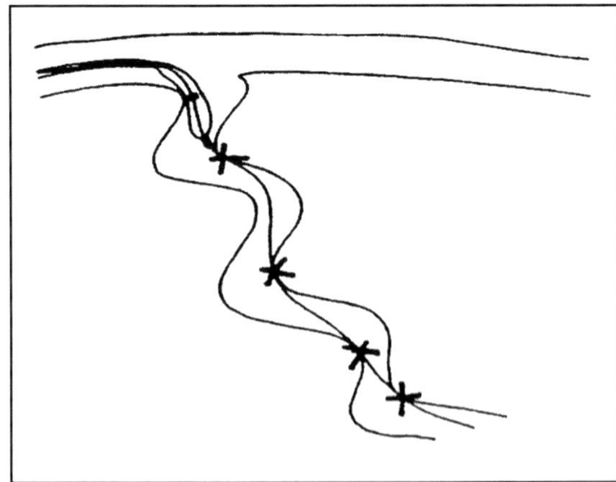

Figure 3 Supportive wire in tortuous vessel for device delivery: Guidewire induced vessel straightening.

property termed steerability is an integral function of guidewire torquability, stiffness, lubricity, tip shapeability, and shaping memory.

Guidewire lubricity

Guidewire lubricity refers to the resistance generated by wire contact with the vessel wall during advancement. As such, it is directly related to the shaft type and surface covering. As already mentioned, coil wires have less lubricity, while polymer sleeve wires are highly lubricious. High-wire lubricity is desirable in tight and calcified lesions, as well as in tortuous vessels. It provides low friction, smooth tracking, and excellent wire movement. However this advantage of hydrophilic wires is offset by their tendency to easily and inadvertently move forward or backward, which can lead to the wire coming back across the lesion or to distal perforation. We, therefore, recommend restricting the use of highly lubricious wires in situations where less lubricious wires have failed, and, if at all possible, to exchange the wire once the distal vessel has been reached. Along with stiffness and support, lubricity is also responsible for the property that is often described as trackability (or tracking).

Shapeability and shaping memory

Shapeability and shaping memory (shape retention) are important guidewire characteristics integral to its distal tip. Shapeability allows the operator to modify its distal tip conformation, while shaping memory is the ability of the tip to return back to its basal conformation after having been exposed to deformation and stress. Guidewires are manufactured either with a preformed "J tip," or a straight tip requiring shaping by the operator. Appropriate tip shaping is paramount in entering side branches and the recanalization of chronic total occlusions. Shapeability and shaping memory do not necessarily go in parallel; wires with stainless steel cores are easier to shape, but shaping memory is better if either nitinol or elastinite is employed. Furthermore, two-piece core wires with an integral shaping ribbon are easier to shape and usually provide better shape retention.

As a general rule, when negotiating through the vessel with the J loop, its distal bend should approximate the diameter of the vessel—more bend increases the chance of the wire tip prolapsing, less bend decreases steerability. The classical review of guidewire tip shaping for negotiating side branches is given by Voda (13), and for chronic total occlusions by Katoh (14) and Ochiai (15).

GUIDEWIRE SELECTION

As a general rule, matching the appropriate guidewire to the intervention under consideration depends on a complex interplay of the vessel morphology, lesion morphology, and device properties. A decision flow chart based on these characteristics is presented in Figure 4. The remainder of the chapter is dedicated to a more in-depth discussion of our approach to wire selection for particular scenarios frequently encountered in day-to-day interventional practice.

Wires for standard lesions

A standard lesion is any lesion that is not:

1. A total occlusion, most probably chronic
2. A side branch originating from a stent
3. A dissection
4. A lesion with heavy calcification
5. A lesion in or beyond a very tortuous segment
6. A situation where a stent does not progress (into the vessel or into another stent)

Nonstandard lesions will be discussed later and for each we will try to highlight specific wires that we consider suitable for each category.

We, therefore, consider a standard lesion to be relatively straightforward and without any complex characteristics. Many manufacturers provide "frontline" or "workhorse" wires that are suitable for such standard lesions. In general, they have floppy, atraumatic tips, and provide low to moderate support, which should be adequate for such lesions. For these types of lesions we recommend one of the following wires.

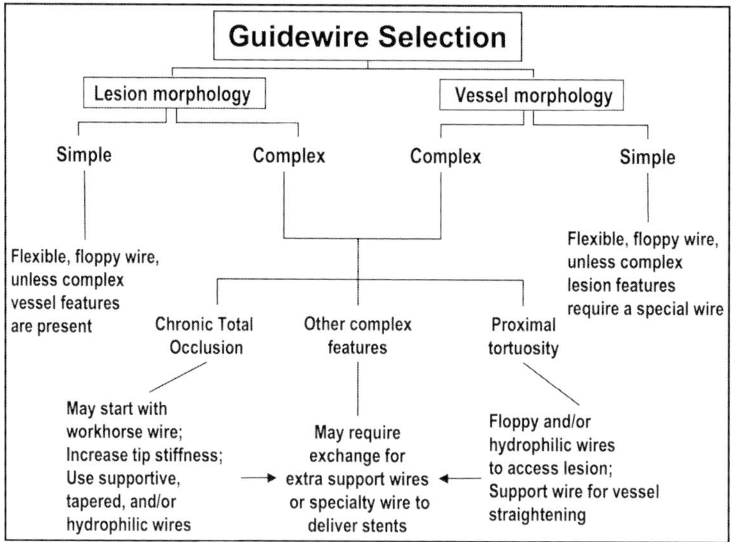

Figure 4 Decision flow chart for guidewire selection.

Balance Middleweight Universal® wire

Balance Middleweight Universal (Abbott Vascular/Guidant, Santa Clara, CA) wire is quite steerable with a gentle distal force. This means that the tip is suitable for bending in a "J" configuration for distal advancement into the distal vessel bed with minimal trauma while still maintaining some torque. As a general rule, when negotiating through the vessel with a J loop, its distal bend should approximate to the diameter of the vessel. The shape retention of the tip of this wire is relatively poor and any J configuration tends to become magnified over time with a consequent loss in steerability. The wire is moderately torquable, and its progression into the distal bed is often aided by the minimal friction provided by its light hydrophilic coating. Dye injection may also be helpful to propagate distal advancement. We consider this wire to be the most user-friendly one currently available and find it suitable for rapid, uncomplicated interventions. In our experience, it carries a low risk to cause either dissections or distal perforations, both of which are much more frequent with polymer sleeve hydrophilic wires such as the Whisper (Guidant, Santa Clara, California, U.S.A.) or PT^2 wires (Boston Scientific, Natick, Massachusetts, U.S.A.). The support provided by this wire is low to moderate.

Balance® and Balance Middleweight® wires

Balance and Balance Middleweight (Abbott Vascular/ Guidant, Santa Clara, CA) wires are from the generation previous to the Universal and lack its light hydrophilic coating at the tip. This means that the tip has more steerability but requires greater effort for distal advancement as it does not have the dye injection facilitation or ability to be rapidly and safely advanced on a "J" configuration. Many interventionists prefer the more direct tactile feedback that these wires may give as compared to the more automatic progression encountered with the Universal wire. An analogy, which summarizes the difference between these wires, is to consider the Universal as a car with power (hydraulic) steering, whereas the Balance is a car with conventional (mechanical) steering. The support of the Balance wire is low while that of the Middleweight is moderate.

IQ® wire

IQ (Boston Scientific, Natick, MA) is the most modern wire from Boston Scientific. In many ways it is similar to the Universal with a light hydrophilic coating and a nitinol core.

Forte® wire

Forte (Boston Scientific, Natick, MA) is a stainless steel core wire available in low and moderate support that is similar to the Balance series of wires. It is available in low and moderate support versions.

Zinger® wire

Zinger (Medtronic, Minneapolis, MN) is equivalent to the Balance—a stainless steel core wire that is available with light, medium, and high support.

Cougar® wire

Cougar (Medtronic, Minneapolis, MN) has a nitinol core with better handling in tortuous anatomy and improved support. This wire is available in medium and light support.

Rinato/Prowater® wire

We consider Rinato/Prowater (Asahi Intecc, Aichi, Japan) wire to be very steerable and stiffer at its tip compared to the Balance series. We use it to aim in a precise direction while maintaining the tip in a straight configuration. This wire should not be used with a J tip configuration and it is often a second choice when a Universal or Balance has failed to progress because of insufficient tip strength or suboptimal steerability. The support of this wire is moderate and superior to that of the Balance wires.

Runthrough NS® wire

Runthrough is a new Terumo wire intended to be a frontline wire, particularly for multilesion interventions. It has a unique dual core design, with the main shaft core of stainless steel and a distal core of nitinol alloy, which extends into a nitinol shaping ribbon. Like the Universal, the distal tip is hydrophilic coated.

Wires for crossing total occlusions

There can be no doubt that our Japanese colleagues are the world leaders in the percutaneous recanalization of occluded coronary arteries with their development and refinement of techniques for this challenging lesion subset. Fundamental to these techniques are guidewires specifically designed for crossing occlusions. The key difference to standard lesions is the need to find (or create) a true lumen through the tissue (which is often fibro-calcific) that comprises the occlusion. As such, wires for chronic occlusions have increased stiffness and excellent torque control compared to frontline or workhorse wires. The stiffness of these wires is measured on a scale quoted in grams, whereby the distal force applied by the wire tip is measured under standardized conditions. Specific wires used in attempting to cross occlusions provide at least 3 g of distal force. To help put this in context, the frontline wires for standard lesions outlined earlier will typically provide less than 1 g of distal force. The finer details of techniques for crossing occlusions are beyond the scope of this chapter, but suffice it to say that several wires, usually of increasing stiffness, may need to be tried during the procedure. We recommend using an over-the-wire balloon or catheter to facilitate wire exchange in these cases.

In our opinion, the Japanese Asahi Intecc family of wires is the current gold standard for crossing total occlusions. We tend to start with the intermediate wire first. This provides 3 g of distal force and moderate support. It is otherwise a conventional stainless steel core wire with 30 mm of tip radio-opacity and 0.014 in. diameter. If this wire fails to cross, we move on to the Miracle series. These 0.014 in. wires have been specifically designed for chronic occlusions and feature 110 mm of distal tip radio-opacity for optimal visualization, and come in four versions of increasing distal force: 3 g, 4.5 g, 6 g, and 12 g. The next evolution is the tapered tip Conquest wire (called Confianza in the U.S.A. and U.K.), which has a distal tip diameter of only 0.009 in. The distal tip is radio-opaque for 200 mm and provides 9 g of distal force. Finally, Asahi has the Conquest Pro (Confianza Pro), which is also tapered to 0.009 in. and provides 9 g of force like the Conquest, but is hydrophilic-coated for the distal 20 cm apart from the extreme distal 2 mm tip. Tip tapering is proposed to help the wire find and navigate microchannels in the occluded segment, while the hydrophilic coating of the Conquest Pro reduces the tip friction by about one-third. It should always be kept in mind that, while such stiff wires undoubtedly have the capacity to penetrate and cross occlusions, this also means that they can easily penetrate and cross other structures such as the arterial wall. Their potential for producing an "extra-arterial experience" is, therefore, significant and they must be used with the utmost vigilance. For laboratories that do not stock the Asahi wires, a reasonable alternative is the Cross-it XT series (Abbott Vascular/Guidant, Santa Clara, CA). These are available with different degrees of distal support (from 3 to 20 g) and like the Conquest are tapered to 0.010 in. at the distal tip.

We consider hydrophilic-coated wires to be a last resort for total occlusions. Indeed, we often refer to them as "terminator wires," as they will either cross the occlusion or create an extensive dissection. Unfortunately, either outcome is in large part beyond the operator's immediate control, hence their designation is as a "last resort." Among these, the Whisper, Pilot 50, Pilot 150, and Pilot 200 (Abbott Vascular/Guidant, Santa Clara, CA), Crosswire NT (Terumo), Shinobi and Shinobi Plus (Cordis, Johnson & Johnson, Miami, FL) are the most commonly used wires. These wires should be reserved for occlusions with a tapering entrance and with extensive calcification. The Pilot series (Abbott Vascular/ Guidant, Santa Clara, CA) are hydrophilic-coated wires of increasing tip stiffness with a durasteel core. The Crosswire NT has the following features: the hydrophilic coating covers only the distal 40 cm of wire, the very tip (1 cm) is made from gold for enhanced radio-opacity, and its double-tapered distal tip has moderate shapeability and tip stiffness of 8 g. The Shinobi family wires are stiff, torquable, steerable PTFE-coated wires. The tip is radio-opaque, 3 cm long and can be shaped by the operator. The Shinobi Plus has higher tip stiffness and higher torque response compared with the ordinary Shinobi wire.

Watchful control of the distal tip of all hydrophilic wires is warranted during the procedure, and their substitution with regular wire, once the occlusion or severe stenosis is passed, is recommended.

For the subintimal tracking and re-entry (STAR) technique (16), hydrophilic wires with a large J configuration at the tip are used to propagate the subintimal dissection plane that the technique relies upon.

A unique device that is not a wire but deserves mention as an alternative for crossing resistant occlusions is the Asahi Tornus catheter (Asahi Intecc, Aichi, Japan) (17). It is an over-the-wire device with screw-like threads at the distal 2 cm of the shaft. These threads allow a screw-like advancement into lesions that cannot be crossed by ordinary balloons. The device is advanced with a counter-clockwise rotation and pulled back with a clockwise rotation. The Tornus catheter is tapered over its distal 150 mm, with the distal tip constructed from a stainless-platinum alloy, which provides strength and radio-opacity. The shaft is silicone coated on both inner and outer surface to reduce friction. The catheter is available in two sizes: 2.1 and 2.6 French. After successfully crossing the lesion with the Tornus catheter, it is usually possible to advance a balloon or, in very calcific lesions, to perform a wire exchange for further rotablation. However, it should be noted that it is not always successful and we recall some heavily calcified lesions that could not be crossed by the device.

Wires for crossing stent struts into side branches

With the high incidence of bifurcation lesions in contemporary interventional practice, it is common for an operator to need to cross stent struts into a jailed side branch. Depending on the technique used, it may even be necessary to re-cross multiple layers of stents such as when the crush technique has been performed. As a general rule, we find that floppy wires often have difficulty advancing into the side branch as they often prolapse into the main branch when the operator tries to advance the wire. Nevertheless, we recommend trying a frontline floppy wire (such as a Universal) if one is already available on the table before reaching for one of the more specialized wires discussed later. However, in order to advance the wire beyond the friction generated by the stent struts, a greater degree of tip strength is often required. After failure of a Universal we move to a

Rinato/Prowater (Asahi Intecc Aichi, Japan), followed by an Intermediate.

If these fail, one can consider using hydrophilic wires such as the Pilot 50 or Pilot 150 (Abbott Vascular/Guidant, Santa Clara, CA). However, we prefer to limit usage of these wires because they may cross the struts between the struts and the vessel wall rather than at the true side branch ostium. This, therefore, creates the potential both for significantly deforming the stent if a balloon is inadvertently inflated at this point and also entering a false lumen in the side branch.

A very final resort, which may enable the operator to keep the success rate for crossing into side branches close to 100%, is the usage of a fixed-wire balloon such as the ACE balloon (Boston Scientific, Natick, MA). In few rare conditions this type of balloon is the only one able to cross into the side branch.

Wires for negotiating through a dissection

The Universal or the Balance Middleweight wires (Abbott Vascular/Guidant, Santa Clara, CA) will be the initial wires to use. As a second choice, more steerable wires such as the Rinato/Prowater followed by an Intermediate (both by Asahi Intecc, Aichi, Japan) should be used. In these situations the operator should not hesitate to use the parallel wire technique, developed for total occlusions when she/he perceives that they have entered a dissection plane. It can be considered one of interventional cardiology's unwritten paradigms—that every time the operator suspects that they have entered a dissection plane, they are highly likely to be correct. On each occasion that the wire seems to have passed the dissected area but does not progress, or every time there is a decrease in the distal flow pattern, the operator should suspect that the wire is in a false lumen.

We almost always try to avoid any type of hydrophilic wire when trying to cross a dissection. Even if, occasionally, these wires can successfully advance into the true distal lumen, the risk of extending the dissection significantly with closure of the residual lumen and multiple side branches is high. As a very last resort, and only when other approaches have failed, the operator can consider implementing the STAR technique (16) to purposefully enter and extend the dissection plane with a hydrophilic wire with the intention (and hope) of spontaneously regaining the lumen distally. This approach should only be considered for very distal branches, for the right coronary artery, and for some obtuse marginal branches. It should be avoided for the left anterior descending artery.

Lesions with heavy calcification

If the Universal (Abbott Vascular/Guidant, Santa Clara, CA) fails to cross a calcified lesion, the next choice is to try a floppy hydrophilic wire such as the Whisper and the Pilot 50 (both from Abbott Vascular/Guidant, Santa Clara, CA), Choice PT (Boston Scientific, Natick, MA), or Fielder (Asahi Intecc Co., Asahi, Japan). When we use these wires we almost always utilize an over-the-wire balloon or catheter such as the Transit (Cordis, Johnson & Johnson, Miami, FL), which has the advantage of being hydrophilic coated also. Assuming that the balloon or catheter also crosses the lesion, this approach allows exchange to a less hydrophilic one in order to reduce the risk of distal perforation. Alternatively, if it is felt that the lesion requires rotational atherectomy, the dedicated 325 cm wire for use with the rotablator device (RotaWire, Boston Scientific, Natick, MA) can be easily placed through the over-the-wire catheter. In many situations the RotaWire can be advanced across the lesion in the conventional manner. However, it is not unusual for this uncoated wire to fail to progress in calcified vessels and it may be necessary to either exchange it as described previously or try to advance another wire first (such as a Universal) before attempting to advance the RotaWire in a parallel fashion. Two types of rotablator wires are currently available: the floppy RotaWire and the extra-support RotaWire. Our practice is to exclusively use the floppy wire as it gives less bias to the burr while performing atherectomy, which in our experience reduces the risk of vessel perforation or rupture. Rotational atherectomy should never be performed unless there is absolute certainty that the wire is in the true lumen throughout its course.

In very calcific arteries the operator may need to use a second, so-called "buddy" wire in order to advance the stent to the lesion. Most of the time, we advance the stent over the less supportive wire with the more supportive wire used as a buddy to stabilize the guiding catheter, and at least partially straighten any vessel tortuosity. Occasionally, the buddy wire may need to be very supportive indeed, such as the Iron Man wire (Abbott Vascular/Guidant, Santa Clara, CA). However, please note that there are no hard and fast rules regarding the use of such buddies, and occasionally we have seen stents that failed to advance over the low support wire, being successfully advanced on the high support wire. Finally, we have occasionally found the Wiggle wire (Abbott Vascular/ Guidant, Santa Clara, CA) to be helpful in this situation. This wire has a series of preformed small bends in a "zigzag" pattern up to 6 cm from the tip. The aim of these bends is to partially divert the tip of the balloon or stent from the wall of the artery, thereby facilitating advancement in difficult anatomies.

Lesions in, or beyond, a very tortuous or angulated segment

With the exclusion of the utilization of rotational atherectomy, most of the considerations stated earlier for calcific vessels also apply to very tortuous vessels. In these circumstances, we often find hydrophilic wires such as the Whisper (Abbott Vascular/Guidant, Santa Clara, CA) may provide the solution. However, as always, we would counsel utmost vigilance in monitoring the distal position of the wire tip, as it will not infrequently perforate the distal vessel if allowed to migrate too distally or into small side branches.

The usage of a buddy wire can be a very important aid and occasionally even the usage of a buddy balloon (1.5 mm) on the buddy wire may provide additional support. As already mentioned, the Wiggle wire (Abbott Vascular/Guidant, Santa Clara, CA) may also be helpful here. In some situations, the operator can obtain better stabilization of the guiding catheter by advancing the buddy wire into another vessel when there are problems to advance the wire in the target vessel.

As a last resort, the operator can consider other techniques such as using a selective 5 French guiding catheter (teleguide) inside a larger 8 French guiding catheter. To do this, the larger catheter needs to be shortened by about 10 or 15 cm in order to allow the smaller internal catheter to advance selectively into the target vessel. Alternatively, the Proxis proximal protection device (St Jude Medical, St Paul, MN) can also be used for the same selective anchoring purpose.

Recently, a new deflectable tip wire has become available (Steer-it, Cordis, Johnson & Johnson, Miami, FL). This wire can be used to negotiate tight or acute bends, even in a retrograde direction, into side branches or beyond bypass graft anastomoses. Theoretically, this wire may also have a role in some total occlusions or in regaining the true lumen from a dissection, but we have no personal experience of successful utilization in such scenarios. As an alternative to the Steer-it wire, the Venture wire control catheter (St Jude Medical, St Paul, MN), has a deflectable tip and allows the use of any guidewire within its central lumen (18).

A situation where a stent does not progress through another stent

This situation is often best dealt with by a buddy wire or with the Wiggle wire (Abbott Vascular/ Guidant, Santa Clara, CA). The proximal stent may rarely need further dilatation (provided it has been implanted during the same procedure). If the stent still fails to progress in such circumstances, the only option may be to switch to a highly trackable stent with a ring design such as the Driver or Endeavour (Medtronic, Minneapolis, MN).

A CLOSING REMARK

To conclude this overview of guidewires and our approach to selecting an appropriate wire for the intervention under consideration, we would like to remind you of the wise words of Charles Dotter and Melvin Judkins: "The guide is passed across the atheromatous block without going through the wall more by the application of judgment than of force" (19).

AUTHORS' NOTE

Our initial intention was to provide a comparative table presenting essential characteristics of the contemporary guidewires available from the major international manufacturers. However, even a basic table would overflow any reasonable space allocation in this book. In addition, the guidewire market is likely to be a fluid one, such that any comparison would in practice have limited relevance. For that reason we decided to provide the links to the web presentations of all relevant guidewire manufacturers, which can be found at the www.jim-vascular.com, whereby comprehensive product information may hopefully be found. Accordingly, we are of the opinion that it is important for the operator to focus on selected set of devices rather than trying to use all wires that are on the market at the same time.

REFERENCES

1. Gruntzig A. Transluminal dilatation of coronary-artery stenosis. Lancet 1978; 1:263.
2. Simpson JB, Baim DS, Robert EW, Harrison DC. A new catheter system for coronary angioplasty. Am J Cardiol 1982; 49:1216–1222.
3. Gruentzig AR, Meier B. Current status of dilatation catheters and guiding systems. Am J Cardiol 1984; 53:92C–93C.
4. Cournand AF. Control of the pulmonary circulation in man with some remarks on methodology. Nobel lecture, December 11, 1956. In: Nobel Lecture, Physiology of Medicine 1942–1962. Amsterdam: Elsevier, 1964:529–542.
5. Stillabower ME. Longitudinal force focused coronary angioplasty: a technique for resistant lesions. Catheter Cardiovasc Diagn 1994; 32:196–198.
6. Meier B, Rutishauser W. Coronary pacing during percutaneous transluminal coronary angioplasty. Circulation 1985; 71:557–561.
7. Meier B. Emergency pacing during cardiac catheterization: it is all there already. Catheter Cardiovasc Interv 2004; 61:501–502.
8. Mixon TA, Cross DS, Lawrence ME, Gantt DS, Dehmer GJ. Temporary coronary guidewire pacing during percutaneous coronary intervention. Catheter Cardiovasc Interv 2004; 61:494–500; discussion 502–503.
9. Hoorntje JC. How to change an over-the-wire PTCA balloon over a normal short guidewire. Catheter Cardiovasc Diagn 1989; 18:284.
10. Agarwal R, Shah D, Mathew S. New technique for exchanging an "over-the-wire" balloon dilatation catheter. Catheter Cardiovasc Diagn 1995; 36:350–351.
11. Meier B. Chronic total occlusion. In: Topol EJ, ed. Textbook of Interventional Cardiology. Philadelphia: WB Saunders, 1990: 300–326.
12. Angelini P. Chapter 3: The procedure. In: Angelini P, ed. Balloon Catheter Coronary Angioplasty. Mt Kisco: Futura Publishing Co., 1987.
13. Voda J. Angled tip of the steerable guidewire and its usefulness in percutaneous transluminal coronary angioplasty. Catheter Cardiovasc Diagn 1987; 13:204–210.
14. Katoh O. Basic wire-handling strategies for chronic total occlusions. CCT, 2004. Http://Www.Cct.Gr.Jp/2003/Wirehand/Index.Html.
15. Ochiai M. Guide wire technique I: shaping the tip and strategies for successful penetrating and crossing the lesion. TCT, 2005. Http://Www.Tctmd.Com/Csportal/Appmanager/Tctmd/Ctocoe?_Nfpb=True&_Pagelabel=Ctocentercontent&Hdcon=1435271&Srcid=64&Destid=65.
16. Colombo A, Mikhail GW, Michev I, et al. Treating chronic total occlusions using subintimal tracking and reentry: the STAR technique. Catheter Cardiovasc Interv 2005; 64:407–411; discussion 412.
17. Tsuchikane E, Katoh O, Shimogami M, et al. First clinical experience of a novel penetration catheter for patients with severe coronary artery stenosis. Catheter Cardiovasc Interv 2005; 65:368–373.
18. Mcclure SJ, Wahr DW, Webb JG. Venture wire control catheter. Catheter Cardiovasc Interv 2005; 66:346–350.
19. Dotter CT, Judkins MP. Transluminal treatment of arteriosclerotic obstruction. Description of a new technic and a preliminary report of its application. Circulation 1964; 30:654–670.

3

Treatment of unprotected left main stenosis

Antonio Colombo and Alaide Chieffo

- **Techniques** • **References**

Despite improvements in the safety and long-term efficacy of percutaneous coronary intervention (PCI), the presence of a significant narrowing in the unprotected left main coronary artery (LMCA) has remained one of the last bastions of surgical dominance. Concerns are mainly due to poor long-term outcome (i.e., restenosis, which in this anatomic location may present as either recurrent angina or sudden death). Accordingly, current guidelines consider unprotected LMCA stenosis, a class IIa or IIb indication for PCI if coronary artery bypass graft surgery (CABG) is not a viable option and a class III indication if CABG is eligible (1–3).

With the availability of drug-eluting stents (DES) and the dramatic reduction in restenosis rates, the results of left main stenting have further improved. Encouraging results have been reported in some observational registries with elective DES implantation in LMCA with a one-year mortality of 0% to 5% in patients (4–7). In these registries, the need for target lesion revascularization (TLR) varied from 0% to 14% and target vessel revascularization from 0% to 19%. In a compassionate registry in which all patients had contraindication to CABG and where distal lesion location was present in 94% of the patients, TLR was 38% (14% if only ischemia-driven TLR is considered) (8). From these preliminary results, it is clear that patient selection as well as lesion location could be responsible for the differences in outcome reported in the different experiences (9,10). Another important finding from these registries is the fact that in all of them, the major contributor to major adverse cardiac events (MACE) is the need for a repeat procedure with no apparent increase in the incidence of myocardial infarction or death, albeit with the limitations of one-year followup and a total of only 489 patients. There is no doubt that further progress has been made: 6- to 12-month mortality rates of 2% to 4% following PCI are now similar to the ones reported for surgery for left main disease in-hospital (1.7–7.0%) and at 1 year (6–14%) (11–14).

Another important finding is that DES-treated lesions in the ostial or mid-left main have a very low (<5%) rate of angiographic or clinical restenosis with DES (4,5,7–9,15). The frequency of LMCA stenosis in the ostium and/or the shaft not involving the distal segment was 6% to 34% (5,7,8,15).

An important limitation is that the majority of left main lesions treated are located in the distal left main bifurcation associated with worse clinical outcome (16), and for which we still do not have an ideal stenting approach. The ostium of the left circumflex is a particular issue, accounting for about one-half of the restenosis cases in these series.

The improved short- and intermediate-term outcomes beg the question of whether drug-eluting stenting is a viable alternative to bypass surgery in patients with left main stenosis.

Recently, two observational studies evaluating DES versus CABG have been reported (4,6). Both studies found no difference in the occurrence of MACE between patients treated with DES compared to the ones treated with CABG. The most important limitations of these registries were the different baseline clinical characteristics of the two populations (PCI and CABG) and the duration of followup (limited to one year). At the present time, there are two ongoing randomized trials with extended followup to at least five years intended to evaluate the outcome of paclitaxel-eluting stent or sirolimus-eluting stent (SES) versus CABG in patients with LMCA stenosis. The Synergy between Percutaneous Intervention with TAXUS® and Cardiac Surgery (the SYNTAX) trial will include 710 patients with LMCA lesions out of a total cohort of 1800 patients with surgical disease. The COMparison of Bypass surgery and AngioplasTy (the COMBAT) trial will evaluate only patients with unprotected LMCA. This study will include 1730 patients with LMCA randomized to SES versusCABG. The primary endpoint of the SYNTAX study is all major adverse cardiac and cerebrovascular adverse events including repeat revascularization at one year, whereas the COMBAT study has the composite of death, myocardial infarction, and cerebrovascular events at two years as its primary endpoint.

TECHNIQUES

Most of the time in this discussion we refer to unprotected LMCA (non-functioning venous or arterial graft to the circumflex or left anterior descending artery). Techniques for stenting the LMCA can be described in relation to the location of the lesion: (*i*) ostial, (*ii*) body, and (*iii*) bifurcation.

Ostial

Stenting an ostial LMCA is no different from stenting any aorto-ostial lesion. The general principles are the same: minimal usage of direct stenting and check for full predilatation unless the operator is prepared to deal with an occasional undilatable stent.

One specific feature of ostial LMCA lesions is the size of the reference vessel, which very frequently may be above 4.0. As with all aorto-ostial lesions, it is important to allow the stent to protrude into the aorta for about 1 or 2 mm in order to succeed in this task, and it is important to check for positioning in multiple views, such as the cranial right anterior oblique and the caudal left anterior oblique, these being the most frequently utilized. Another important caveat is to use a short stent to avoid fully covering the distal bifurcation; still, the operator should be careful not to use a stent that is too short, running the risk that it could be dislodged during postdilatation or while maneuvering the guiding catheter, with the consequent risk of it being embolized in the ascending aorta.

In order to obtain an optimal final result, we suggest usage of intravascular ultrasound (IVUS) whenever possible.

Due to the fact that aorto-ostial lesions are associated with a high restenosis rate, sometimes even if the reference vessel size is large, we advocate the use of DES whenever possible.

Treatment of most aorto-ostial lesions rarely requires prophylactic support with aortic balloon counterpulsation.

Body

Lesions located at the body of the LMCA should be treated as ostial lesions, trying not to compromise the distal bifurcations. This goal is not always achievable, because the lesion may extend very close to the bifurcation and some plaque shift may occur. If there is any doubt about this possibility, a reasonable strategy is to extend the stent into the left anterior descending artery (LAD). When stenting extends over the LAD, it may be necessary to dilate the circumflex and to perform final kissing inflation.

As already said for ostial LMCA, the final stent sizes are usually 4 mm or above.

If 4 mm is the target size, it is possible to utilize a 3.5-mm stent with postdilatation with a 4-mm balloon.

As for ostial lesions, most of the LMCA lesions located in the body of the vessel are relatively straightforward, and rarely there is a need for prophylactic usage of aortic balloon counterpulsation.

Bifurcation

Treatment of an LMCA bifurcation lesion remains one of the most challenging types of lesions.

It is important to evaluate at the time of starting the procedure if the disease at the bifurcation only involves one branch of the bifurcation [LAD or the left circumflex (LCX)], or if it extends into both branches or into three distal branches such as ramus intermedius ("true" bifurcation). In all these situations, we suggest the use of prophylactic aortic balloon counterpulsation.

When the disease is limited to one branch, the best strategy is to stent from the left main into the diseased branch. Following stent placement over the lesion, some evaluations will be done according to the magnitude of plaque shift toward the unstented vessel and if the unstented vessel is the LAD.

The decision to place a second stent should be made only after having dilated the unstented branch and after having performed the final kissing balloon inflation. The threshold to place a second stent will be lower if the unstented vessel is the LAD. When there is a need to place a second stent, the operator can decide according to the angle between the LAD and the LCX and according to his/her personal experience among the following four stent techniques: (*i*) T-stenting, (*ii*) reverse crush, (*iii*) culotte, and (*iv*) T-stenting with slight protrusion (TAP). The first three techniques are fairly well known and are discussed in the section on bifurcation; therefore, we will describe in more detail the most recent TAP technique. This recently developed technique is basically a simplification of the reverse crush technique. The steps of the TAP technique are: (*i*) a second stent is advanced in the side branch in a way to minimally protrude (1 or 2 mm) into the main branch where a stent has been already implanted, (*ii*) a balloon is advanced in the main branch, and (*iii*) the side branch stent in deployed as usual (about 15 atm or above) and the main branch balloon is simultaneously inflated at 15 atm or above.

Despite some concerns about stent protrusion from the side branch, we have been able to perform intravascular ultrasound (IVUS) in both branches and, when needed, to advance additional stents distally in any of the branches.

When the disease involves the origin of the LCX and especially when it extends a few millimeters distally to the ostium, we think it is appropriate to consider implanting two stents as intention to treat.

In this case, we recommend an 8 French guiding catheter even if a 7 French is acceptable with some new generation DES. We think that the 8 French guide will give better visualization and it will decrease friction during advancement of the stents. The main techniques we apply when we decide to implant two stents as intention to treat are: (*i*) the crush, (*ii*) the culotte, or (*iii*) the V. All these techniques have been described in the section dealing with bifurcations. Important to note are the following considerations:

- The crush technique is the one that will give the most rapid patency of both branches and should be applied in conditions of instability or when the anatomy appears complex.
- The culotte technique will give the best immediate angiographic result and theoretically it may guarantee a more homogeneous distribution of the struts and of the drug at the site of the bifurcation. The limitations of the culotte technique are its complexity and the fact that it can only be used with a stent that has an open cell design, allowing opening of the stent struts toward the side branch to a diameter larger than 3 mm. At present, we have no data regarding the outcome of the culotte technique versus the crush technique.
- The V-technique is probably the easiest and the one that will give immediate patency and access to both branches, faster than the crush. We prefer to apply this approach only when the disease does not extend proximally to the bifurcation. The need to implant a more proximal stent demands conversion of the V-technique into a crush.

Table 1 Guidelines left main CAD—2005

ESC 2005 PCI: Class IIb (Level C)

- The use of PCI for patients with significant unprotected LMCA stenosis is indicated in the absence of other revascularization options.

AHA/ACC 2005: Class IIa (Level B)

- The use of PCI for patients with significant unprotected LMCA stenosis of a reasonable revascularization in patients not elegible for CABG and in carefully selected patients.
- It is reasonable that patients undergoing PCI to unprotected left main coronary obstructions be followed up with coronary angiography between two and six months after PCI (Level C).

AHA/ACC 2005: Class III

- Left main disease and eligibility for CABG
- Level of Evidence C in patients with SA
- Level B in patients with UA or NSTEMI.

Abbreviations: AHA/ACC, American Heart Association–American College of Cardiology; CABG, coronary artery bypass graft surgery; LMCA, left main coronary artery; PCI, percutaneous coronary intervention; STEMI, ST segment elevation myocardial infarction.
Source: From Refs. 2, 3, and 5.

Study	Site(s) Patients	Years	Patients	Stent	DCA(%)	Comment
Park et al.	Asan Medical Center, Seoul, Korea	2003–2004	102	SES	2.9%	EF≤40% excluded
Valgimigli et al.	Erasmus Medical Center, Netherlands	2001–2003	95	SES or PES	3.1%	Acute MI and bail-out included
Chieffo et al.	Columbus Hospital and San Raffaele Hospital, Milan	2002–2004	85	SES or PES	2.3%	45% poor surgical candidates
De Lezo et al.	Reina Sofia Hospital, Cordoba, Spain	2002–2004	52	SES	-	45% poor surgical candidates

Figure 1 Published unprotected left main percutaneous coronary intervention drug-eluting stents series. *Abbreviations*: MI, myocardial infarction; PES, paclitaxel-eluting stent; SES, sirolimus-eluting stent.

Series	Procedure success (%)	Death
Chieffo et al.	100	0
Park et al.	100	0
Valgimigli et al.	99	1.0
De Lezo et al.	96	0
Gershlick et al.	100	0

Figure 2 In-hospital outcomes: drug-eluting stents in left main percutaneous coronary intervention series.

In our experience and according to IVUS studies performed at the end of most procedures involving distal left main bifurcations, one of the main reasons why there is restenosis at followup is incomplete stent expansion at the ostium of the side branch (LCX).

Table 1 and Figures 1 to 15 are an attempt to summarize the field LMCA stenting with some of the available results and some typical examples. We would like to highlight the last case (Case 4) that shows an acute intraprocedural thrombosis with the possible message, according to our judgment, to give high weight to optimal pharmacological antithrombotic therapy (glycoprotein IIb/IIIa inhibitors or bivalirudin) when treating these lesions located in such a critical area.

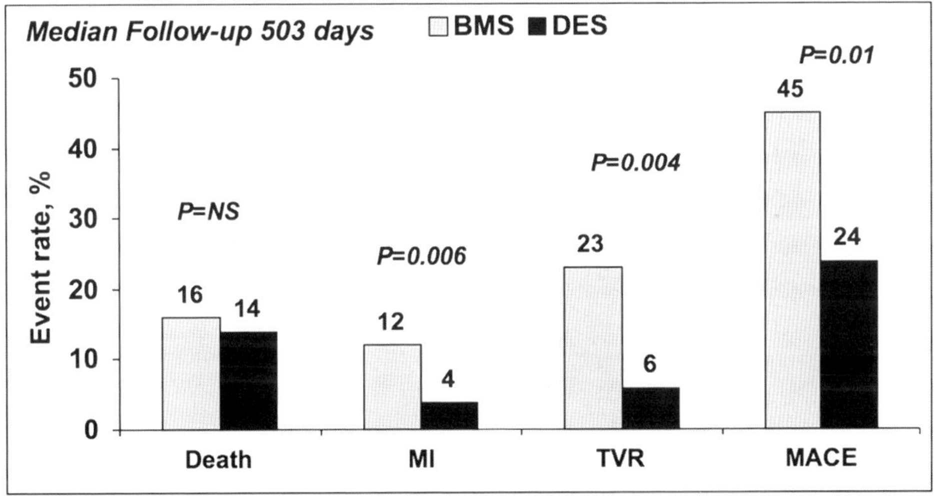

Figure 3 Drug-eluting stents versus BMS in left main percutaneous coronary intervention Research and T-search registries. *Abbreviations*: BMS, bare-metal stents; DES, drug-eluting stents; MI, myocardial infarction; TVR, target lesion revascularization. *Source*: From Ref. 16.

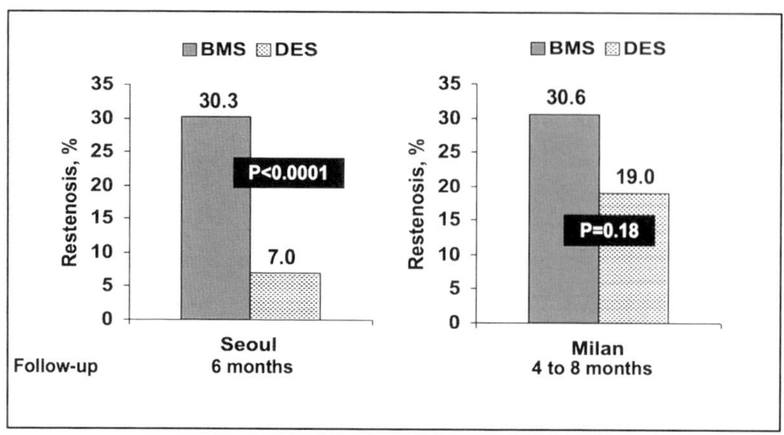

Figure 4 Angiographic restenosis in drug-eluting stents versus BMS in left main coronary artery percutaneous coronary intervention. *Abbreviations*: BMS, bare-metal stents; DES, drug-eluting stents. *Source*: From Refs. 5 and 7.

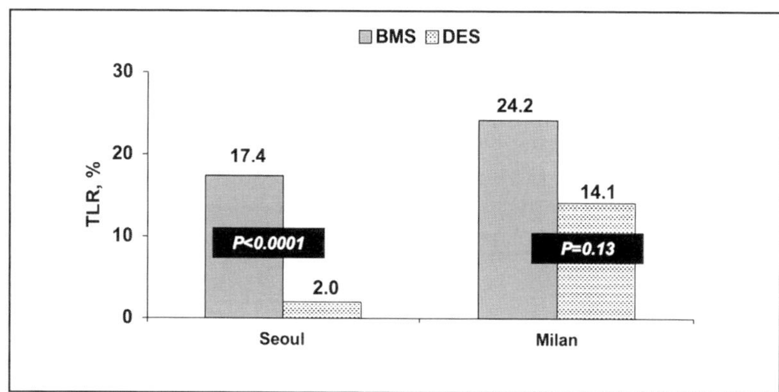

Figure 5 Drug-eluting stents versus BMS in left main coronary artery percutaneous coronary intervention target lesion revascularization. *Abbreviations*: BMS, bare-metal stents; DES, drug-eluting stents; TLR, target lesion revascularization. *Source*: From Refs. 5 and 7.

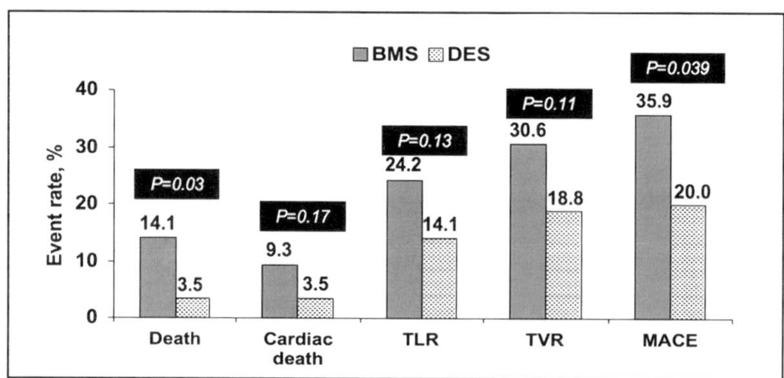

Figure 6 Six-month follow-up in drug-eluting stents versus BMS left main coronary artery percutaneous coronary intervention. *Abbreviations*: BMS, bare-metal stents; DES, drug-eluting stents; TLR, target lesion revascularization; TVR, target vessel revascularization. *Source*: From Ref. 5.

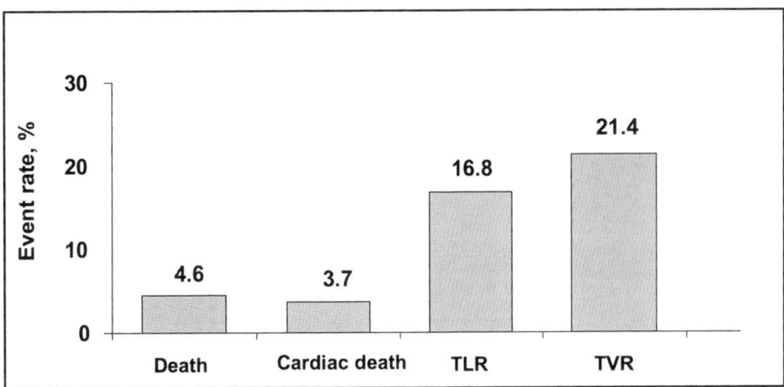

Figure 7 Two-years follow-up in drug-eluting stents left main percutaneous coronary intervention (Milan experience). *Abbreviations*: TLR, target lesion revascularization; TVR, target vessel revascularization.

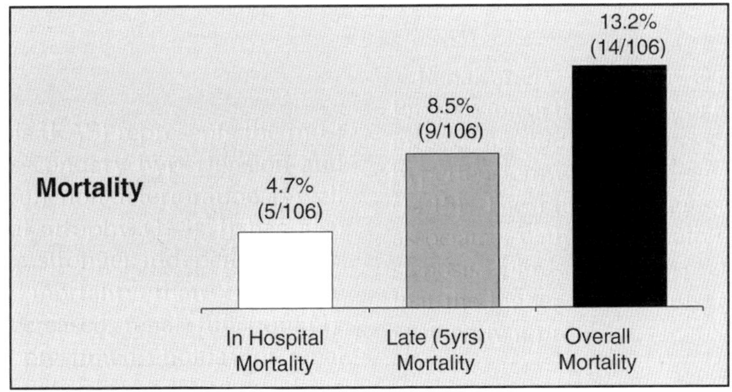

Figure 8 Isolated left main stenosis treated with surgery. *Note*: Of 106 patients with isolated LM stenosis treated with coronary artery bypass graft elective surgery was performed in 100 patients (94.4%) and emergency surgery in 6 (5.6%). *Source*: From Ref. 12.

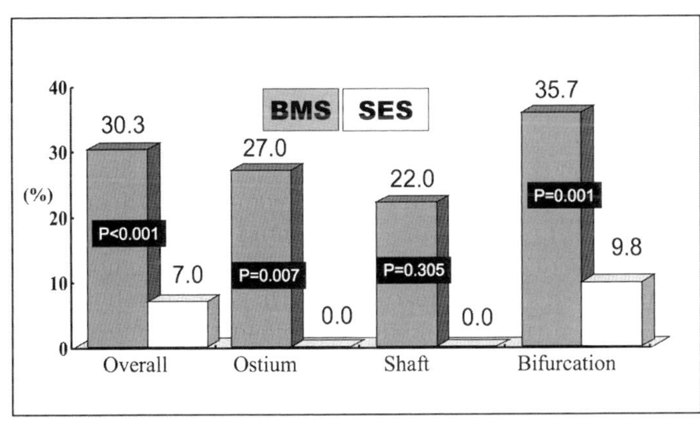

Figure 9 ULM treated with sirolimus-eluting stent (Korean experience)—restenosis rate. *Note*: 102 patients treated with SES verus 121 with BMS for ULM lesions. *Abbreviations*: BMS, base-metal stents; SES, sirolimus-eluting stent. *Source*: From Ref. 7.

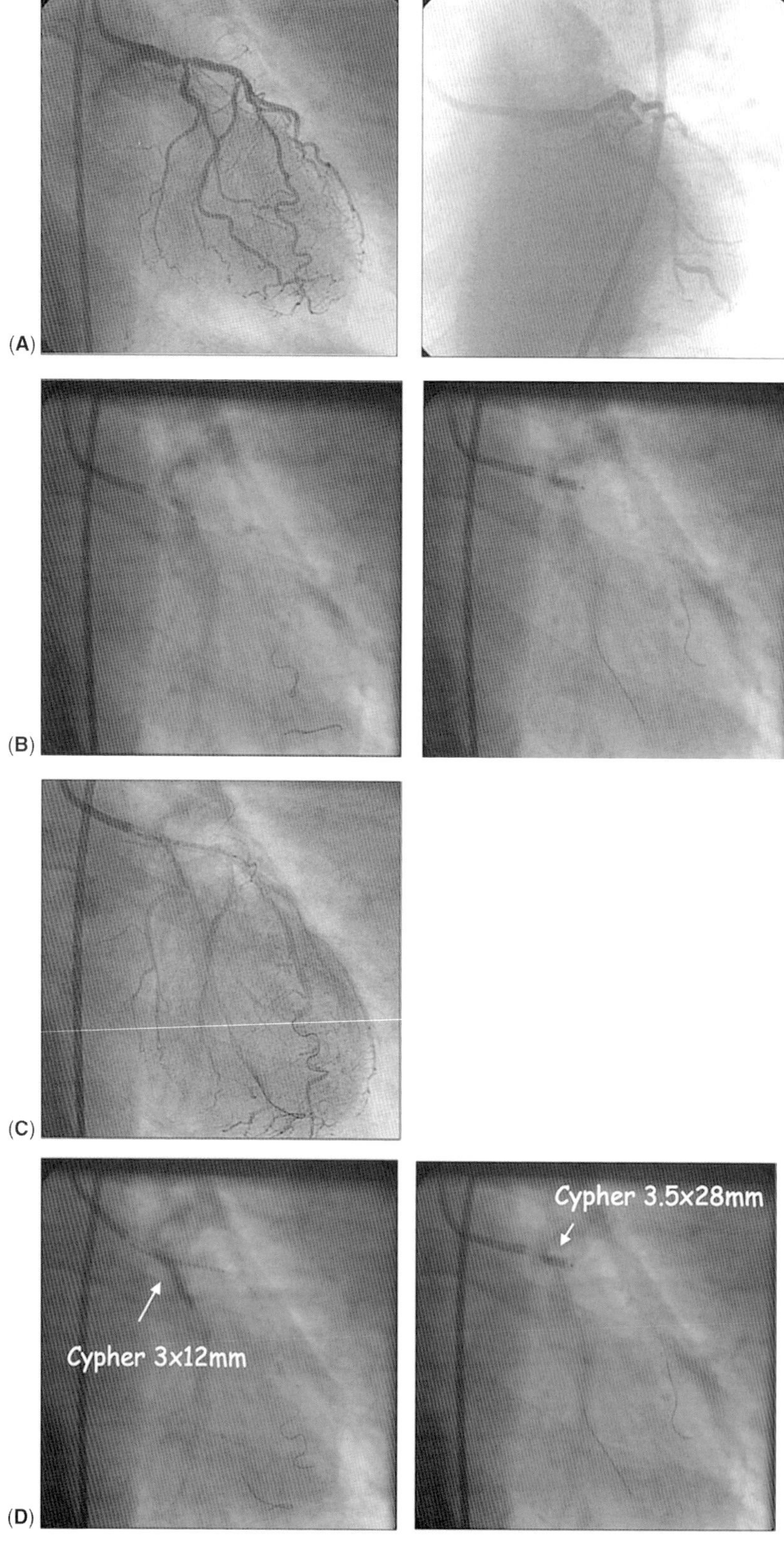
(A)
(B)
(C)
(D)
Cypher 3x12mm
Cypher 3.5x28mm

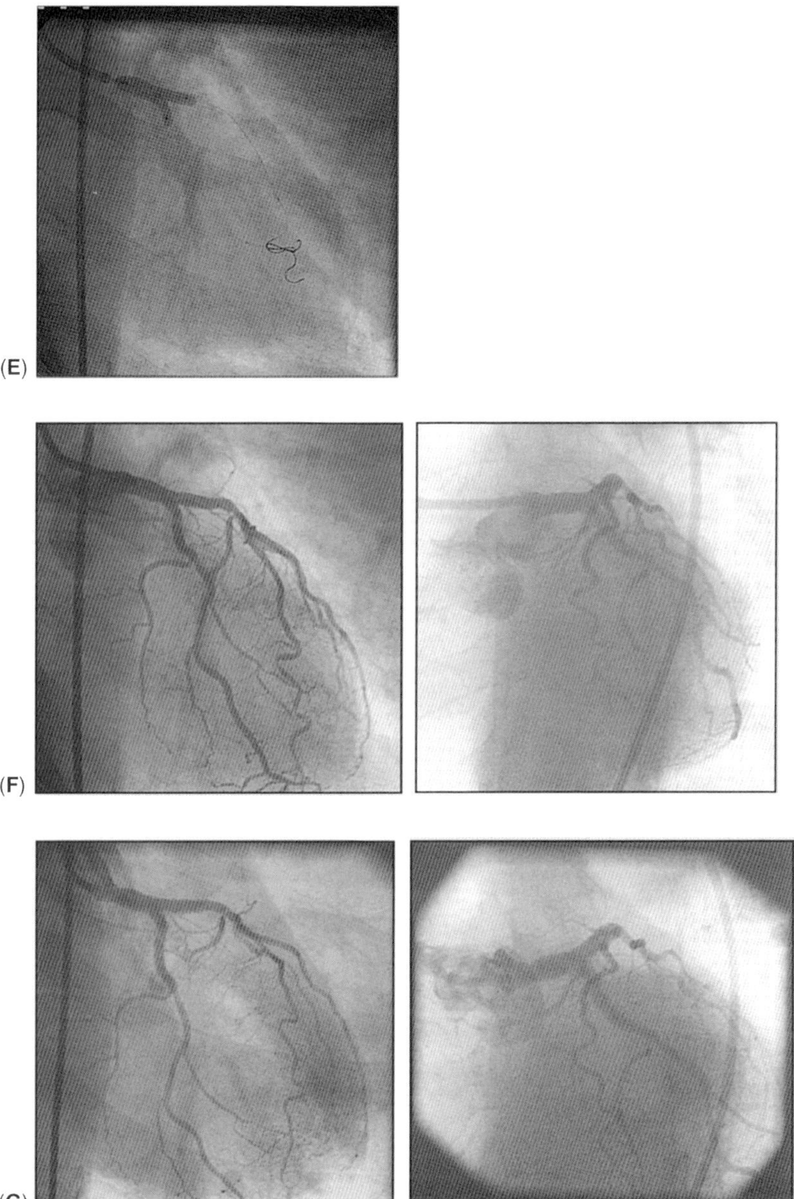

Figure 10 Case 1: Distal left main coronary artery stenosis. (Very favorable follow-up.) (**A**) Distal left main coronary, artery stenosis; (**B**) predilatation of both branches; (**C**) and (**D**) positioning of cypher stents-crush technique; (**E**) kissing balloon inflation; (**F**) final angiograms; (**G**) six-month angiographic followup.

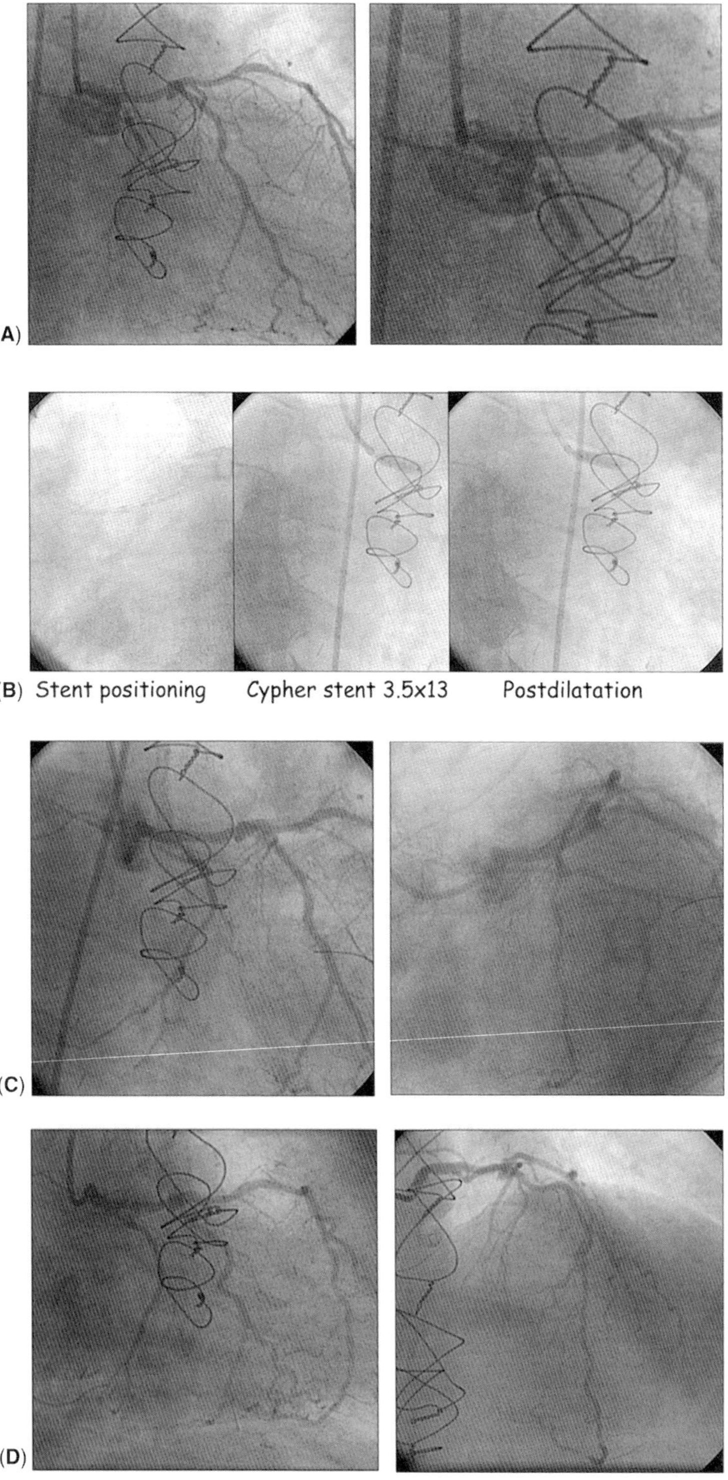

Figure 11 Case 2: Ostial left main coronary artery stenosis. (Very favorable follow-up.) (**A**) Coronary artery bypass graft surgery tends to RIMA on left anterior descending artery and LIMA on diag both accluded. (**B**) Stent Implantation. (**C**) Final angiograms. (**D**) Six-month followup.

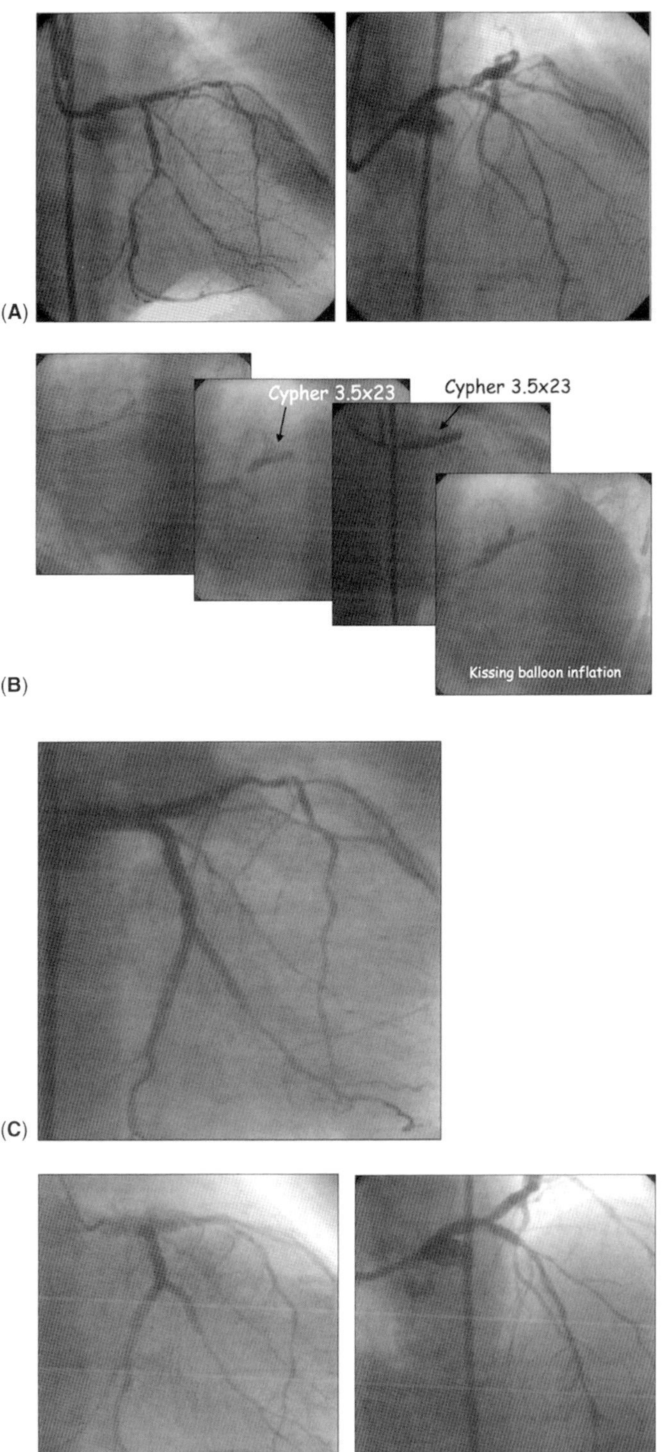

Figure 12 Case 3: Distal left main coronary artery stenosis. (Mediocre angiographic result at follow-up.) (**A**) Distal left main coronary artery stenosis; (**B**) crush technique; (**C**) final angiogram; (**D**) six-month angiographic followup.

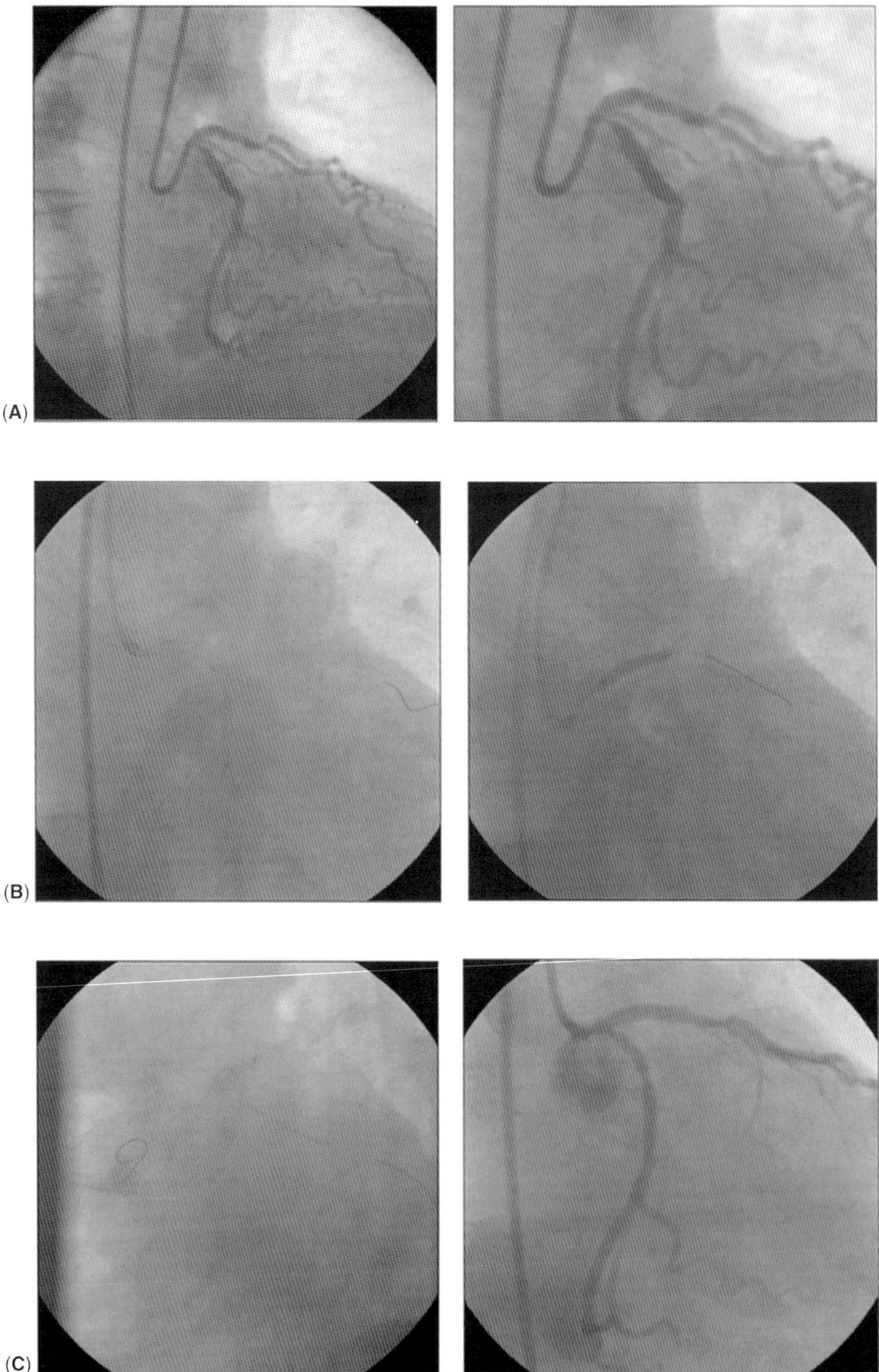

Figure 13 Case 4: Distal left main coronary artery stenosis. Intraprocedural stent thrombosis (preprocedural aspirin and clopidogrel loading; intraprocedural heparin 70 μ/kg).

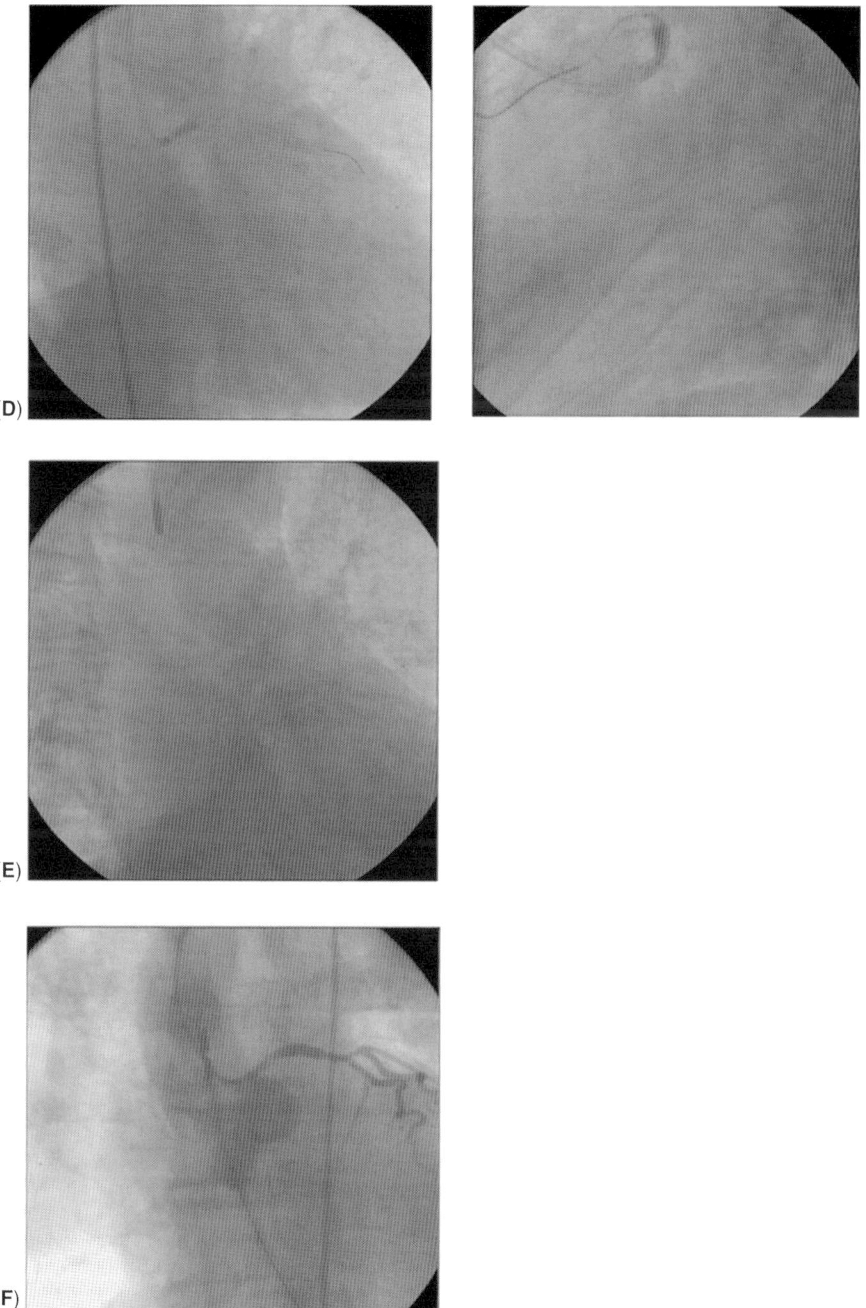

(**A**) Distal left main coronary artery stenosis; (**B**) predilatation of both branches; (**C**) Taxus 3.0 × 16 mm "T" stent implantation in left circumflex (LCX) (*left*) and after Taxus implantation in LCX (*right*); (**D**) Taxus 3.5 × 20 mm stent implantation in LMCA/left anterior descending artery (*left*) and postdilatation (*right*); (**E**) thrombosis in LMCA tends to cardiogenic shock (IABP + CPR); (**F**) thrombosis in LMCA (final angiogram).

	DES n = 107	CABG n = 142	On Pump n=86	Off Pump n=56
MI	10 (9.3%)	37 (26.05%)	29 (33.7%)	8 (14.3%)
Q- MI	0	5	4	1
TVR	0	3 (2.1%)	1 (1.2%)	2 (3.5%)
CVE	0	2 (1.4%)	1 (1.2%)	1 (1.7%)
Death	0	3 (2.1%)	2 (2.3%)	1 (1.7%)

Figure 14 Percutaneous treatment with drug eluting stent implantation versus bypass surgery for unprotected left main stenosis: In-hospital outcome. *Abbreviations*: CABG, coronary artery bypass graft surgery; CVE, cerebrovascular events; DES, drug-eluting stents; MI, myocardial infarction; TVR, target vessel revascularization. *Source*: From Ref. 17.

	DES n = 107	CABG n = 139	On Pump n=84	Off Pump n=55
MI	1 (0.9%)	2 (1.4%)	1 (1.2%)	1 (1.7%)
TLR	17 (15.8%)	5 (3.6%)	2 (2.4%)	3 (5.4%)
TVR	21 (19.6%)	5 (3.6%)	2 (2.4%)	3 (5.4%)
CVE	1 (0.9%)	1 (0.7%)	1 (1.2%)	0
Death	3 (2.8%)	9 (6.4%)	5 (5.9%)	4 (7.2%)

Figure 15 Percutaneous treatment with drug eluting stent implantation versus bypass surgery for unprotected left main stenosis: One-year outcome. *Abbreviations*: CABG, coronary artery bypass graft surgery; CVE, cerebrovascular events; DES, drug-eluting stents; MI, myocardial infarction; TVR, target vessel revascularization. *Source*: From Ref. 17.

REFERENCES

1. Eagle KA, Guyton RA, Davidoff R, et al. ACC/AHA 2004 Guidelines update for coronary artery bypass graft surgery. Circulation 2004; 110: 1168– 1176.
2. Silber S, Albertsson P, Aviles FF, et al. Guidelines for percutaneous coronary interventions. The task force for percutaneous coronary interventions of the European Society of Cardiology. Eur Heart J 2005; 26:804–847.
3. Smith SC Jr, Feldman TE, Hirshfeld JW Jr III, et al. ACC/AHA/SCAI 2005 guideline update for percutaneous coronary intervention—summary article: a report of the American College of Cardiology/ American Heart Association Task Force on Practice Guidelines (ACC/AHA/SCAI Writing Committee to update the 2001 guidelines for percutaneous coronary Intervention). Circulation 2006; 113:156–175.
4. Chieffo A, Morici N, Maisano F, et al. Percutaneous treatment with drug-eluting stent implantation versus bypass surgery for unprotected left main stenosis. A single-center experience. Circulation 2006; 113:2542–2547.
5. Chieffo A, Stankovic G, Bonizzoni E, et al. Early and mid-term results of drug-eluting stent implantation in unprotected left main. Circulation 2005; 111:791–795.
6. Lee MS, Kapoor N, Jamal F, et al. Comparison of coronary artery bypass surgery with percutaneous coronary intervention with drug-eluting stents for unprotected left main coronary artery disease. J Am Coll Cardiol 2006; 47:864–870.
7. Park SJ, Kim YH, Lee BK, et al. Sirolimus-eluting stent implantation for unprotected left main coronary artery stenosis Comparison with bare metal stent implantation. J Am Coll Cardiol 2005; 45: 351–356.
8. Price MJ, Cristea E, Sawhney N, et al. Serial angiographic follow-up of sirolimus-eluting stents for unprotected left main coronary artery revascularization. J Am Coll Cardiol 2006; 47:871–877.
9. Baim DS, Mauri L, Cutlip DC. Drug-eluting stenting for unprotected left main coronary artery

disease: are we ready to replace bypass surgery? J Am Coll Cardiol 2006; 47:878–881.
10. Chieffo A, Colombo A. Treatment of unprotected left main coronary artery disease with drug-eluting stents: is it time for a randomized trial? Nat Clin Pract Cardiovasc Med 2005; 2:396–400.
11. Beauford RB, Saunders CR, Lunceford TA, et al. Multivessel off-pump revascularization in patients with significant left main coronary artery stenosis: early and midterm outcome analysis. J Card Surg 2005; 20:112–118.
12. d'Allonnes FR, Corbineau H, Le Breton H, Leclercq C, Leguerrier A, Daubert C. Isolated left main coronary artery stenosis: long term follow up in 106 patients after surgery. Heart 2002; 87:544–548.
13. Holm F, Lubanda JC, Semrad M, et al. Main clinical and surgical determinants of in-hospital mortality after surgical revascularization of left main coronary artery stenosis: 2 year retrospective study (1998– 1999). J Mal Vasc 2004; 29:89–93.
14. Lu JC, Grayson AD, Pullan DM. On-pump versus off-pump surgical revascularization for left main stem stenosis: risk adjusted outcomes. Ann Thorac Surg 2005; 80:136–142.
15. Valgimigli M, van Mieghem CAG, Ong ATL, et al. Short- and long-term clinical outcome after drug-eluting stent implantation for the percutaneous treatment of left main coronary artery disease. Circulation 2005; 111:1383–1389.
16. Valgimigli M, Malagutti P, Rodriguez-Granillo GA, et al. Distal left main coronary disease is a major predictor of outcome in patients undergoing per-cutaneous intervention in the drug-eluting stent era: an integrated clinical and angiographic analysis based on the Rapamycin-Eluting Stent Evaluated At Rotterdam Cardiology Hospital (RESEARCH) and Taxus-Stent Evaluated At Rotterdam Cardiology Hospital (T-SEARCH) registries. J Am Coll Cardiol 2006; 47:1530–1537.
17. Chieffo A, Morici N, Maisano F, et al. Percutaneous treatment with drug-eluting stent implantation versus bypass surgery for unprotected left main stenosis: a single-center experience. Circulation 2006; 113:2542–2547.

4

Bifurcation lesion stenting

Yves Louvard and Thierry Lefèvre

• Coronary bifurcation lesions occur frequently • What is a bifurcation lesion? • Can side branch deterioration during main branch stenting be predicted? • Role of the angle between both branches • Practical definition of bifurcation lesions • Available techniques and classification • Bifurcation stenting in a bench test • Bifurcation stenting using bare stents • Bifurcation stenting using drug-eluting stents • How to stent a bifurcation lesion • Systematic double stenting strategies • The "big to small" inverted techniques • Approach to trifurcation lesions • Approach to distal left main • Conclusion • Acknowledgment • Editor's comments • References

Like chronic coronary occlusions, coronary bifurcation lesions are still considered a challenging technical issue in contemporary interventional cardiology. However, considerable progress has been achieved over the past few years, and the main difficulty is now more of a strategic than purely technical nature. Indeed, the approach to bifurcation lesions should integrate several requirements: a bifurcation lesion must be identified prior to the procedure and be viewed optimally in order to visualize the origin of the side branch. The selection of an appropriate strategy must include a bail-out option in case of failure. The efficacy of the technique implemented should be measured by the immediate procedural success and the midterm restenosis rate, and its safety not only by procedure outcome but also by the long-term outcome, including the risk of stent thrombosis, which is associated with a high risk of mortality.

CORONARY BIFURCATION LESIONS OCCUR FREQUENTLY

Bifurcations are frequent in nature, and ramifications are ruled by complex laws of mathematics (1). Consequently, bifurcation lesions are frequently observed in routine practice. Atheromatous plaque is located in areas of turbulent flow, mainly to be found at the level of bifurcations, in the main branch opposite the side branch, and in the side branch opposite the carina (2). In a population of patients undergoing percutaneous coronary interventions, the rate of coronary bifurcation lesions is higher in patients with multiple vessel disease. Currently, coronary bifurcation lesions are still a common indication for coronary artery bypass grafting surgery. In our center between 1996 and 2003 we observed a decrease in surgery and an increase in the percentage of coronary bifurcations treated by percutaneous coronary intervention (PCI) from less than 5% in 1996 to more than 15% after 2003 (3). In the PRESTO study, the reported percentage of bifurcation lesions treated was 12.3% (4). The percentage of bifurcation lesions treated at the Thoraxcentrum (Rotterdam, The Netherlands) with bare-metal stents (BMS) was 8% and increased in one year to 16%, when it was decided to use DES as a default strategy (5).

In the ARTS II study (PCI with the CYPHER stent in patients with multivessel disease), the percentage of patients treated for at least one bifurcation lesion was 53% and the percentage of bifurcation lesions among the total of coronary lesions treated was 22% (6). Interventional cardiologists are, indeed, routinely confronted with

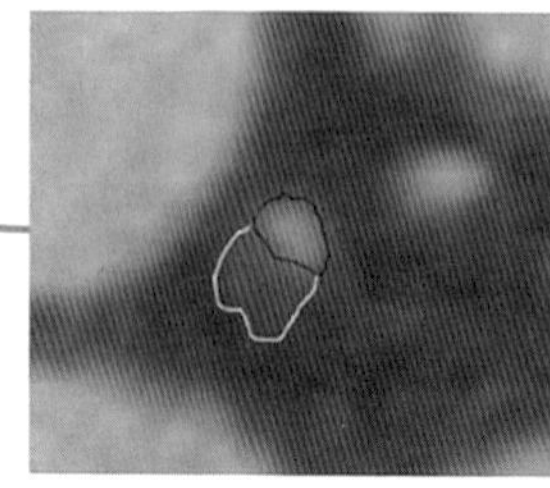

Figure 1 Bifurcation anatomy on coronary computed tomography scan.

the issue of bifurcation lesions and the challenge of finding optimal strategies for treating them.

WHAT IS A BIFURCATION LESION?

Coronary angiography provides two-dimensional visualization of a three-dimensional environment, especially in bifurcations where the main vessel and its side branches are in distinct planes. Operators should obtain optimal angiographic views in order to be able to visualize, describe, and classify bifurcation lesions. Appropriate visualization should allow them to select the most "comfortable" view for unhindered guidewire insertion and easy identification of the side branch ostium, without foreshortening. A lesion involving a coronary bifurcation may be overlooked due to inadequate angiographic views that fail to show the two branches distinctly and render a superimposed image. Three-dimensional reconstruction from two angiographic views or coronary computed tomography (CT) scan may assist in visualizing the bifurcation anatomy more accurately and even pinpoint the location and size of the plaque (Fig. 1) in order to anticipate the inherent risk of redistribution of the incompressible plaque after stenting.

Indeed dilation, and to an even greater extent, stenting of a lesion involving only one branch of a coronary bifurcation may well cause a significant narrowing or occlusion in the other branch. This can be accounted for by the axial plaque shifting phenomenon described by Lemos (7), the increase in the arterial lumen diameter being commensurate with the increase in the external vessel diameter, as well as the result of the longitudinal shifting of the incompressible plaque (Fig. 2). Circular plaque redistribution may also occur, which could explain the fact that a main branch lesion located opposite the side branch origin may occlude the side branch as a consequence of stent placement in the main branch. There is another phenomenon that may lead to the deterioration of the side branch ostium as a result of main branch stenting, namely the collapsing of the carina toward the side branch.

Clearly it appears that the angle between the distal main branch and the side branch (8) is a predictor of side branch occlusion (the more acute the angle, the higher the risk of side branch occlusion). In the most complex lesions, these various mechanisms (and probably others such as thrombus) interact and generate a "bifurcation issue," which did not exist at the beginning of the procedure. This goes to show that anticipation is a key aspect of bifurcation lesion management.

Side branch occlusion has long been considered to be a relatively insignificant occurrence, resulting only in transient chest pain and mild creatinine increase (9–12). However, the NIRVANA study (13) demonstrated a significant risk of myocardial infarction with or without Q waves (CPK >5 times the normal value) associated with side branch occlusion (40%) and this is why "significant" side branches should be respected.

Index of bifurcation lesions

Coronary bifurcation lesions have been the subject of several classifications with the underlying

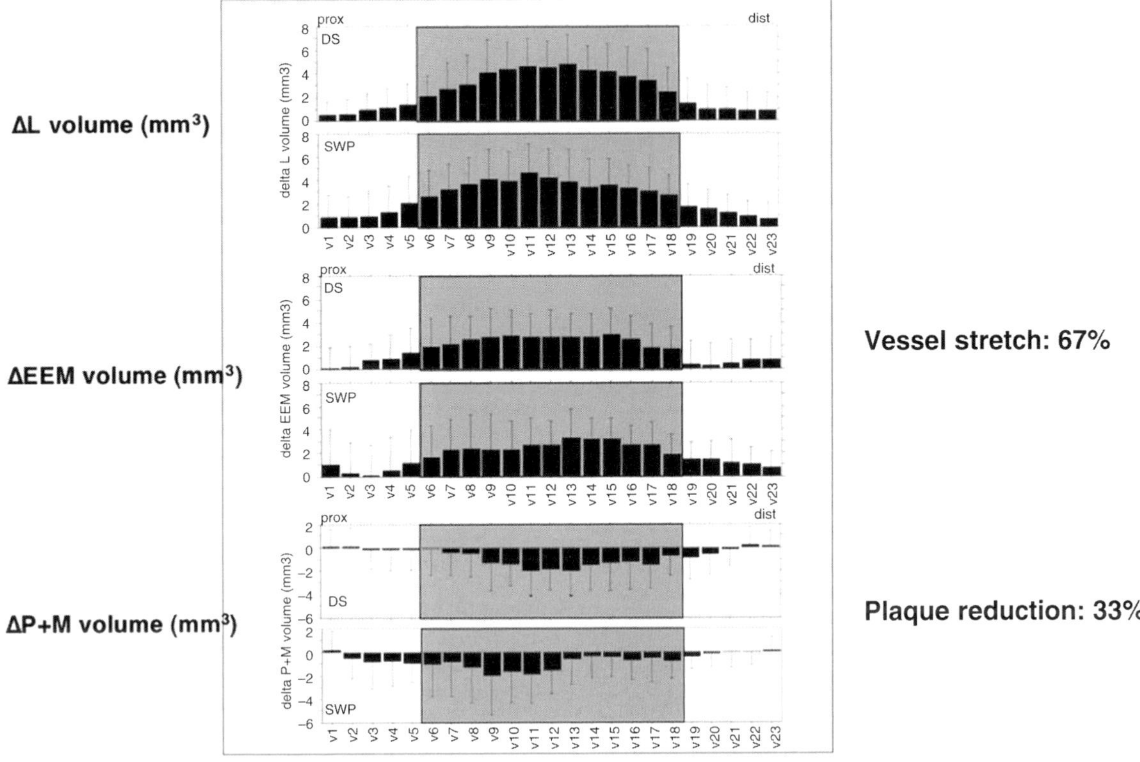

Figure 2 The axial plaque shifting phenomenon.

assumption that each type could be associated with a specific treatment. The Institut Cardiovasculaire Paris Sud (ICPS) classification that we published in 1996 (14) was regarded as useful, though requiring good memorization skills. In this lesion index, two types (1 and 4) were labeled true bifurcation lesions and the remaining types (2, 3, 4a, and 4b) labeled false bifurcation lesions. The classification recently proposed by Medina (Fig. 3) at the PCR meeting is extremely simple, accurate, and exhaustive. It consists of writing three consecutive figures sepaated by commas with only two values: 0 (<50% stenosis) or 1 (>50% stenosis). The first figure represents the proximal main branch, the second figure the distal main branch, and the third the side branch ostium. Other important parameters are the distribution of plaque in the bifurcation and the length of the side branch lesion. Moreover, in the current era of drug-eluting stents (DES), the reference diameters of the main vessel and side branch remain predictive factors of restenosis. The degree of stenosis in each branch as well as the presence of calcification and sinuous proximal segments are factors that increase complexity.

CAN SIDE BRANCH DETERIORATION DURING MAIN BRANCH STENTING BE PREDICTED?

Acute coronary syndromes are clinical predictors of side branch occlusion during main branch stenting. A side branch originating in the main branch lesion, a lesion at the side branch ostium, a small side branch reference diameter, and a high stent diameter/artery ratio are considered angiographic predictors of occlusion (9–15). In the corelab analysis of the TULIPE study (15), only the angle between the side branch and the main branch distal to the bifurcation was found to be predictive of side branch occlusion and, to a lesser degree (P = NS), the presence of an ipsilateral lesion in the main vessel.

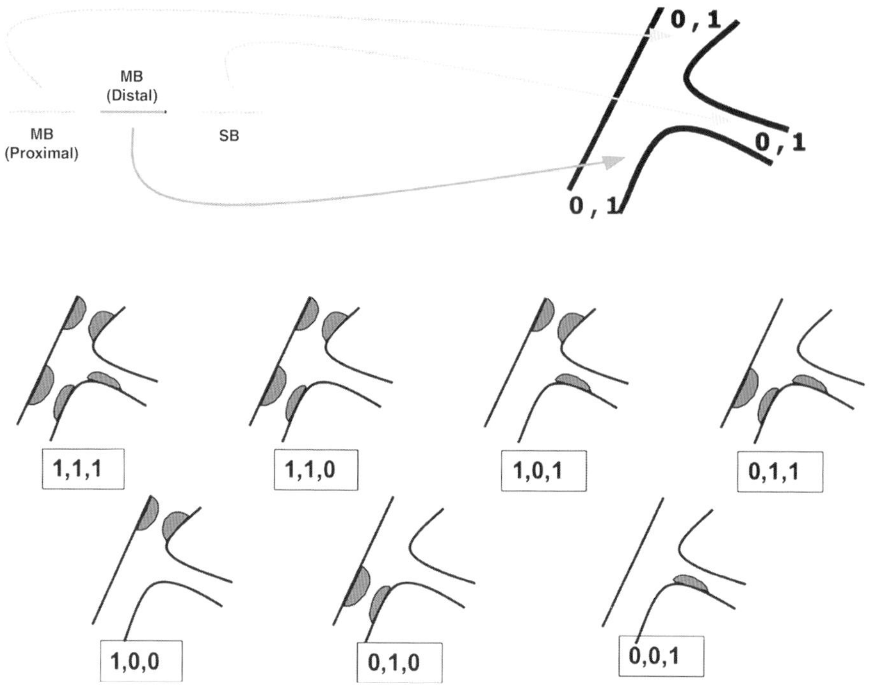

Figure 3 Medina classification of bifurcation lesions.

ROLE OF THE ANGLE BETWEEN BOTH BRANCHES

The angle between the branches of a bifurcation may influence not only the outcome of angioplasty after stenting but also the angiographic success rate. The proximal (A) and distal (B) angles should be considered separately, as they are not complementary because the main branch does not form a straight line. Angle A when <110° may complicate guidewire insertion into the side branch. Once in place, the wire may favorably modify this angle (Fig. 4) (8), which accounts for the usefulness of the jailed wire technique at the beginning of the procedure. Angle B is a predictive factor of side branch occlusion as mentioned earlier (15). In this case,

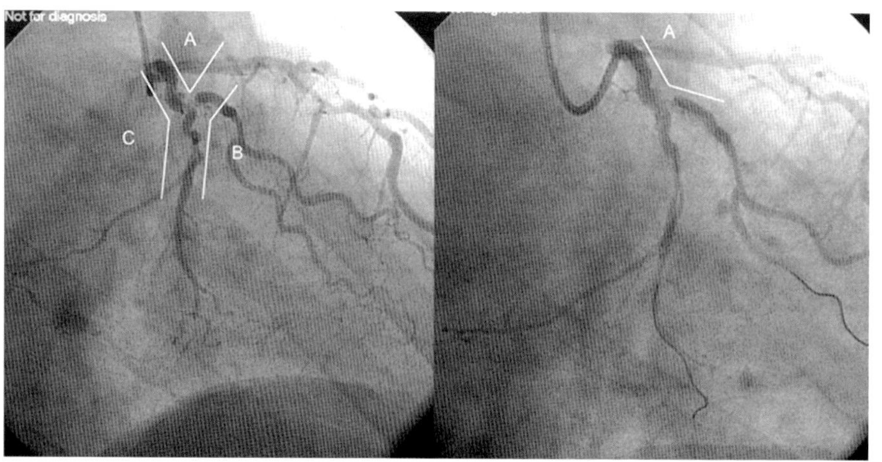

Figure 4 The proximal (*A*) and distal (*B*) angles of bifurcation lesion and main branch angle (*C*).

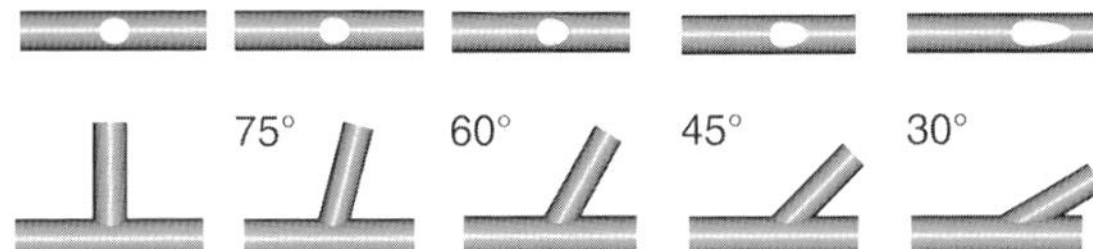

Figure 5 Impact of various bifurcation angles on side-branch ostium anatomy.

the jailed wire keeps the branch open and serves as a marker in cases of occlusion. Thus, whatever the angle, the jailed wire technique seems to be beneficial in all cases. The only caveat is that the wire should not be excessively jailed by using high pressures or balloons of too large a size during stent placement in the main branch. Furthermore, Choice PT® wires should be avoided due to their inherent risk of rupture, which is not the case with BMW wires. Angle B may also impact the acute and long-term results. Indeed, very acute angles require the placement of a stent with optimal strut opening potential in the main branch (Fig. 5). Conversely, when the angle is 90°, the crush technique is associated with a high risk of stent malapposition in the side branch. The angle formed by the two proximal and distal segments of the main branch on each side of the bifurcation (C) may be an important parameter when using dedicated stents, as shown recently by Amador et al. (16). Indeed, when <180°, this angle may prevent the successful placement "in phase" of the Frontier® stent (and probably other dedicated devices).

PRACTICAL DEFINITION OF BIFURCATION LESIONS

A bifurcation lesion is a coronary lesion involving two branches, the main branch and a significant side branch. A significant side branch may be a large and long branch vascularizing a broad territory of viable myocardium, but also a smaller branch clinically and functionally significant, generating collateral branches in a viable territory, or a branch vascularizing a viable territory in a patient with prior history of myocardial infarction or significant left ventricular dysfunction. In routine practice, a coronary bifurcation lesion is defined as a lesion involving a side branch that must be preserved.

AVAILABLE TECHNIQUES AND CLASSIFICATION

In the 1980s, bifurcation lesions were treated by balloon angioplasty with a low rate of success and a high incidence of complications and re-interventions, despite a relatively early introduction of the kissing balloon technique (17,18). Directional atherectomy was also used, but did not result in a higher rate of success and a lower rate of reintervention (19,20).

Many stenting techniques for bifurcation lesions have been described (21–31). In 1996, we proposed an indexed management of bifurcation lesions (14) including four treatment types. Type A consisted of stenting the side branch ostium and then the main branch over the side branch. Type B is also a T-stenting technique starting with the main branch. Type C or "culotte" stenting consisted of implanting a stent in the proximal segment of the main branch covering each of the two branches (double proximal stenting). Type D involved the stenting of the distal main branch and side branch ostia with or without proximal stenting. A classification of techniques provides an accurate definition of the strategies used allowing analysis and comparison of clinical results in homogeneous patient populations. The numerous techniques that have been described since then may be classified into categories derived from the four original types.

A FAMILY

Side-branch stenting (SBS) is ideal in T-shape bifurcations in which the proximal angle is close to 90° (Fig. 6). This type of bifurcation is very rare (especially after side branch wire placement). In fact, due to the angle between both branches, the placement of a stent at the SBS may theoretically result in a gap between the two stents. In order to fill this gap, the SBS may be implanted so as to involve part of the main branch; however, this entails a risk of hindering the subsequent placement of the MBS. The modified T-stenting technique consists of leaving a second stent undeployed in the main branch while implanting the SBS. The MBS is then deployed after removal of the side branch wire and balloon. The crush technique is an "extreme" modified

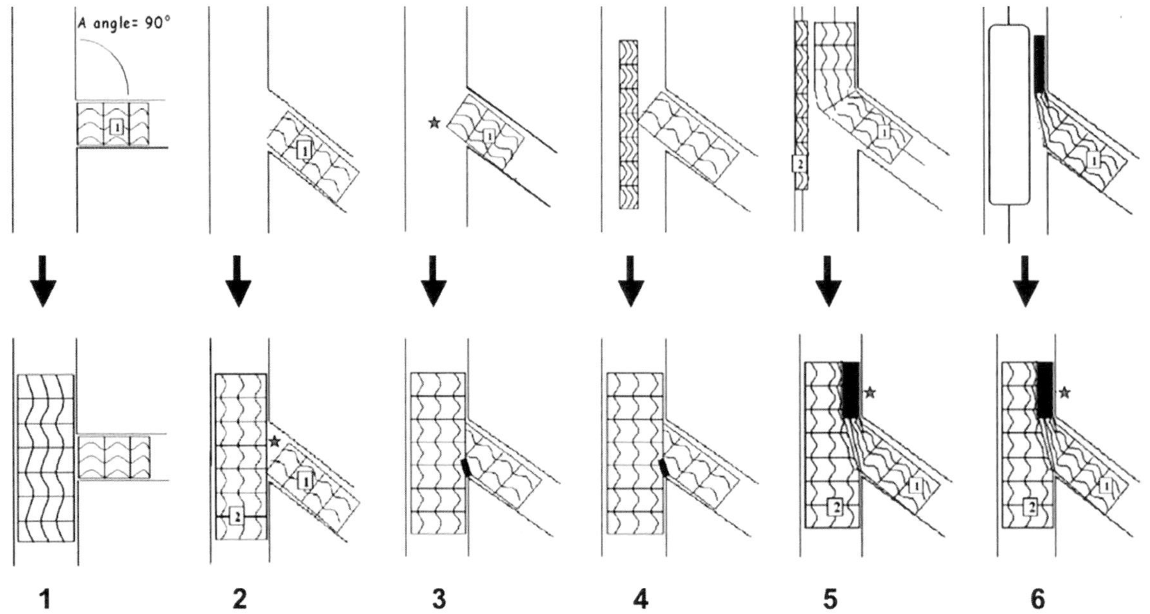

Figure 6 Type A bifurcation stenting technique. * = Drawbacks.

T-stenting approach, where the SBS is partially deployed in the main branch, with the MBS already in place. Then, the side branch balloon and wire are removed and the MBS is deployed, crushing the proximal part of the SBS. The crush technique may include an additional step in order to allow the use of a 6 French guiding catheter: the SBS is crushed by a balloon previously inserted in the main branch, while deploying the SBS. Then, the MBS is deployed (balloon crush technique or step crush technique).

B family

The first strategy deriving from the type B technique is the provisional T stenting of the side branch followed by kissing balloon inflation and is now the "gold standard" strategy with the majority of bifurcation-dedicated devices allowing permanent access to both branches as well as provisional stenting of the side branch ostium (Fig. 7). This strategy has been further simplified in order to allow basic protection of the side branch by means of a wire ("protection wire") or by predilatation of the side branch, followed by stent placement in the main branch, with or without protection. The SBS may also be implanted so as to protrude slightly into the main branch, with subsequent balloon crushing defined as internal crush or reverse crush.

C family

This treatment is still limited to the conventional "culotte" technique (Fig. 8).

D family

The conventional technique has a shortcoming in instances requiring stenting of the main branch proximal to the two stents deployed in the ostia in that it leaves a gap (Fig. 9). Distal deployment of the stent over the main branch wire may cause crushing of the SBS. Several solutions to this technical difficulty have been described. One of them consists of the systematic placement of a proximal stent before stenting the two distal branches simultaneously (Helqvist technique). This D technique was originally carried out with two stents manually crimped onto two balloons before stenting the distal branches ("skirt" technique) or after ("trouser legs and seat" technique). The skirt technique is now used with the DEVAX dedicated device.

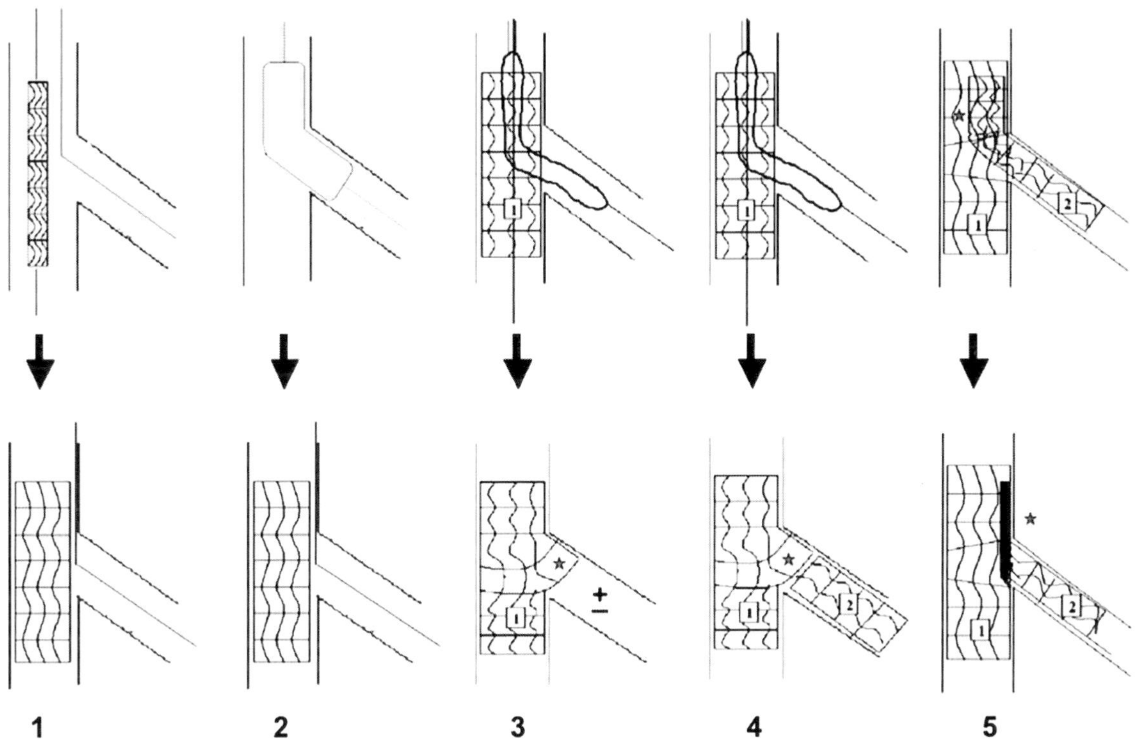

Figure 7 Type B bifurcation stenting technique. * = Drawbacks.

Inverted techniques

Inverted techniques involve the placement of a stent from the main branch toward the side branch (Fig. 10). This does not apply to cases in which the side branch is larger than the distal "main branch," for instance the circumflex and a marginal artery. These strategies could be called the "big (large) to small" techniques.

BIFURCATION STENTING IN A BENCH TEST (32–35)

Bench testing of bifurcation stenting has allowed us to analyze potential stent deformation resulting from the opening of struts opposite the side branch. These distortions vary according to the stent type, the quality of stent coverage (density, evenness), and the technical difficulties associated with each individual strategy.

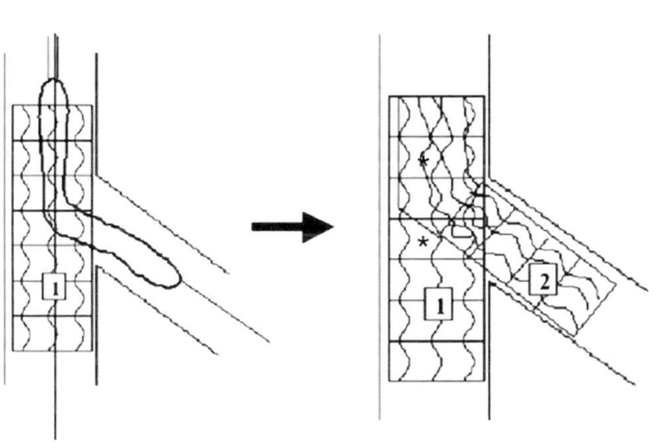

Figure 8 Type C bifurcation stenting technique. * = Drawbacks.

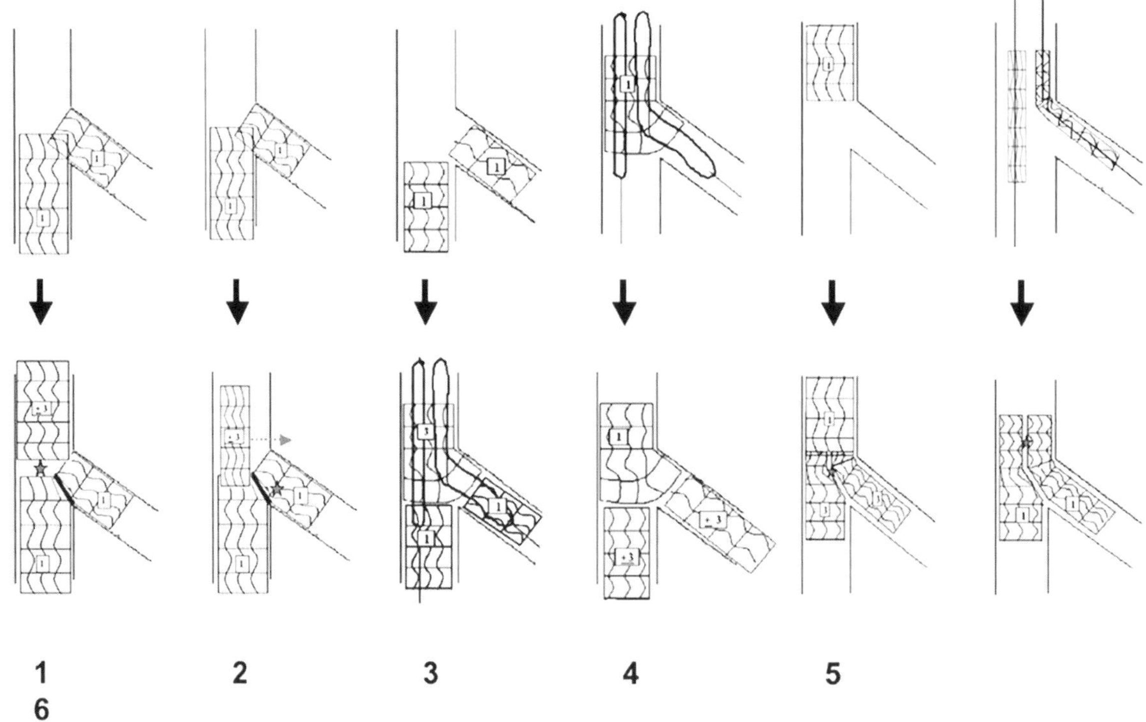

Figure 9 Type D bifurcation stenting technique. * = Drawbacks.

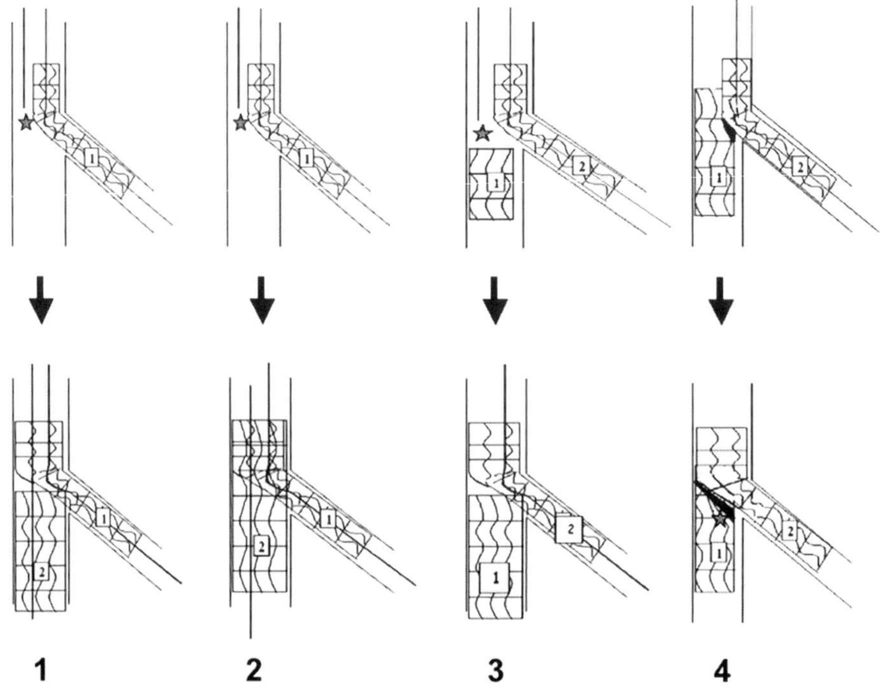

Figure 10 Inverted stenting techniques. * = Drawbacks.

The opening of a stent strut toward the side branch has two types of consequences: strut expansion (*i*) may be adequate and involve solely the origin of the side branch or (*ii*) may cause stent dislodgment and attract the struts facing the side branch toward the center of the main lumen. This phenomenon depends on the stent expansion potential and, consequently, on the size of the vessel in which the stent is deployed. It is also related to the strut through which the side branch balloon is inserted. When angle A is open, the contralateral distortion of the stent is commensurate with the size of the side branch and the distal location of the strut. This detrimental occurrence is associated with a beneficial phenomenon, namely the projection of one or two struts of the MBS onto the wall of the side branch ostium, which may prove sufficient for stenting short ostial lesions of the side branch (Fig. 11). These two interrelated phenomena are obviously well controlled in a bench test but remain completely unpredictable in a patient, resulting in leaving the ostium of the side branch unstented. The untoward effect of this double phenomenon may be corrected while the SBS strut is kept in place by kissing inflation.

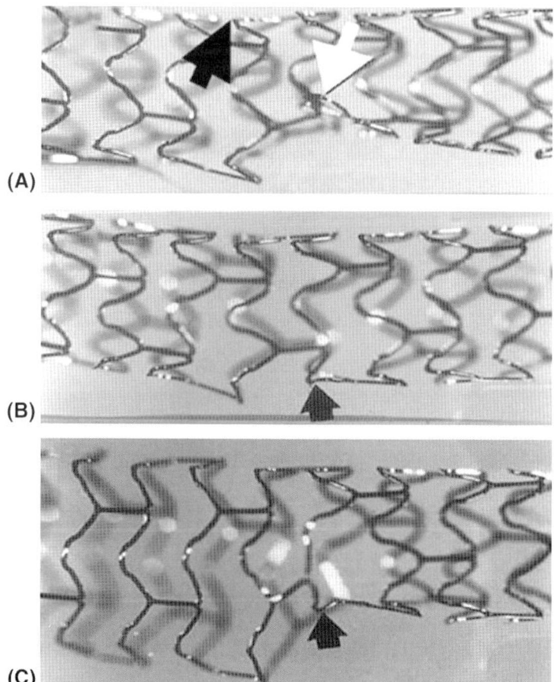

Figure 11 Provisional side-branch stenting: bench model.

The crush technique has been well studied in bench tests. As the stent is implanted in the side branch so as to protrude into the main branch, it is "crushed" by the MBS.

Due to its longitudinal stability, the SBS is subsequently stretched between two anchoring points: the distal side branch where it is deployed and the proximal main branch where it is crushed. As a result, the stent struts located in the side branch ostium are pushed away from the carina wall (and no biological effect can occur on the unstented wall if a DES is used). This can be partially corrected by kissing-balloon inflation optimizing the longitudinal and circular expansion ability of the SBS. Complete correction can be achieved by high-pressure inflation of a balloon in the side branch that allows adequate repositioning of one or both anchoring points. The latter maneuver should be completed by kissing balloon inflations of adequate size ($\geqslant$ deployment balloons) to avoid insufficient crushing of the SBS, which may result in stent thrombosis as well as protrusion of the SBS toward the carina (Figs. 12 and 13).

Use of high-pressure balloons for kissing inflation with the crush technique may result in the destruction of the polymer coating of DES (Fig. 13) and partially explain the relatively high risk of side branch restenosis and stent thrombosis associated with this technique.

BIFURCATION STENTING USING BARE-METAL STENTS

All BMS studies (36–44) have shown that, whatever the technique used, the use of two stents was not associated with a better outcome compared to the implantation of a single stent in the main branch followed by kissing dilatation of the two branches (Fig. 14) with provisional stenting of the side branch. No conclusion can be drawn in the absence of randomized studies. One may assume that patients treated with two stents had more complex lesions. However, the implantation of two stents has been evaluated as a strategical approach without evidence of a clear benefit. As things currently stand, a

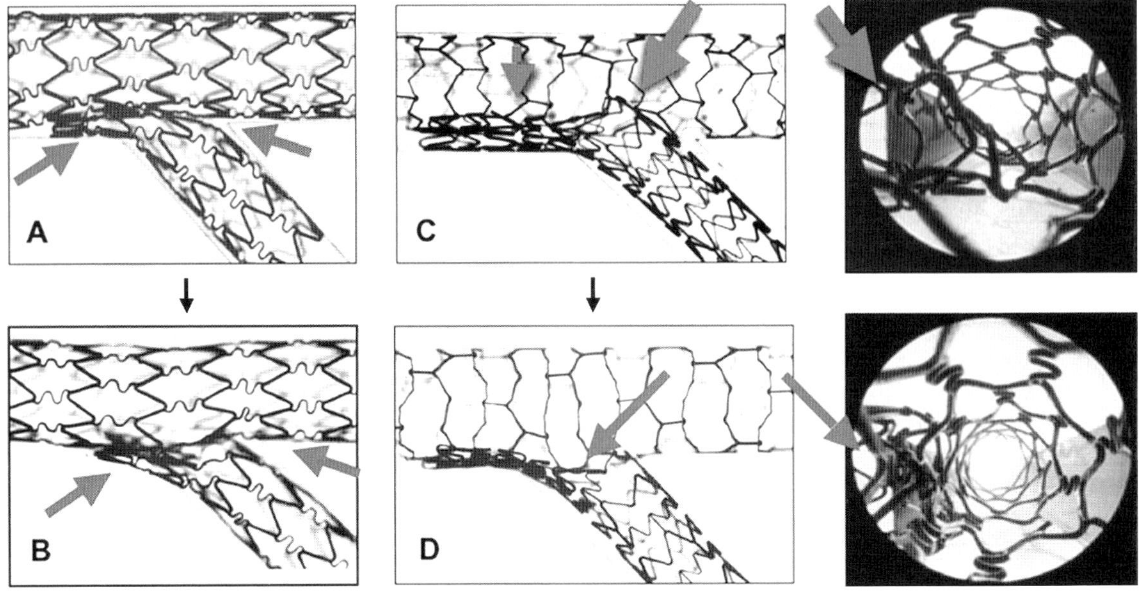

Figure 12 Bench model of a crush technique before and after kissing balloon inflation.

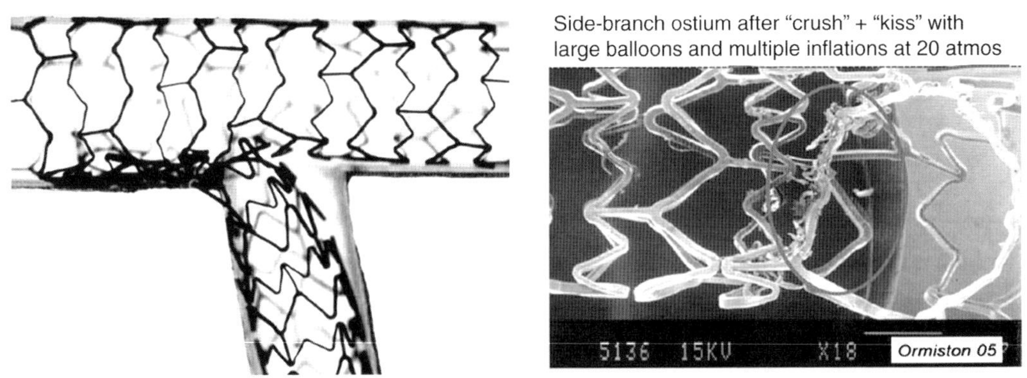

Figure 13 Destruction of the polymer coating following high pressure kissing inflation with the crush technique.

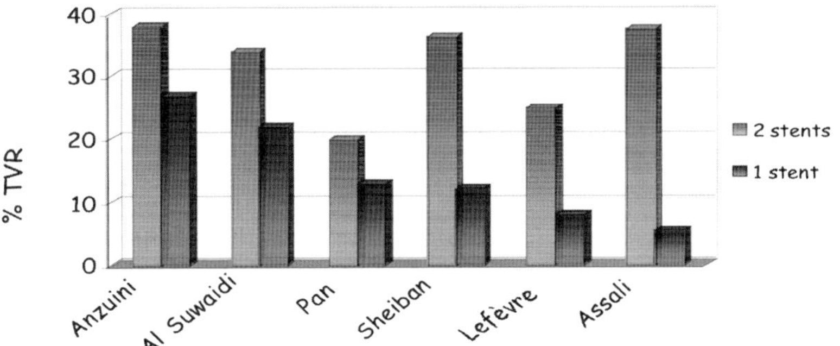

Figure 14 Target vessel revascularization rates in studies comparing two stent strategy vs. single stent strategy with bare metal stents. *Abbreviation*: TVR, target vessel revascularization. (*See color insert.*)

consensus has been reached in favor of provisional T stenting with BMS, including dedicated stents such as Frontier® and Twin Rail®, designed for provisional T stenting of the side branch.

BIFURCATION STENTING USING DRUG-ELUTING STENTS

In fact, apart from a dramatic reduction in the re-intervention rate (6,45–53), the advent of DES has not brought about any other major changes. The results observed in bench tests remain unchanged and the data published in the literature still show a favorable trend toward the use of a single stent (Fig. 15). Indeed, two randomized studies (46,47) have not shown any benefit associated with the systematic use of two drug-eluting stents compared to a strategy of using one stent for treating the main branch with side branch provisional T stenting. Although unpublished, Steigen et al. presented the six-month results of the Nordic Bifurcation Study at American College of Cardiology Meeting in Atlanta in 2006. In this study, 413 patients were randomized to both branches ($n = 206$) with "crush," "culotte," "Y," or other techniques or provisional stenting ($n = 207$) using SES implantation. The cross over from provisional to double branches stenting was allowed only if TIMI flow following side branch dilation was zero. Procedural success was achieved in 97% of cases in the provisional versus 95% in both branch stenting groups. The side branch was stented only in 4.3% of the patients in the provisional stenting group; FKB balloon was performed, respectively, in 32% and 74% of the patients ($P < 0.001$). At six months, there was no difference between the two groups regarding cardiac death, myocardial infarction (MI), index lesion MI, target vessel revascularization (TVR), and stent thrombosis.

Nevertheless, the importance of final kissing inflation has been emphasized in recent evaluations of the crush technique (50) and the increased risk of thrombosis resulting from the use of two stents has also been underlined (52,53).

HOW TO STENT A BIFURCATION LESION?

In routine practice, bifurcation stenting techniques may be classified into three main strategies: all subsequent steps are guided by the initial treatment intent, the results of the first steps or the occurrence of more or less predictable events.

Simultaneous stenting of the two branches

Both stents are deployed simultaneously in both branches following or followed by proximal stenting when necessary. The main issue lies in implanting the stent according to the position of the carina V stenting or simultaneous kissing stents (SKS). Simultaneous double stenting requires also the use of 8 French guiding catheters as well as aggressive predilatation of both branches.

Stenting of the side branch ostium first

It consists of systematic double stenting, starting with the side branch and usually requires predilatation of both branches and 8 French guiding catheters in the majority of cases—systematic T stenting, modified T stenting, inverted culotte (big to small culotte), or the crush technique.

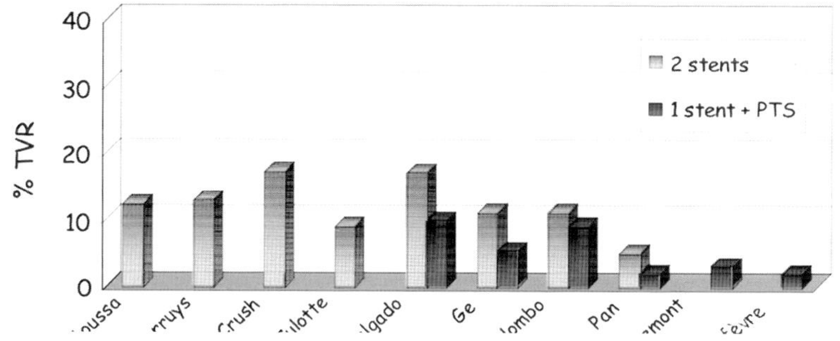

Figure 15 Target vessel revascularization rates in studies comparing two stent strategy versus single stent strategy with drug-eluting stents. *Abbreviations*: PTS, provisional T stenting; TVR, target vessel revascularization. (*See color insert.*)

Provisional side branch stenting

It consists of stenting the main branch over the side branch after dilatation of the side branch when necessary, or in opening of MBS struts facing the side branch, followed or not by kissing balloon inflation. In the presence of inadequate results, SBS can be performed with T-stenting, internal crush or culotte, followed by optional kissing balloon inflation. This approach can be performed with a 6 French guiding catheter via the femoral or radial approach whatever the technique used. We believe that this is the most rational strategy in the management of bifurcation lesions, given the fact that most side branch lesions, when present, are short. Thus, stent placement in the side branch is performed only in the presence of a significant lesion in the side branch ostium after kissing-balloon inflation.

STEP BY STEP PROVISIONAL SIDE BRANCH STENTING

Is it a bifurcation lesion?

The first step is to determine the importance of the side branch. Therefore the question becomes "is this side branch significant"? In instances when the operator judges the side branch as unimportant and not worth preserving, the lesion is not considered to be a bifurcation lesion and can be treated as a simple lesion.

Is the patient well prepared?

As bifurcation lesion treatment constitutes a predictive factor of stent thrombosis, the patient should have received appropriate antithrombotic treatment of adequate duration.

Access site approach

The vascular approach can be either femoral or radial through 6 French guiding catheters whatever the size of the two branches including the left main coronary artery (6 French guides are compatible with kissing-balloon inflation using 2 × 3.5 balloons). If the operator feels more comfortable with 7 French guides, he may decide to use a 7 French guide.

Guiding catheter selection

If selected, 6 French guiding catheters should have a wide internal lumen (0.071 in.). The shape must provide good support at the ostium (coaxial catheterization) or active support by deep-seated intubation (6 French). Left Amplatz catheters, when appropriately handled, may facilitate selective access to the circumflex or give good support for angioplasty of the distal right coronary artery. However, these catheters should not be used for distal left main angioplasty due to potential difficulties associated with ostial stent positioning.

Optimal views

Angiography must provide information on the side branch ostium and proximal segment of the main branch. The most useful views are as follows:

1. *Distal left main*: Working view is usually RAO 0–30°, caudal 25–30°. Side branch ostium visualization: LAO 30–60°, caudal 25–35° LM. Ostial positioning RAO 0–10°, cranial 40°.
2. *LAD/diagonal or septal bifurcation*: Working view is usually RAO 0–10°, cranial 40°. Side branch ostium visualization: LAO 40–45°, cranial 25–30° or LAO 45–55°, caudal 25–30°.
3. *Circumflex/marginal*: Working view RAO 0–15°, caudal 25°. Side branch ostium visualization: LAO 45–55° + caudal 25–30°. In cases, of dominant circulation, RAO 0–15°, cranial 25°.
4. *Mid RCA*: Working view LAO 40°. Side branch ostium visualization lateral view, RAO 30°.
5. *Distal RCA*: Working view LAO 35–50°. Side branch ostium visualization: LAO 0–15°, cranial 20°, lateral view.

Side branch wire protection

Our strategy is to systematically wire the side branch at the beginning of the procedure. The main advantages are that wire protection may help prevent side branch occlusion (15) and has been shown to be a predictor of PCI success in the side branch (54). When angle A is difficult, it favorably modifies the angle between the proximal segment of the main branch and the side branch (8) and facilitates subsequent wire exchange, balloon insertion, and potential placement of a second stent (Fig. 4). When angle B is sharp, it may help prevent side branch occlusion. Systematic placement of a side branch protective wire at the beginning of the procedure can be a rapid process. In cases where it should prove more time-consuming, the operator should keep in mind that this may turn into a real difficulty if performed after MBS.

Wire selection and wire shaping

Selection of the side branch wire must take into account the fact that the wire will be jailed between the stent and the main vessel wall. All peelable wires should be avoided, especially the PT choice wire, as there is a risk of its distal part coming loose and remaining in the side branch during withdrawal. In order to facilitate the procedure, all successive wire maneuvers and functions should be anticipated. Thus, the side branch wire should have a short tip adapted to the initial diameter of the main branch and also be loop-shaped so as to allow easy passage of the stent along the main branch without crossing the stent struts. The main branch wire should also be shaped according to the configuration of the main branch lesion. Nevertheless, the shape should also allow easy wire insertion into the side branch after stent placement in the main branch through the struts. The tip should be longer that the main branch diameter after adequate dilatation. Double shaping is sometimes necessary (long primary shape and short distal) (Fig. 16).

Wire insertion and manipulation

One of the difficulties generated by the use of two wires is the crisscrossing of wires that may hinder balloon and stent advancement. A number of "tricks" may reduce the risk of guidewire crisscrossing:

- Insert the first wire into the branch that seems to be the least accessible to catheterization and where wire rotation will be required.
- Limit second wire rotation to <180° by using wrist rotation.
- Keep wires separately on the table in the same position throughout the procedure even after wire exchange.

Another potential issue is side branch wiring. Several progressive methods may be implemented:

- Shaping of the wire to form a loop distal to the side branch. The loop is then pulled and the wire resumes its normal shape in the side branch.
- In cases of failed attempts to engage the side branch, the main branch should be dilated with balloons of gradually increasing diameters. The use of rotablator or directional atherectomy has been suggested. Deep breathing may modify the angulation of the distal branches of the RCA and facilitate wire insertion in the PDA.
- Stenting of the main branch over the side branch followed by selective catheterization of the side branch. In such cases, the risk of side branch occlusion may be significant and should lead the operator to reconsider the angioplasty option.

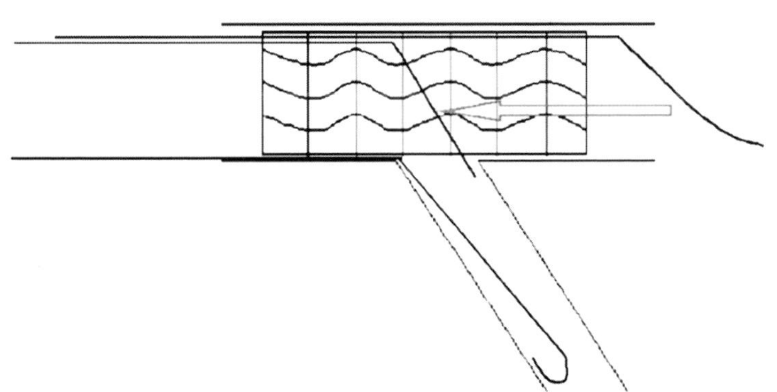

Figure 16 Guidewire tip shape.

- The use of an orientable micro catheter allowing guidewire insertion into the side branch may be another option though it has not yet been evaluated.

Predilatation

As for single branch lesions, predilatation of the main branch is indicated in the presence of distal lesions, sinuous segments, calcification, long lesions, and circumflex artery. The degree of stenosis is not a predictive factor of direct stenting failure. Direct stenting or undersized balloons may be useful in preventing dissection from spreading to the side branch.

Predilatation of the side branch remains controversial—it may be part of the provisional SBS strategy as suggested by Pan et al. (38). This very simple strategy consists in predilating the side branch followed by a simple stent implantation in the main branch, and nothing else in the presence of adequate results in the side branch.

In our opinion, predilatation should be avoided as it does not seem to prevent the risk of side branch occlusion during MBS. In the occurrence of side branch dissection, the operator can either opt for another strategy (SBS first), or be faced with the difficulty of crossing not only the struts of the MBS but also the dissection. The impossibility of performing guidewire exchange and side branch wiring after stent implantation in the main branch is a rare occurrence even when the side branch is occluded. For the same reasons, kissing predilatation of both branches is unnecessary and risky.

Stenting of the main branch

Selection of the stent type must obviously comply with national guidelines and regulations. However, DES have been clearly shown to improve the outcome of patients with bifurcation lesions. The wider the angle between the proximal segment of the main branch and the side branch (angle A) or the narrower the angle between the two distal branches (angle B), the larger the side branch ostium area, hence the necessity for the operator to select a large-cell stent for the main branch.

The length of the MBS should be selected according to the lesion length. It is important to remember that the stent should be implanted from one healthy arterial segment to another healthy arterial segment and that, conversely, stent length is a predictive factor of stent thrombosis. Consequently, stent length is always a compromise.

Stent diameter should be selected according to the diameter of the distal main branch segment with a 1:1 stent/artery ratio in order to avoid the occurrence of dissection or distal arterial rupture. A large side branch or the implementation of the "big to small" technique result in a diameter discrepancy between the stent and the proximal main vessel segment (distal left main), which must be corrected in order to ensure adequate stent/arterial wall apposition, and allow easy guidewire exchange without passage outside the proximal stent segment. In such cases, the operator may need to expand the proximal stent segment fully with a larger short balloon before the guidewire exchange (Fig. 17).

Stent deployment pressure can be used to adjust the diameter to the main branch distal and proximal segments. Care should be taken in the presence of hard or calcified lesions when a wire has been jailed.

At this stage of the procedure, assessment of the results according to the initial objectives is essential:

- When the side branch diameter is small and the vessel patent with adequate flow, and,

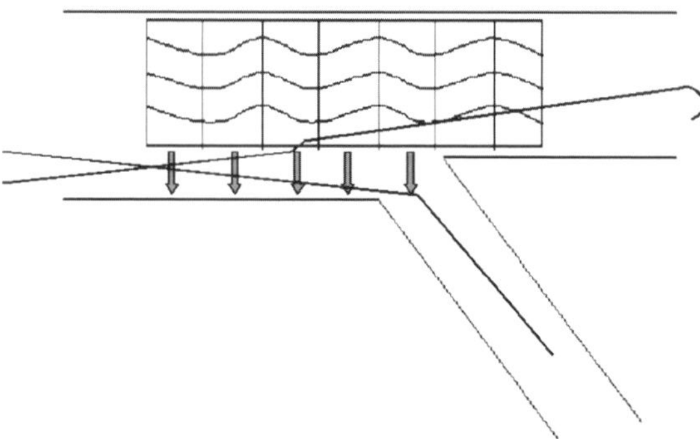

Figure 17 Problems with under-expanded proximal stent segment.

in the absence of chest pain or ECG changes, the result can be considered acceptable even if suboptimal and the procedure stopped at this level.

- In the presence of a lesion at the ostium of a larger side branch, guidewire exchange should be performed for subsequent PCI of the side branch. In this setting, the usefulness of a functional analysis of the side branch (FFR) may be discussed.

Two free wires

In order to free the wire in the side branch and carry on with the procedure, a third wire can be used. However, experience shows that it may be preferable to use the main branch wire secured by the stent. This wire has been pre-shaped to enter the side branch after withdrawal from the main branch (Fig. 16), through the most distal strut of the stent covering the ostium. In cases of access failure, the guidewire should be withdrawn and reshaped or exchanged for a hydrophilic wire. In cases of persistent failure, deployment of the MBS can be optimized opposite the ostium with a larger short balloon in order to modify cell geometry.

The subsequent maneuver consists in freeing the wire from the side branch. The guidewire should be gently withdrawn to avoid the risk of deep intubation of the guiding catheter leading to a potentially serious dissection. In such cases, the guiding catheter can be pulled back in the aorta with the left hand, while the right hand is pulling back the jailed wire simultaneously.

The wire retrieved from the side branch is then inserted into the distal main branch sometime after being shaped into the form of a short loop in order to avoid passage through the struts (Fig. 16).

Opening the side branch and performing kissing balloon inflation

The next step is the opening of the MBS strut toward the side branch. We prefer to perform directly kissing balloon inflation by inflating the main branch balloon first to avoid plaque or carina shifting toward the main branch (Fig. 18) and to correct stent distortion caused by the opening of a strut. This also allows optimization of the stent diameter in the proximal part of the bifurcation.

Selection of the side branch balloon is made according to the usual 1:1 balloon/artery ratio. The balloon length should match the length of the lesion. In the presence of plaque shifting, a very short balloon should be used in order to reduce the risk of geographical miss.

The size and length of the main branch balloon should be identical to that of the balloon used for stent deployment (in certain cases, the balloon delivery system of the stent can be used).

Balloons selected for kissing inflation must be 6 French compatible with an optimal profile.

The passage of a balloon in the side branch through the MBS may prove difficult. In case of failure, a 1.5 mm balloon can solve the problem in the majority of cases. In cases of persistent failure and anticipated difficulties, guidewires should be uncrossed (by retrieving and re-inserting the main branch wire). If balloon insertion through the strut still proves impossible, the stent should be further dilated or another strut should be selected. Another attempt should be made with a 1.5 mm coaxial balloon. Once the balloon is in the cell, it should not be inflated distal to the strut to avoid "balloon jailing" (a few cases have been described in the literature).

Passage of the main branch balloon may also pose problems usually related to guide wire crisscrossing.

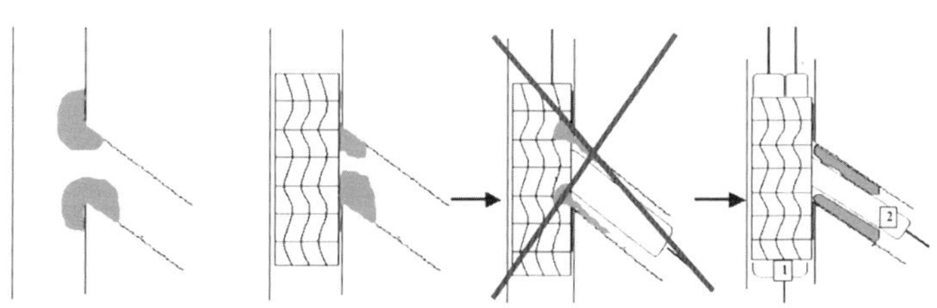

Figure 18 Plaque shifting toward the main branch following side branch balloon inflation. (*See color insert.*)

We start kissing inflation with the main branch balloon (Fig. 18), which does not require high-inflation pressures since the stent has already been deployed. However, pressure can be used for diameter adjustment. We inflate the side branch balloon (until disappearance of the balloon print) until it is fully expanded. We never use devices allowing simultaneous inflation of both balloons.

Assessment of the procedure outcome following kissing inflation is the key moment of the provisional SBS strategy. The results are evaluated according to the initial objective of side branch patency with good flowing or absence of significant stenosis in an anatomically or functionally important vessel. The interesting aspect of this strategy is the fact that, after stenting the most significant vessel, the operator may decide either to stent the side branch or not, and even choose from several implantation techniques for the second stent.

Side branch stenting

If the decision has been made to stent the side branch, T-stenting is the only technique that we use. It is, moreover, the only strategy that has been adequately evaluated. Stent selection is made according to artery size and the length of the lesion to be covered. Stent placement must be performed using the angiographic view(s) providing optimal visualization of the side branch ostium. The balloon marker should be positioned in the lumen of the MBS on the carina side without causing the stent to protrude. Low-pressure inflation of a balloon in the main branch may facilitate the accurate placement of the SBS. After stent deployment, another kissing inflation should be performed in accordance with the guidelines mentioned previously (no inflation outside the stents).

If the decision is to perform a reverse crush (or internal crush), the most important aspects are:

- The positioning of a balloon in the main branch next to the stent, which is subsequently deployed in the side branch and in the proximal segment of the main branch. This balloon is used to "crush" the SBS in the main branch after removal of the side branch wire.
- The limitation of the crushed stent length in order to reduce the risk of thrombosis (absence of or delayed endothelization)
- Kissing balloon inflation has not been shown to be indispensable with the reverse crush technique, though it may prevent the occurrence of restenosis and, possibly, thrombosis (recrossing of three stent layers with a wire and a balloon).
- Opening of the side branch with a large balloon prior to kissing inflation has been recommended in order to ensure optimal apposition to the carina.

This technique is sometimes involuntarily applied in cases when stent advancement in the side branch proves difficult. The superiority of the reverse crush over the culotte technique in this setting has not yet been debated.

If the decision is to perform a culotte technique, this involves the partial deployment of the SBS in the proximal segment of the main branch followed by the opening of a strut toward the distal segment of the main branch.

The procedure should be completed with kissing balloon inflation in order to achieve proximal deployment and apposition of both stents. One of the problems inherent in this technique lies in diameter discrepancy between the proximal segment of the SBS deployed in the proximal main branch and the artery diameter, which may generate further difficulties during wire insertion into the distal main branch. Immediate optimal expansion of the proximal segment of the SBS with a larger balloon may facilitate passage of the wire and balloon. Another difficulty is the performance of kissing balloon inflation, though this is indispensable with this very "metallic" technique.

SYSTEMATIC DOUBLE STENTING STRATEGIES

All these strategies require predilatation of both bifurcation vessels. When simultaneous double stenting is performed, prior kissing predilatation is preferred in order to facilitate stent passage and positioning as well as reduce the risk of plaque shifting from main branch to side branch after stenting (Fig. 18).

When simultaneous stenting techniques are used (V stenting, SKS) the length of the new carina should be limited to a minimum (lesion coverage) in order to reduce the risk of stent thrombosis and facilitate wire re-crossing maneuvers.

In strategies of initial stent deployment in the side branch (Fig. 19), the SB wire should be retrieved before stent implantation in the main branch in order to avoid wire jailing between two stents. The same maneuver is recommended for T-stenting in order to restore the original angle between the SB and the proximal main branch.

Prior to performing the indispensable kissing balloon inflation upon completion of a crush procedure, the operator must ensure that the SBS is adequately deployed and apposed to the vessel wall by dilating the ostium at high pressure with a balloon of appropriate size. Kissing balloon inflation should be subsequently performed using moderate pressure.

THE "BIG TO SMALL" INVERTED TECHNIQUES

These techniques can be implemented in type 1,0,1 or 0,0,1 lesions. The inherent difficulties arise from the discrepancy in diameter between the proximal segment of the main vessel and the side branch, the associated risk of side branch dissection when the side branch is overdilated, and the risks related to stent under-deployment in the main vessel (Fig. 11).

The best solution is to select a "big to small" stent matching the side branch diameter. Any subsequent maneuver should be preceded by the optimal deployment of the proximal segment of the stent using a bigger balloon.

APPROACH TO TRIFURCATION LESIONS

The same treatment strategies may be implemented in coronary trifurcations with increased attention to the handling of the wires. The post-stenting results can be optimized by the simultaneous inflation of three balloons (requiring at least 7 French guidewires).

Certain "metallic" techniques do not seem very reasonable (double crush, double culotte, triple simultaneous stenting).

APPROACH TO DISTAL LEFT MAIN

All techniques used in simple bifurcations have been shown to be applicable to the distal left main trunk using either bare stents or drug-eluting stents. Even the simplest techniques (stenting over the side branch with basic protection, provisional SBS strategy) have been used with very promising results.

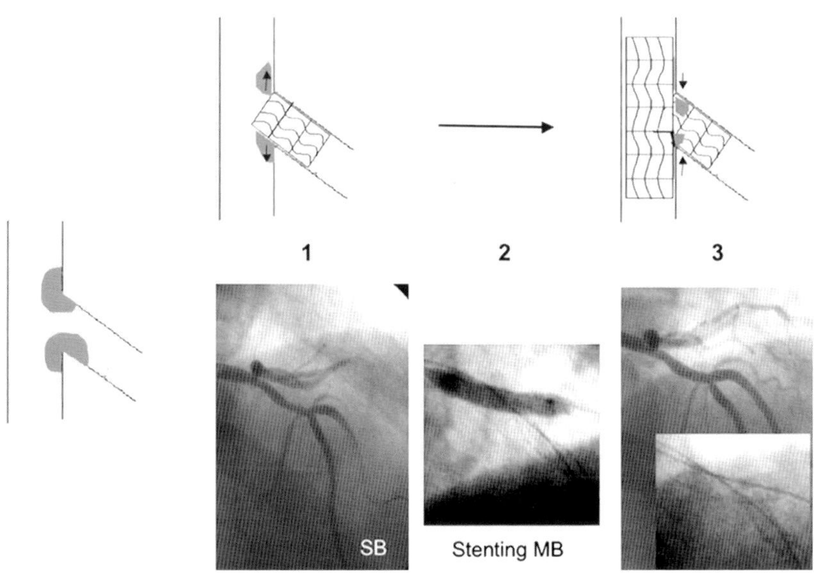

Figure 19 Plaque shifting toward the main branch following initial stent deployment in the side branch. (*See color insert.*)

The left main coronary artery is a large-diameter vessel. The stents that are currently on the market are not ideally suited to this vessel. The size of the cells may be inadequate for the side branch and the maximal expansion capacity of the stent may be suboptimal for the left main or for partial coverage of the side branch ostium. This inadequacy may result in clinical complications (thrombosis and reinterventions)

Whatever the technique used in short or long left main trunks, the ostium must be covered in order to prevent the risk of restenosis. The vulnerability of the ostium is increased by kissing dilatation and guiding catheter insertion.

CONCLUSION

In the era of DES, the treatment of coronary bifurcation lesions has become relatively consensual. Most specialists agree that provisional SBS is the optimal strategy in the presence of a short stenosis in the side branch (70–80% of bifurcation lesions). When basic guidelines are adequately followed, this strategy is associated with excellent short- and midterm outcome, a low risk of thrombosis and a one-digit rate of reintervention (Fig. 20). Moreover, though the optimal strategy has not yet been defined in more complex instances where the side branch lesion is more than 3 to 5 mm in diameter, provisional stenting of the side branch remains a valid option.

It is likely that in the near future, drug-eluting dedicated stents will become available and will help solve the controversy between the provisional SBS option and the systematic use of two stents.

EDITOR'S COMMENTS

Louvard and Lefevre give a superb overview of this field and very little needs to be added except to emphasize a few points:

With difficult access into the side branch, do not hesitate to change projection or wire. Hydrophilic wires can solve the problem in two ways—access the side branch or close the side branch. Sometimes the only strategy to allow access into the side branch is to predilate the main branch.

You do not need to become familiar with all techniques. Try to stay with the approach that has given you the best results and using which you feel comfortable and safe.

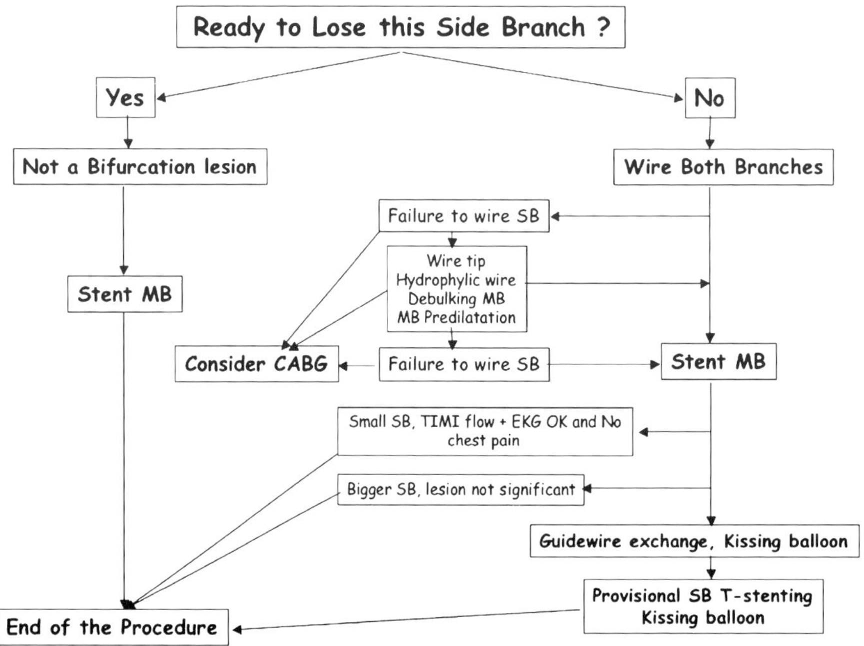

Figure 20 Provisional side branch stenting strategy algorithm.

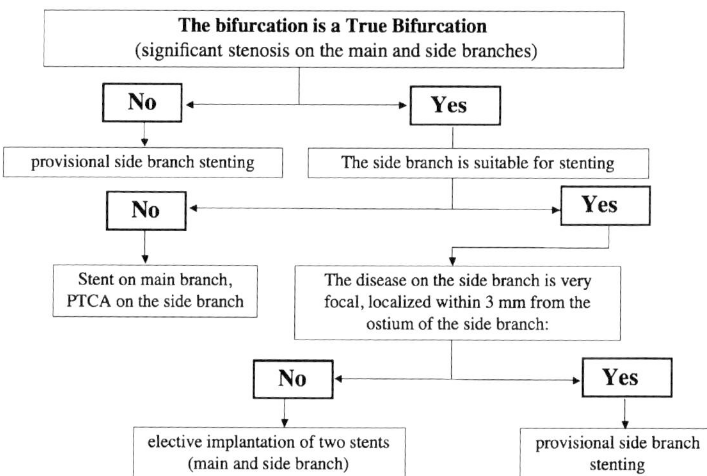

Figure 21 Editor's approach to bifurcation lesion treatment.

Never forget that many side branches just need to stay open and a residual stenosis is many times clinically not relevant.

If you have any doubt about the need to protect a branch this means that the branch needs protection.

We conclude by proposing the algorithm in Figure 21 to help in selecting the best approach (according to the Editors) to treat bifurcational lesions.

ACKNOWLEDGMENT

We thank Mrs Catherine Dupic for help in preparation of the manuscript.

REFERENCES

1. Zhou Y, Kassab GS, Molloi S. On the design of the coronary arterial tree: a generalization of Murray's law. Phys Med Biol 1999; 44:2929–2945.
2. Mallus MT, Kutryk MJ, Prati F, et al. Extent and distribution of atherosclerotic plaque in relation to major coronary side-branches: an intravascular ultrasound study in vivo. G Ital Cardiol 1998; 28:961–969.
3. Lefèvre T, Morice MC, Sengottuvel, et al. Influence of technical strategies on the outcome of coronary bifurcation stenting. Eurointervention 2005; 1:31–37.
4. Garot P, Lefevre T, Savage M, et al. Nine-month outcome of patients treated by percutaneous coronary interventions for bifurcation lesions in the recent era a report from the Prevention of Restenosis with Tranilast and its Outcomes (PRESTO) trial. J Am Coll Cardiol 2005; 46(4): 606–612.
5. Lemos PA, Serruys PW, van Domburg RT, et al. Unrestricted utilization of sirolimus-eluting stents compared with conventional bare stent implantation in the "real world": the Rapamycin-Eluting Stent Evaluated at Rotterdam Cardiology Hospital (RESEARCH) registry. Circulation 2004; 109:190–195.
6. Colombo A, Keichi, Lefèvre T, et al. Efficacy of sirolimus-eluting stent in the treatment of patients with bifurcation lesions in multivessel coronary artery disease: A substudy of the ARTS II trial [abstr]. Circulation 2005; 112(suppl II):421.
7. Lemos PA, Serruys PW, van Domburg RT, et al. Unrestricted utilization of sirolimus-eluting stents compared with conventional bare stent implantation in the "real world": the Rapamycin-Eluting Stent Evaluated At Rotterdam Cardiology Hospital (RESEARCH) registry. Circulation 2004; 109:190–195.
8. Louvard Y, Lefèvre T, Cherukupalli R, et al. Favorable effect of the "jailed wire" technique when stenting bifurcation lesions. Am J Cardiol 2003; 6(abstr. suppl).
9. Prasad N, Ali H, Schwartz L. Short- and long-term outcome of balloon angioplasty for compromised side branches after intracoronary stent deployment. Catheter Cardiovasc Interv 1999; 46:421–424.
10. Fischman DL, Savage MP, Leon MB, et al. Fate of lesion-related side branches after coronary artery stenting. J Am Coll Cardiol 1993; 22:1641–1646.

11. La Vecchia L, Bedogni F, Finocchi G, et al. Troponin T, troponin I and creatine kinase-MB mass after elective coronary stenting. Coron Artery Dis 1996; 7:535–540.
12. Aliabadi D, Tilli FV, Bowers TR, et al. Incidence and angiographic predictors of side branch occlusion following high-pressure intracoronary stenting. Am J Cardiol 1997; 80:994–997.
13. Bhargava B, Waksman R, Lansky AJ, Kornowski R, Mehran R, Leon MB. Clinical outcomes of compromised side branch (stent jail) after coronary stenting with the NIR stent. Catheter Cardiovasc Interv 2001; 54:295–300.
14. Lefèvre T, Louvard Y, Morice MC, et al. Stenting of bifurcation lesions: classification, treatments, and results. Catheter Cardiovasc Interv 2000; 49: 274–283.
15. Louvard Y, Sashikand G, Lefèvre T, Garot P, Darremont O, Brunel P. Angiographic predictors of side branch occlusion during the treatment of bicurcation lesions. Catheter Cardiovasc Interv 2005 (abstr. suppl).
16. Amador C, Delgado A, Medina A, et al. Immediate and long-term findings in bifurcation lesions treated with the dedicated Stent system Frontier [Abstr]. Circulation 2005; 112(suppl II):422.
17. Meier B. Kissing balloon coronary angioplasty. Am J Cardiol 1984; 54:918–920.
18. George BS, Myler RK, Stertzer SH, et al. Balloon angioplasty of bifurcation lesions: the kissing balloon technique. Catheter Cardiovasc Diagn 1986; 12:124–138.
19. Brener SJ, Leya FS, Apperson-Hansen C, Cowley MJ, Califf RM, Topol EJ. A comparison of debulking versus dilatation of bifurcation coronary arterial narrowings (from the CAVEAT I Trial). Coronary angioplasty versus excisional atherectomy trial-I. Am J Cardiol 1996; 78:1039–1041.
20. Dauerman HL, Higgins PJ, Sparano AM, et al. Mechanical debulking versus balloon angioplasty for the treatment of true bifurcation lesions. J Am Coll Cardiol 1998; 32:1845–1852.
21. Colombo A, Gaglione A, Nakamura S, Finci L. "Kissing" stents for bifurcation coronary lesion. Catheter Cardiovasc Diagn 1993; 30:327–330.
22. Carrie D, Karouny E, Chouairi S, Puel J. "T"-shaped stent placement: a technique for the treatment of dissected bifurcation lesions. Catheter Cardiovasc Diagn 1996; 37:311–313.
23. Schampaert E, Fort S, Adelman AG, Schwartz L. The V-stent: a novel technique for coronary bifurcation stenting. Catheter Cardiovasc Diagn 1996; 39:320–326.
24. Khoja A, Ozbek C, Bay W, Heisel A. Trouser-like stenting: a new technique for bifurcation lesions. Catheter Cardiovasc Diagn 1997; 41:192–196.
25. Kobayashi Y, Colombo A, Akiyama T, Reimers B, Martini G, di Mario C. Modified "T" stenting: a technique for kissing stents in bifurcational coronary lesion. Catheter Cardiovasc Diagn 1998; 43: 323–326.
26. Carrie D, Elbaz M, Dambrin G, et al. Coronary stenting of bifurcation lesions using "T" or "reverse Y" configuration with Wiktor stent. Am J Cardiol 1998; 82(11):1418–1421.
27. Sheiban I, Marsico F, Pagnotta P, et al. Modified "T"-stenting technique for kissing stents in bifurcational coronary lesions: clinical feasibility and immediate angiographic results. Am J Cardiol 1998; 84:50S.
28. Alberti A, Missiroli B, Nannini C. "Skirt" technique for coronary artery bifurcation stenting. J Invasive Cardiol 2000; 12:633–636.
29. Kobayashi Y, Colombo A, Adamian M, Nishida T, Moussa I, Moses JW. The skirt technique: A stenting technique to treat a lesion immediately proximal to the bifurcation (pseudobifurcation). Catheter Cardiovasc Interv 2000; 51:347–351.
30. Sheiban I, Albiero R, Marsico F, et al. Immediate and long-term results of "T" stenting for bifurcation coronary lesions. Am J Cardiol 2000; 85:1141–1144, A9.
31. Carlier SG, Colombo A, de Scheerder I, et al. Stenting of bifurcational coronary lesions: results of the multicentric European culottes registry. Eur Heart J 2001; 22(Abstr. Suppl):348.
32. Pomerantz RM, Ling FS. Distortion of Palmaz-Schatz stent geometry following side- branch balloon dilation through the stent in a rabbit model. Catheter Cardiovasc Diagn 1997; 40: 422–426.
33. Ormiston JA, Webster MW, Ruygrok PN, et al. Stent deformation following simulated side-branch dilatation: a comparison of five stent designs. Catheter Cardiovasc Interv 1999; 47:258–264.
34. Stankovic G, Martini G, Ferraro M, et al. An in-vitro assessment of stent geometry for bifurcation lesions after kissing balloon inflation. Am J Cardiol 2001; 88(suppl 5A):60G.

35. Brunel P, Leurent B, Banus Y, et al. Stent mesh access and deformation in the treatment of coronary bifurcation lesions: an in vitro–in vivo study. Am J Cardiol 2002; 90(suppl 6A):78H.
36. Louvard Y, Lefèvre T, Morice MC. Percutaneous coronary intervention for bifurcation coronary disease. Heart 2004; 90:713–722.
37. Al Suwaidi J, Yeh W, Cohen HA, Detre KM, Williams DO, Holmes DR Jr. Immediate and one-year outcome in patients with coronary bifurcation lesions in the modern era (NHLBI dynamic registry). Am J Cardiol 2001; 87:1139–1144.
38. Pan M, Suarez de Lezo J, Medina A, et al. Simple and complex stent strategies for bifurcated coronary arterial stenosis involving the side branch origin. Am J Cardiol 1999; 83:1320–1325.
39. Yamashita T, Nishida T, Adamian MG, et al. A. Bifurcation lesions: two stents versus one stent–immediate and follow-up results. J Am Coll Cardiol 2000; 35:1145–1151.
40. Anzuini A, Briguori C, Rosanio S, et al. Immediate and long-term clinical and angiographic results from Wiktor stent treatment for true bifurcation narrowings. Am J Cardiol 2001; 88:1246–1250.
41. Lefèvre T, Guyon P, Brunel P, et al. Stenting of bifurcation lesions using the BX velocity stent: a multicenter french study. Am J Cardiol 2001; 88(supp1 5A):21G.
42. Pan M, Suarez de Lezo J, Medina A, et al. A step-wise strategy for the stent treatment of bifurcated coronary lesions. Catheter Cardiovasc Interv 2002; 55:50–57.
43. Gobeil JF, Lefevre T, Guyon P, et al. Stenting of bifurcation lesions using the Bestent: A prospective dual center study. Catheter Cardiovasc Interv 2002; 55:427–433.
44. Koning R, Huret B, Caussin C, et al. Coronary stenting in bifurcated lesions: clinical and angiographic results of a french multicenter study. Am J Cardiol 2002; 90(suppl 6A):43H.
45. Colombo A, Stankovic G, Orlic, et al. Modified T-stenting technique with crushing for bifurcation lesions: immediate results and 30-day outcome. Catheter Cardiovasc Interv 2003; 60: 145–151.
46. Colombo A, Moses JW, Morice MC, et al. Randomized study to evaluate sirolimus-eluting stents implanted at coronary bifurcation lesions Circulation 2004; 109:1244–1249.
47. Pan M, de Lezo JS, Medina A, et al. Rapamycin-eluting stents for the treatment of bifurcated coronary lesions: a randomized comparison of a simple versus complex strategy. Am Heart J 2004; 148(5):857–864.
48. Sharma SK, Choudhury A, Lee J, et al. Simultaneous kissing stents (SKS) technique for treating bifurcation lesions in medium-to-large size coronary arteries. Am J Cardiol 2004; 94: 913–917.
49. Tanabe K, Hoye A, Lemos PA, et al. Restenosis rates following bifurcation stenting with sirolimus-eluting stents for de novo narrowings. Am J Cardiol 2004; 94(1):115.
50. Ge L, Airoldi F, Iakovou I, et al. Clinical and angiographic outcome after implantation of drug-eluting stents in bifurcation lesions with the crush stent technique importance of final kissing balloon post-dilation. J Am Coll Cardiol 2005; 46(4):613–620.
51. Ge L, Tsagalou E, Iakovou, et al. In-hospital and nine-month outcome of treatment of coronary bifurcational lesions with sirolimus-eluting stent. Am J Cardiol 2005; 95:757–760.
52. Ong L, Hoye A, Aoki J, et al. Thirty-day incidence and six-month clinical outcome of thrombotic stent occlusion after bare-metal, Sirolimus, or paclitaxel stent implantation. J Am Coll Cardiol 2005; 45:947–953.
53. Iakovou I, Schmidt T, Bonizzoni, et al. Incidence, predictors, and outcome of thrombosis after successful implantation of drug eluting stents. JAMA 2005; 293:2126–2130.
54. Brunel P, Lefèvre T, Darremont O, et al. Provisional T-stenting in the treatment of coronary bifurcation lesions. Results of the French Multicentre "Tulipe" study. Catheter Cardiovasc Interv 2006; 68:67–73.

5

Chronic total occlusion: A recipe for success

Giora Weisz and Jeffrey W. Moses

Successful recanalization and percutaneous revascularization of coronary arteries with chronic total occlusion (CTO) is one of the "last frontiers" in coronary interventions. Conquering this objective will enable complete percutaneous revascularization in an increasing number of patients. Revascularization of CTOs carries multiple theoretical advantages, like improvement in wall motion abnormality and left ventricular function and, ultimately, increased long-term survival. In the long term, when the coronary disease may progress, having an open artery may increase the tolerance to future coronary events. Reducing or abolishing myocardial ischemia improves electrical stability, and reduces predisposition to arrhythmic events. A review of the definitions, clinical relevance, indication for treatment, and results were recently summarized in a consensus document (1,2).

Learning and mastering the skills to recanalize CTO is an advanced-stage procedure that is left for an experienced operator. There is a wide variety of CTO cases, and special expertise is needed to differentiate between different anatomic situations, selecting the appropriate devices, being able to change strategies as the cases progresses, and keeping it safe—avoiding and taking care of potential complications. Needless to say that the success rate of CTO treatment is related to the accumulative general percutaneous coronary intervention (PCI) experience of the operator in general, and CTO cases in particular. The operator who takes on CTOs should approach cases of increasing difficulty, gradually going from tapered to flash occlusions, from short occlusions to longer ones, from straight segments to more tortuous vessels and, in time, to being able to tackle long-standing complete CTOs.

ANGIOGRAPHY

Meticulous angiography is the key point for success in treating CTOs. Correct evaluation of the occluded segment, vessel course, CTO morphology, edges, and bifurcations will enable the operator to select the appropriate strategy and devices, leading to high success rates. Features that are considered as favorable (increased success rate of recanalization) include occlusion of less than three months, occlusion segment less than 1.5 cm, some antegrade blood flow, and visible stump (dimple). Unfavorable features are long-standing occlusion, long segment, TIMI 0 flow, and bifurcating branches at either the proximal or distal edge of the occlusion segment.

Although the duration of occlusion may be unknown, some parameters can help the operator to determine for how long the artery has been occluded. Clues from the clinical history—prior myocardial infarction (MI) and reviewing old angiograms—can be very helpful. The presence of bridging collaterals is an indication of long-standing occlusion, but exceptions happen.

Important anatomical characteristics that should be noticed by the operator include the vessel shape and tortuosity, the proximity of the lesion to the ostium, and the CTO morphology. One of the most important features is the existence or absence of a dimple (tapering CTO). This has a significant impact on the success rate. It is important not to overlook the dimple, and multiple projections should be examined to avoid side branch overlapping as well. Careful investigation of the cine runs, sometimes going frame by frame, may yield additional important information such as small channels inside the CTO. In cases of bridging collaterals, it is important to distinguish between inside channels and out-of-the-vessel collaterals.

Bends or tortuosity inside the occluded segment is important but hard to appreciate, especially in long CTOs. Here, experience with the coronary anatomy plays a major role, and some clues may be helpful. Calcification, as seen during fluoroscopy prior to contrast injection, is the best way to understand the vessel course. Another potential clue is the movements of the proximal and distal segments of vessel. If they move in different directions, this is a sign of tortuosity inside the CTO. New, innovative strategies are using the computed tomography (CT) angiogram to follow the epicardial vessel anatomy. The three-dimensional reconstruction combined with coregistration of other imaging techniques, like the magnetic assisted navigation system (Stereotaxis, St. Louis, MO), can be helpful in evaluating the anatomy and vessel course.

Dual injection

The documentation of collaterals serves to evaluate the segments of the artery, distal to the occlusion, which is essential to CTO success. In addition to the valuable information like the size of the ischemic territory, the operator can evaluate the length of the occluded segment, and the size and location of the run-off. One should never blindly cross an occlusion without clearly knowing where the wire should be directed and whether it is inside the lumen or in a dissection plane. Having a simultaneous contralateral injection can simplify the procedure and increase the chances of successful and safer procedure if ipsilateral collaterals are insufficient. The contralateral injection is done by using a 4 to 5 French diagnostic catheter inserted through an additional arterial access, usually the contralateral groin. The retrograde injection is done a few heartbeats before the antegrade injection, to allow optimal documentation of both sides of the occlusion segment's adjacent branches and to evaluate its actual length, occasionally demonstrating an unsuspected lumen. The best view is one that does not foreshorten the occlusive segment and the immediate segment distal to it.

While crossing the occlusion with the wire, retrograde test injections or full cine angiograms are performed to verify that the wire is in the correct plane, and after crossing the occlusions that the wire is inside the true distal lumen of the artery.

After the initial predilatation of the occlusion, when antegrade flow is confirmed, there is no further need for the retrograde injection, and the diagnostic catheter may be removed.

GUIDING CATHETERS

As is true in regular interventions, the guiding catheter is of paramount importance in providing safe access of interventional tools to the treatment area, while providing support. In CTO cases, extra support is usually needed in greater force for delivery of devices. This is especially important after crossing with the wire. Many times, there is significant resistance to cross the lesion even with a very low profile balloon, and having an extra support guiding catheter can be of help. When the support of the guiding catheter is insufficient, the success rate is lower, especially in cases with unusual anatomic variability, calcified vessel, and additional complexities. The transfemoral approach usually lends even better support than the transradial approach, beyond the option of having a larger caliber catheter.

In the left coronary artery, good guiding catheter support can be achieved with a broad transition guiding catheter that has a secondary curve that leans against the opposite wall of the aorta (passive backup), usually EBU (Medtronic, Minneapolis, Minnesota), XB (Cordis, Gaithersburg, Maryland), or Voda (Boston Scientific, Natick, Massachusetts) will be sufficient, with rare cases requiring an Amplatz curve catheters.

In the right coronary artery, an excellent support can be achieved with the Amplatz left family of catheters, usually AL1, with AL 0.75 for small aortas and AL 1.5 or 2.0 for dilated roots. The operator should remember that these are relatively aggressive catheters with higher risk of having a dissection. In cases where such a dissection has occurred with inability to cross it with a wire, but the patient has no chest pain or evidence of ischemia, the dissection can usually be left for self-healing and the procedure can be re-attempted in few weeks.

Having a stiff catheter also gives an additional support for the system, with the limitation of reducing the ability for deep engagement, and higher rate of ostial/proximal risk of dissection from the tip. Using a (softer) 6 French guiding catheter may allow for additional support by relatively safe deep engagement of the catheter, deep into the coronary artery (active backup), but 7 to 8 French are generally preferred.

The selection of the guiding catheter is also influenced by the location of the occlusion. With very proximal occlusions, having an AL1 catheter may be counterproductive. The tip of the AL1 will be abutted into the occlusion, which potentially causes subintimal dissection at the occlusion and eventually reduces the chances of steering into the best channel for crossing with the wire. In such cases, Judkins' right shape-guiding catheter may be superior, despite having less support. Taking a higher caliber catheter will compensate for the lack of support, with the option of having additional tricks like an anchoring wire and balloon (see below).

Additional active backup maneuvers can help achieve better support for forward advancement of the hardware.

1. *Anchor wire technique*. If there is a reasonable size side branch proximal to the occlusion [like a proximal diagonal for mid left anterior descending artery (LAD) occlusion, or the left circumflex (LCX) for ostial LAD occlusion], a second wire can be inserted into this branch, helping to fix the catheter position in place. A relatively stiff support wire is preferred.
2. *Anchor balloon technique*. With this technique, a wire, followed by a balloon, is introduced into a side branch proximal to the occlusion. The balloon is inflated to a low pressure and size that are just sufficient to anchor the guiding catheter and enable deeper engagement, while pushing the guide over the balloon catheter shaft. Again, the operator should keep in mind the risk of proximal dissection with this procedure, which may necessitate a longer segment of stenting.

Intravascular ultrasound of the entry point

Sometimes, despite multiple view angiography, it is still difficult to assess the exact entry point of the proximal edge of the CTO. This is typical of any occlusion that takes place immediately after a bifurcating branch. Typical examples are ostial LAD occlusion, or in the right coronary artery (RCA), immediately after a right ventricular branch. In such cases, the location of the entry point can be obtained by wiring the side branch and doing a thorough intravascular ultrasound (IVUS) interrogation, pulling back from the side branch. The IVUS will be less useful in cases of heavy calcification in the vessel wall at the CTO ostium or side branch.

RECANALIZATION

Wire-based techniques

To enable maximal guidewire torquability and pushability, there is a need to have subselective support. We are using an over the wire 1.5-mm balloon system (that can be used also for first predilatation after crossing the occlusion) or a low profile tracking catheter. In the past, we have used exchange length guidewires, so the wires can be easily exchanged during the procedure, even after crossing the occlusion. Short wires are now preferred for better tip control and can be easily exchanged after crossing with the pressure-stabilization technique. In this technique, the 1.5-mm balloon or tracking catheter is pulled back, up to the tip of the wire. The balloon inflator is connected to the support catheter, making sure that no bubbles are introduced.

The balloon or catheter is pulled while having pressure up to 14 to 16 atm, which stabilizes the guidewire inside.

Selection of guidewire

Two groups of wires are usually used for CTOs: polymer-coated and coil wires. The polymer-coated wires have a hydrophilic coating that lowers the resistance in or outside of the lumen, making it move very easily through any tissue, increasing the risk of advancing the wire into subluminal planes, and creating false lumen, long dissections, or perforations. The coil wires have good torquability even inside the CTO segment with good pushability. The harder the wire tip, the higher the torquability of the wire, but the less resistance at the tip felt by the operator and the higher the risk of a false lumen. Coiled wires give more resistance, which may reduce the chance to engage very small channels, making it more likely to create a false lumen. With tapered wires (like the Confienza® 0.014–0.009 in® or Crossit® 0.014–0.010 in®), there is a better chance to get very small channels than with normal sized coil wires. With heavier coil wires like the Crossit® 300 to 400 (Guidant), Miracle 9® and 12 g (Asahi), or Persuader® (Medtronic), the harder tip tends to end up in a false lumen, especially after bends, and it is difficult to feel the resistance if they do so. Using these specific wires requires close attention by the operator to reduce the chance of a false lumen, to recognize when a false lumen is created, and to avoid perforations. These wires should be used only by experienced operators only after attempting more conventional wires.

Selecting a wire is a difficult decision with no straightforward solution. Our practice is to go from light to heavy, always starting with a soft tip, changing to a harder and stiffer wire if the lighter and softer wires do not work. For occlusions that are less than six months old, an intermediate wire will usually work. The Miracle Bro® 3 g (Asahi) has excellent torquability and often will be a good choice. For harder lesions that are older than six months, wires with harder tips will often be needed.

Shaping the tips of the CTO wires is somewhat different. Usually, a short (>2 mm) 45° bend enables torquability and selection of different routes or channels. A larger bend may go more easily into the subintima and create a wider false lumen. Experienced operators use the two-handed technique. With the right hand, they rotate the wire, and with the left, push and pull, sensing resistance from the tip of the wire. This is combined with a fluoroscopic visualization to see if the wire is advancing and to avoid buckling.

Multiple octagonal views should be taken to identify where the proximal fibrous cap should be penetrated. Sometimes, there is a "nipple" or a "dimple" that directs the way for the first few millimeters. While advancing the wire, orthogonal views should again be taken to verify that the wire is advanced intraluminally and not in a dissection plane.

Two wire techniques

In cases where a wire is repeatedly advancing into the wrong plane, it can be left in place (subintimal) to mark the wrong plane and to avoid seperating the problem and a new wire is used to get into the correct way. Using this "parallel-wire method," the first wire is left in the wrong plane, the support catheter is pulled out, and an additional wire is introduced through the support catheter, approaching the occlusion. In modification of the technique called the "seesaw wiring method," the parallel wire is used with the help of two support catheters. This enables alternate use of the wires, easily alternating their roles as markers of the wrong plane and for forward advance through the occluded segment.

Usually the procedure is started with a standard, relatively soft tip guidewire that is used first to transfer the delivery system (small balloon or support catheter) closer to the lesion and to use a safer wire for the first attempt. Failure to cross with the standard wire is followed with stiffer wires in escalating tip stiffness (usually measured in weight scale, signifying the weight force that is needed to buckle the tip). The final attempt is usually to use stiff tapered and/or hydrophilic tips. This is left for the very expert operator, since it involves higher risk of complications.

After successfully crossing the occlusion, the operator should carefully verify that the wire is indeed intraluminal before predilatation. If a stiff wire was used, it should be exchanged for a wire with a soft tip to avoid distal dissection or perforation that may occur while working and concentrating more proximally.

Subintimal tracking and reentry technique

A new promising technique was recently introduced by Colombo, similar to the one utilized in treating some peripheral artery occlusions and aimed at creating a subintimal dissection with distal reentry. A 0.014 in. hydrophilic wire with a J configuration is utilized for this purpose. The hydrophilic wire is pushed through the subintimal dissection plane. When distal to the occlusion, the J tip is directed toward the lumen, attempting reenter the true lumen.

Retrograde wire approach

When antegrade crossing of a CTO fails, the retrograde approach may be considered. In this technique, the operator utilizes the existence of clearly visible straight collaterals, as demonstrated by the bilateral injection angiography. The retrograde diagnostic catheter is replaced with a guiding catheter. Careful selection of the guiding catheter is necessary. A supportive (at least 7 French) short guide (90 cm) should be used to enable a longer coronary segment to pass through. A hydrophilic soft wire of 1.5 mm (1.25 mm in Japan and Europe) over the wire balloon is advanced through the collateral to the retrograde approach of the CTO. This technique is used largely in RCA occlusions, in which the retrograde wire is navigated through a septal branch. The straightest septal branch that seems to be directly connected to the distal RCA is selected; sometimes, a gentle dilatation of the septal branch with the 1.25 to 15 mm balloon is needed to facilitate the further delivery of the support balloon. After advancing the supporting balloon close to the occlusion, the wire can be exchanged for one with a stiffer tip to cross the occlusion. In some cases, especially in those when the antegrade wire was advanced into a false lumen, a retrograde wire can be used to clarify the location of the true lumen, thus helping the operator to correctly direct the antegrade wire forward.

OCR and radio frequency technologies

The OCR technology uses low coherence (near-infrared) light transmission through an optical fiber within a 0.014-in. guidewire. The back-scattered light (reflection time and intensity) from tissue in front of the guidewire is measured, and an algorithm analyzes the back-scattered light to identify the interface between the normal arterial wall and diseased plaques. A visible and audible signal warns the operator when the tip approaches within 1 mm of the outer vessel wall, allowing the operator to redirect the wire before dissecting or perforating. The safe-Cross RF system (IntraLuminal) combines OCR technology with a controlled radio frequency (RF) energy that the operator can discharge through the wire tip when an OCR "green" signal is displayed; that is, the tip of the wire is facing an intraluminal plaque, not the vessel wall. Delivery of a series of RF energy pulses can facilitate crossing hard fibrotic material within the occluded vessel, eliminating the risk of perforation.

Frontrunner® catheter

A second line device to attempt recanalization of CTO is the Frontrunner® (LuMed, Cordis, Johnson & Johnson). It is often used when the protocol of wire-based attempts have failed. This device is designed to create intraluminal blunt micro-dissection to facilitate penetration of the fibrous cap. The Frontrunner catheter is steered and delivered through the coronary artery, just proximal to the occlusion, so that the blunt tip engages the proximal cap of the CTO. The tip is gently pushed forward to displace the plaque. Remote opening of the small forceps separates atherosclerotic plaque in various tissue planes by inducing the blunt dissection. Repetitive opening and steering of the catheter creates a micro-channel through the occlusion, facilitating the placement of a guidewire across the occlusion. The blunt dissection strategy takes advantage of the elastic properties of the adventitia as compared to the inelastic characteristics of the fibroelastic plaque to create the fracture planes. This device may have a special role in refractory in-stent CTO, where the stent serves to confine the device as it passes through the occlusion.

CROSSING THE LESION

Balloon

After exchanging the stiff wire for one with a soft tip, a low profile 1.5-mm balloon is advanced through the lesion and inflated for first predilatation. This is followed by additional predilatations as needed, according to the vessel size.

In some cases, even the 1.5-mm low profile over-the-wire balloon cannot cross the lesion. In such cases, additional support can be gained by deep-sitting the guiding catheter and/or exchanging it for a larger one that may give more support. An additional way to get more support is with an anchoring wire and balloon in a side branch (as described earlier).

Tornus®

The Tornus® device (Asahi, Japan) is a catheter made up of eight stainless steel strands woven together to enhance flexibility and strength in exchanging wires, delivering balloons, and providing support for CTO procedures. It is used after a wire has crossed a chronic occlusion where a balloon will not cross. The Tornus is advanced into the CTO by up to 20 counterclockwise rotations without strong backup support once the tip is encroached. The device can make a smooth channel without dissection, allowing passage for a low profile balloon.

Ablation

When the 1.5-mm balloon cannot be advanced through the lesion despite good support, or when efficient support cannot be achieved, debulking devices such as the Rotoblator® or use of a laser are usually helpful. The use of an excimer laser does not require wire exchange, and can be used with high power (80/80), crossing the lesion and creating a lumen that enables delivery of a balloon. The point 9 X-80 catheter can cross even heavily calcified lesions.

REASONS TO STOP

The most common reason to bring the procedure to an end is failure to recanalize the occlusion. With more experience, the operator learns how to escalate with a thoughtful selection of guidewires and other devices, and knows the point when further attempts are futile and carry more risk than benefit. Avoiding complications is of major importance in mastering the technique of CTO treatment, and the skilled operator should have the tools and knowledge to take care of complications when they occur. Of course when complications occur, the operator should stop the procedure, rectify the situation, stabilize the hemodynamic status if needed, and avoid the temptation to go on with the procedure. An additional attempt may take place a few weeks later when the patient is stable and willing to give it another chance.

In rare cases when the occlusion is crossed with the wire and is predilated but cannot be crossed with a stent, it makes sense to conclude the session even if only partially successful, retaining the option for a reattempt a few weeks later when the vessel recovers, small dissections heal, and a further attempt to deliver a stent can be enhanced by more aggressive predilatation or rotoblation.

CASE DEMONSTRATIONS

Case 1: In stent chronic total occlusion of mid-RCA

In the first attempt, a 7 French AL 1 guiding catheter was used for support, causing a dissection from the tip of the guiding catheter (Fig. 1A). An attempt to get a wire into the true lumen failed. Since the patient was asymptomatic with collateral blood supply through the left coronary system, the procedure was halted. The patient was brought back to the catheter lab after four weeks, demonstrating healing of the dissection (Fig. 1B). Dual injection demonstrated the distal RCA branches, enabling correct direction of the wire through the CTO segment, with excellent angiographic result after stenting (Fig. 1C).

Case 2: Dual wire technique for a bifurcating chronic total occlusion

A 63-year-old man presented with chronic angina and inferior-lateral wall ischemia on stress thallium test. Angiography revealed a chronic occlusion of the distal LCX, with a bifurcation into two OM branches just at the distal

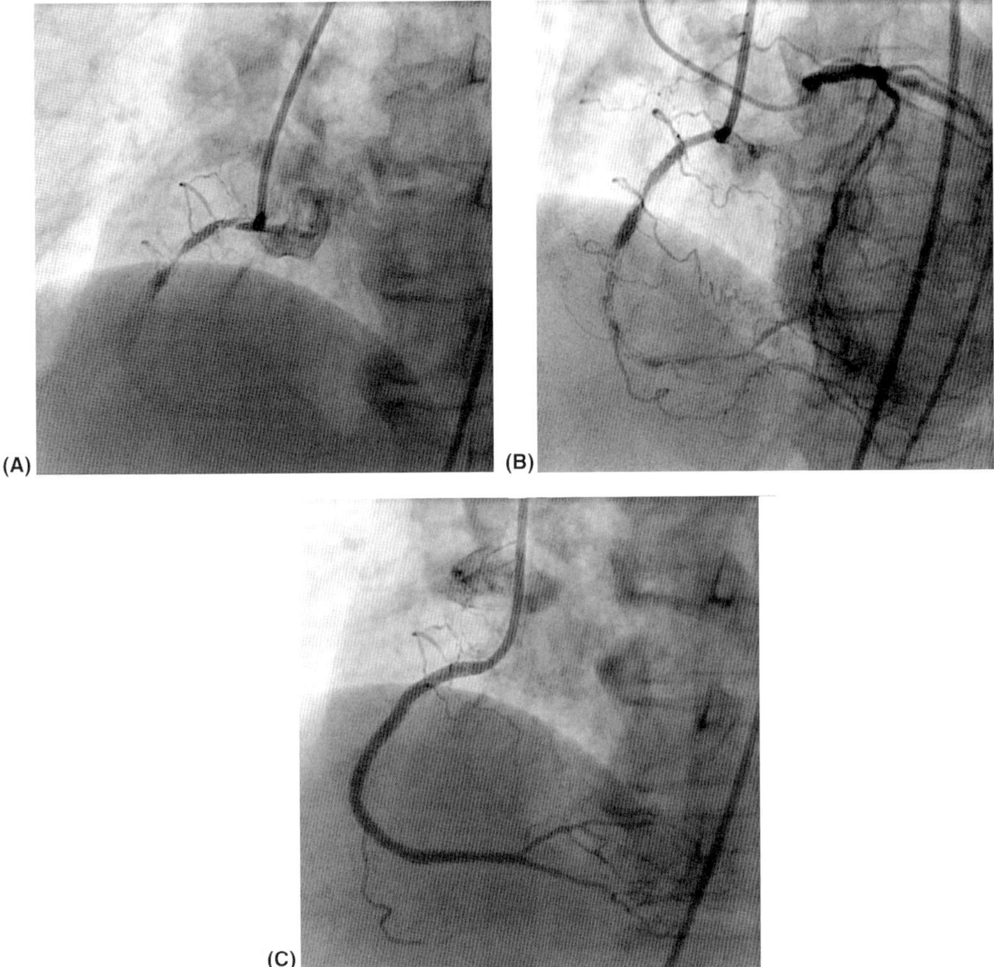

Figure 1A–C Case 1

edge of the lesion (Fig. 2A). A 3.5-EBU 8 French guiding catheter (Medtronic) was used with good support. After getting into the LCX with a soft tip floppy wire, it was exchanged by a Miracle 3 (Asahi) with a 1.5 × 9 mm over the wire balloon for subselective support. The wire repeatedly advanced into a subintimal plane. It was left in the false lumen, and an additional Miracle 3 wire was taken, trying to navigate it through an additional 1.5 × 9 mm similar support balloon to get into a channel in the true lumen (Fig. 2B). The two wires were used in alternating fashion, using the seesaw method. In such a way, they were advanced through the lesion (Figs. 2C–E). First, one of the wires was directed into the distal lower branch (Fig. 2F), and the second was navigated into the upper one (Fig. 2G), enabling successful angioplasty and stenting (Fig. 2H).

Case 3: Anchor wire technique

A 75-year-old man presented with angina and inferior wall ischemia on nuclear stress test. The mid-RCA was known to be occluded, since a similar angiogram that was done a year previously at another hospital, failed the attempt to open it. A dual injection (JR 4, 7 French guiding catheter with side holes in the RCA, diagnostic 5 French JL 4 in the left man coronary artery) demonstrated the length of the occlusion, and the diffuse disease of the distal RCA run-off (Fig. 3A).

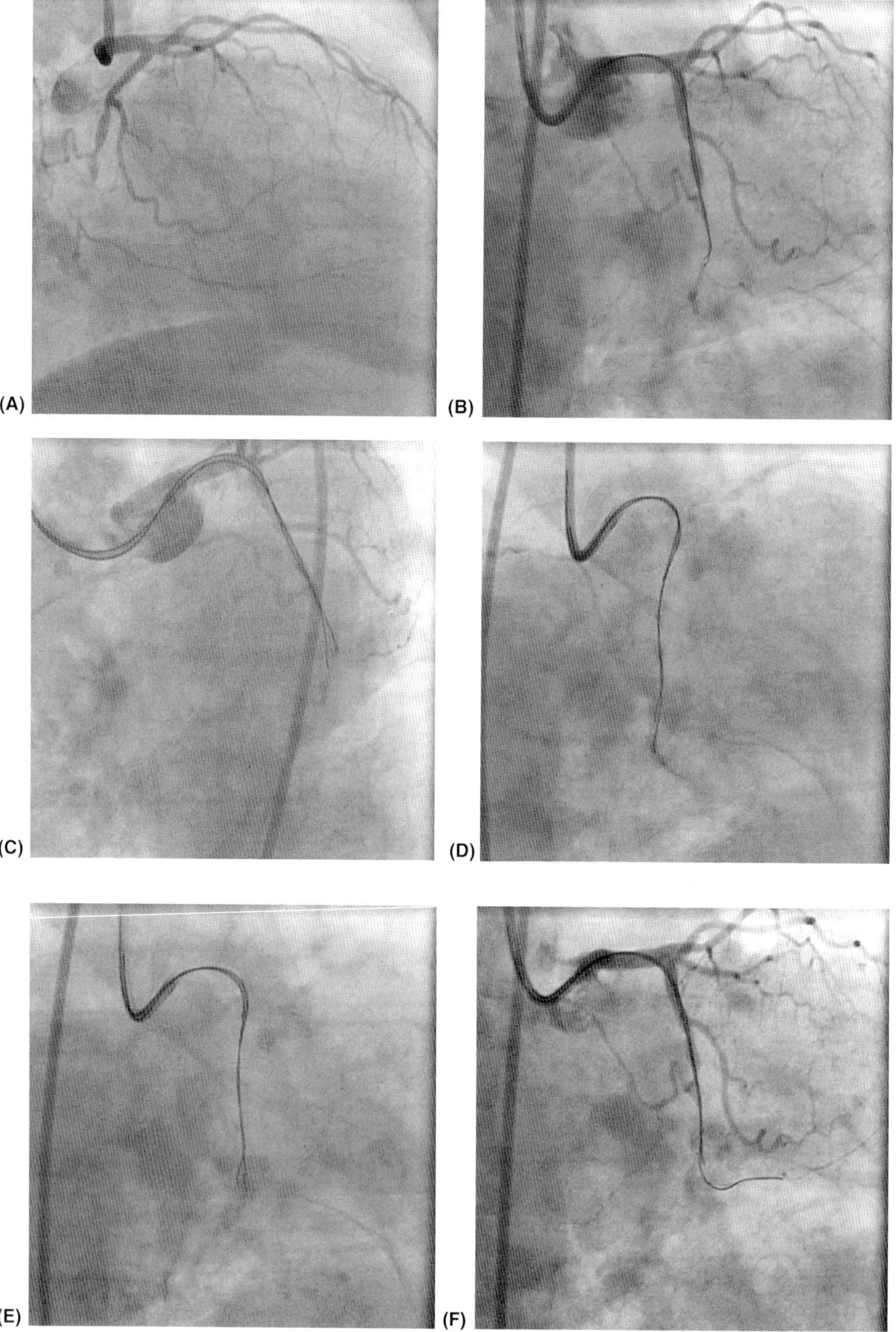

Figure 2A–F Case 2 (*Continued*)

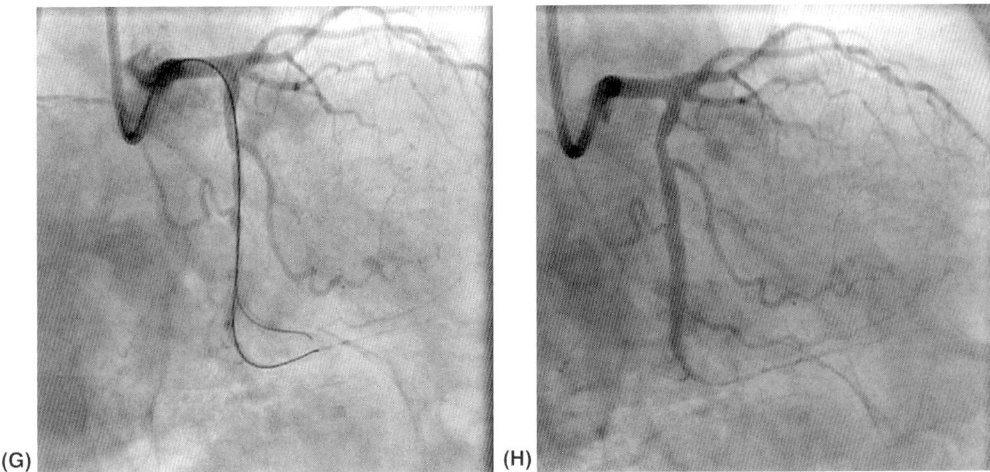

Figure 2G–H Case 2 (*Continued*)

To improve the guiding catheter support, a stiff wire (Extra-support, Guidant) was placed in the first proximal RCA branch (Fig. 3B). A Miracle 3 (Asahi) was used, but was introduced into a subintimal plane. It was left in the wrong plane; the supporting 1.5- × 9-mm balloon (Maverick 2, Boston Scientific) was pulled out, and an identical new wire was introduced through the balloon (Fig. 3C) to get to the correct path (Fig. 3D). An excellent result was achieved after predilatation and stenting (Fig. 3E).

Case 4: Complex occlusion of the RCA with retrograde recanalization

A 76-year-old man with shortness of breath on exertion, who was found to have triple vessel disease, refused to have CABG surgery. The LAD and CTO of the LCX were stented in the first procedure, and the RCA occlusion staged. Despite multiple orthogonal views, no dimple was found to reveal the entrance point of the occlusion (Fig. 4A). The conal branch takes off at this CTO branch. An 8 French JR 4 with side holes was used to enable multiple devices and support. A floppy wire (Prowater, Abbott) was placed in the conal branch and a pull-back IVUS interrogation was done to demonstrate the exact entry point (Fig. 4B). A Miracle 3 (Asahi) wire was manipulated to the identified point of entry, and exchanged with stiffer wires (Miracle 6 and 12, Asahi), using parallel-wire methods, but without success (Figs. 4C and 4D). A 7 French EBU guiding catheter (Medtronic) angiographically demonstrates multiple septal branches that connected directly to the PDA (Fig. 4E). The widest and most straight branch was selected for retrograde wiring. A Ryujin wire (Terumo) was directed to this branch (Fig. 4F), using a 1.5- × 15-mm Maverick 2 balloon (Boston Scientific) that followed the wire as it was advanced (Figs. 4G and 4H). The wire was advanced to the distal cup and the proximal stiff wire was advanced antegrade (Figs. 4I and 4J). The retrograde wire was pulled back, and the antegrade stiff wire was exchanged to a floppy wire (BMW universal, Guidant), using the pressure-stabilizing technique (Fig. 4K). Stenting the RCA resulted in excellent angiographic result (Fig. 4L).

Case 5: Retrograde marking of true lumen

A 61-year-old woman presented with severe angina despite maximal anti-anginal medical therapy. Total occlusion of the RCA had been diagnosed two years earlier, but was not treated at that time. Coronary angiography revealed no obstructive lesions in the left system, and revealed a relatively short occlusion in the proximal RCA with distal flow due to bridging collaterals (Figs. 5A and 5B). Attempts to cross the

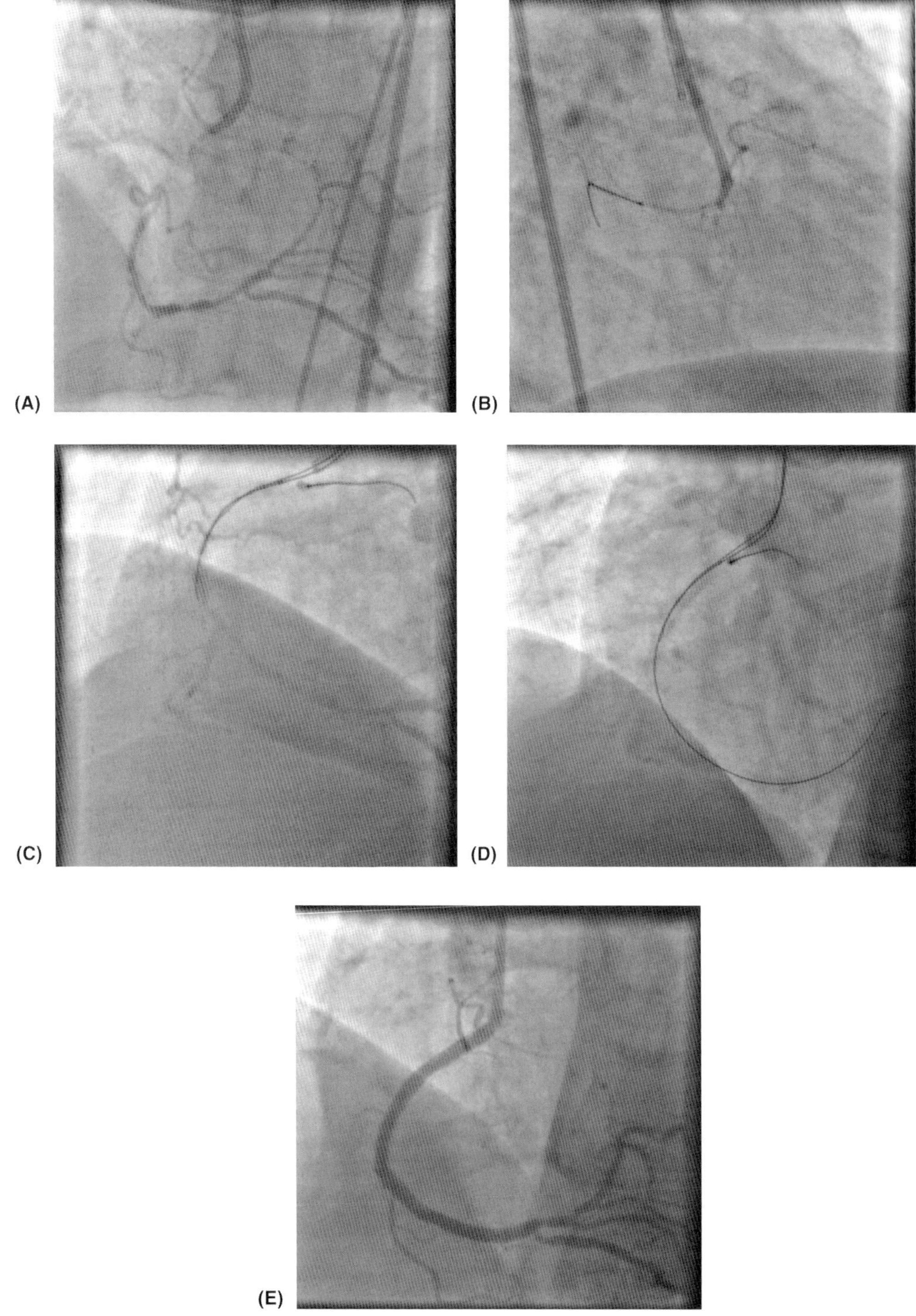

Figure 3A–E Case 3

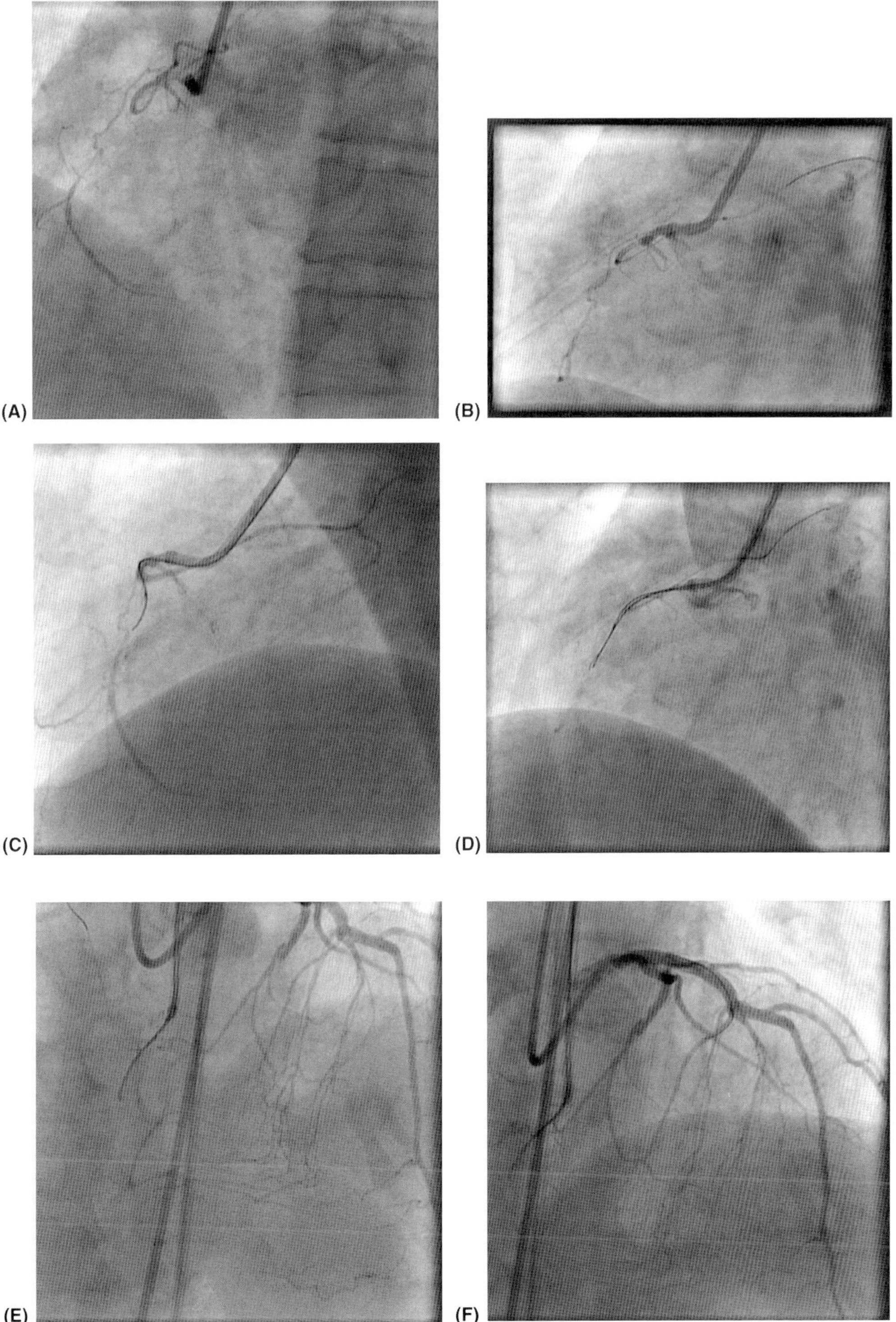

Figure 4A–F Case 4 (*Continued*)

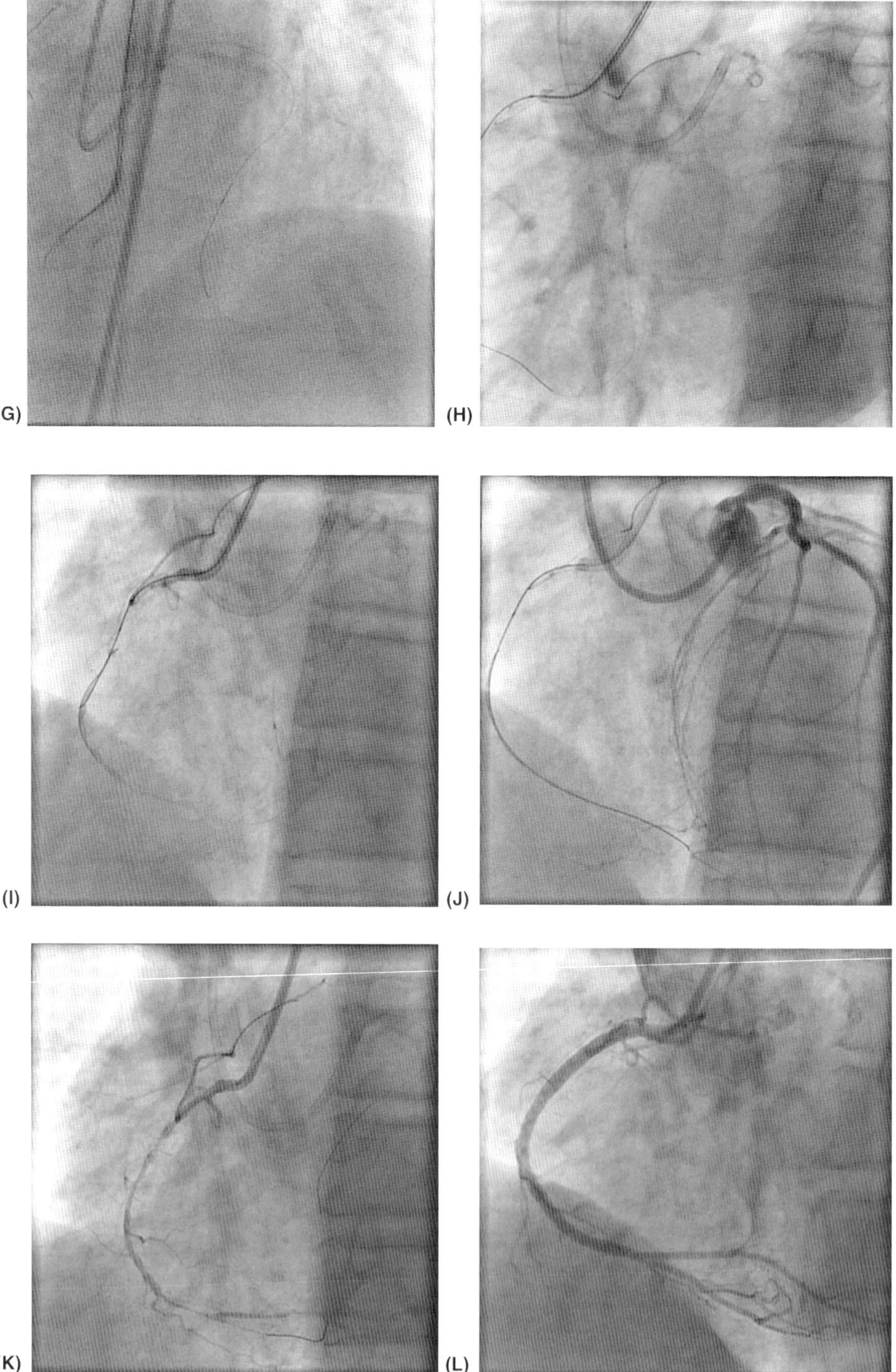

Figure 4G–L Case 4

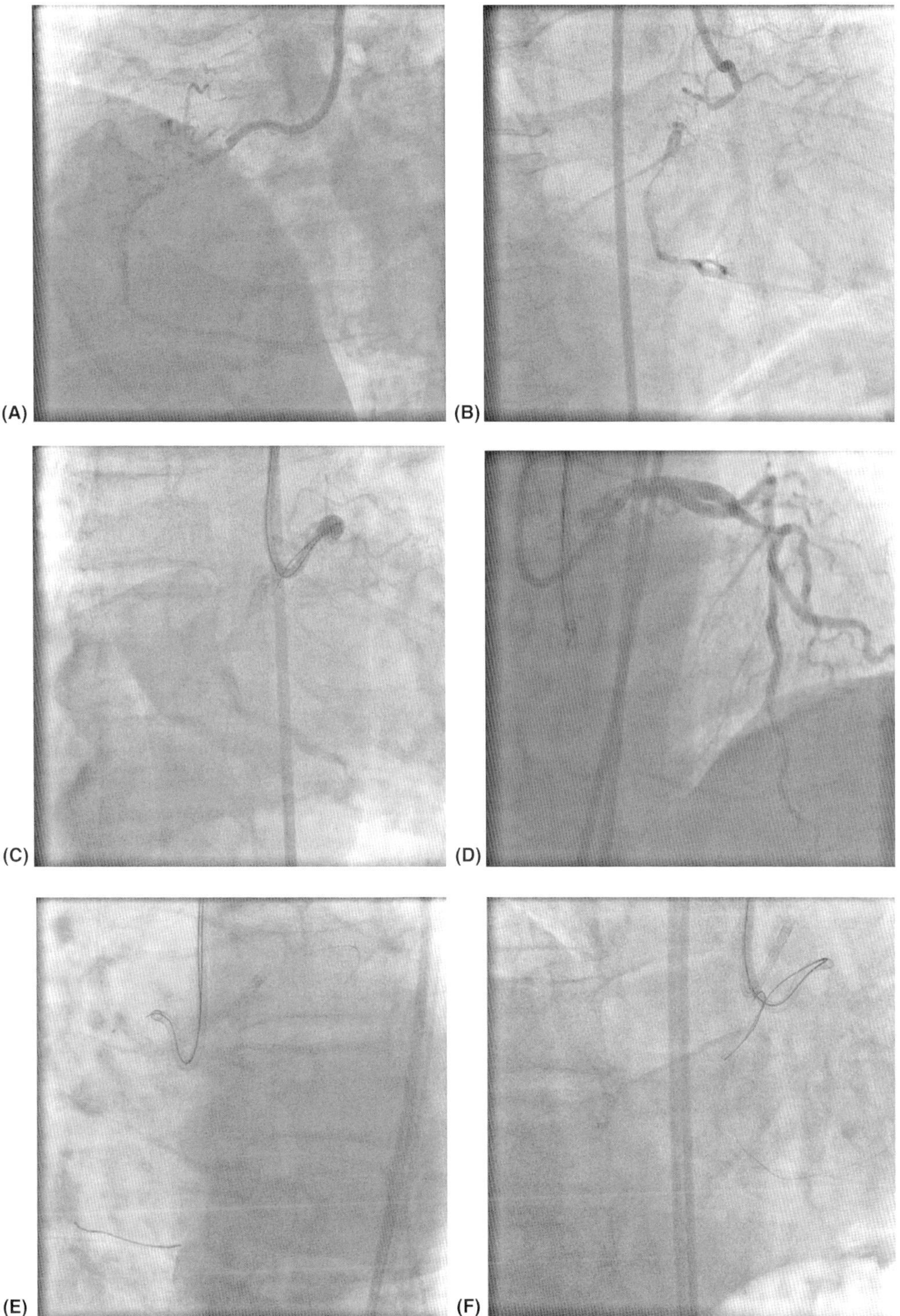

Figure 5A–F Case 5 (*Continued*)

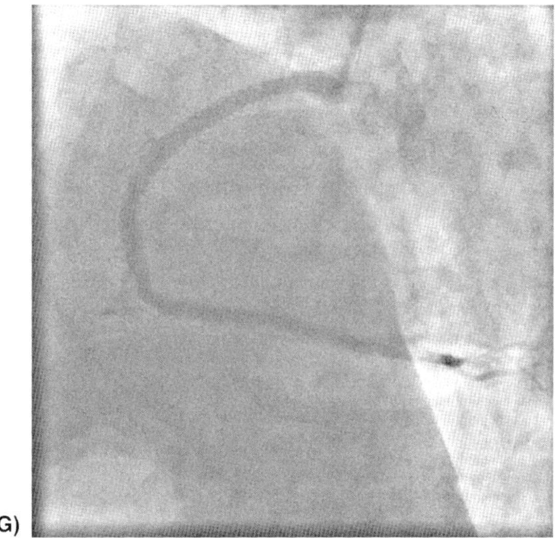

(G)

Figure 5G Case 5 (*Continued*)

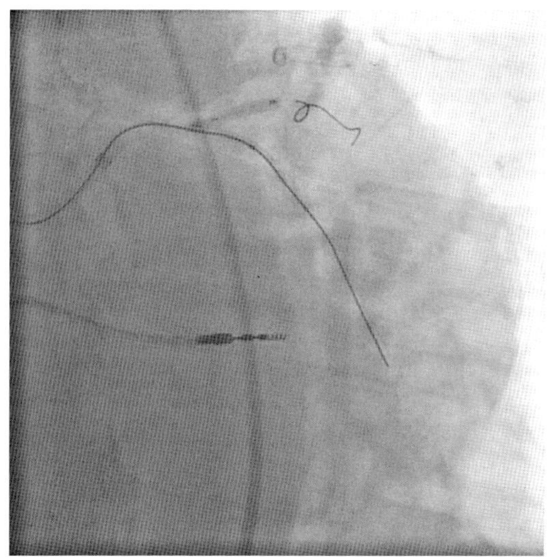

Figure 6 Case 6

occlusion with multiple stiff wires (Mircale 3, Miracle 6, and Confienza, Asahi) were unsuccessful (Fig. 5C). Through an additional arterial access, a 7 French XB guiding catheter (Cordis, Johnson & Johnson) was placed in the ostium of the LMCA and, in contrast, helped to demonstrate a septal branch that directly connected to the distal RCA run-off (Fig. 5D). A hydrophilic wire (Pilot 50, Guidant) was navigated through the LAD and the septal branch into the distal RCA, using an over the wire 1.5- × 9-mm Mavrick 2 balloon (Boston Scientific) for subselective support (Fig. 5E). The retrograde wire was advanced as close as it could get to the distal cup of the occlusive segment, identifying and marking the correct position of the distal true lumen, where a Miracle 3 wire (Asahi) was directed in the antegrade path to cross the CTO (Fig. 5F). After crossing, the retrograde wire was removed, and the procedure completed with stenting of the RCA (Fig. 5G).

Case 6: Anchor balloon technique

In a CTO of a large OM 2 branch (Fig. 6), a 3.5-EBU 8 French guiding catheter (Medtronic) did not give enough support while trying to recanalize the occlusion. A short floppy wire was navigated into a small proximal branch, and a 2.25 × 15 Maverick 2 balloon (Boston Scientific) inflated to give advanced support. A Miracle 6 (Asahi) was used for crossing the CTO.

REFERENCES

1. Stone GW, Kandzari DE, Mehran R, et al. Percutaneous recanalization of chronically occluded coronary arteries: a consensus document: part I. Circulation 2005; 112(15):2364–2372.
2. Stone GW, Reifart NJ, Moussa I, et al. Percutaneous recanalization of chronically occluded coronary arteries: a consensus document: part II. Circulation 2005; 112(16):2530–2537.

6

Long lesions and diffuse disease

Flavio Airoldi

INTRODUCTION

Diffuse coronary artery disease poses a significant therapeutic challenge. The experience gathered in more than ten years of use of bare-metal stents (BMS) has shown that lesion length is an independent predictor of in-stent restenosis (1–3). Full lesion coverage with a stent from the proximal to distal normal segment has provided good immediate outcome, but has been associated with a suboptimal long-term result. A strategy of spot stenting has been proposed as an attractive alternative to the "full covering" strategy with long stent implantation (4). This techniques takes advantage of intravascular ultrasound (IVUS) and limits the use of stenting only in particular segments of a lesion where the luminal result does not meet prespecified IVUS criteria after balloon angioplasty. The use of drug-eluting stents (DES) has markedly reduced the incidence of restenosis in long lesions and has greatly attenuated the relationship between stent length and restenosis (5–8). Furthermore, the pattern of restenosis is, in most cases, focal and responds positively to a second percutaneous procedure (9,10). Still, no information is available about the optimal technique for the treatment of diffusely diseased vessels. Spot stenting is a laborious technique, and its advantages over the complete vessel coverage are not demonstrated. Due to the lack of a dedicated prospective study specifically addressing to this topic, most of the information we report in the following pages does not derive from the "evidence-based medicine"; rather, it reflects our current practice in this complex setting.

TECHNIQUE OF STENTING

The main objective when treating long lesions is to completely cover the diseased segment with fully expanded stents. This goal can be reached with various techniques according to operator's experience and lesion characteristics. Whatever strategy the operator chooses, the intervention should be performed following three mandatory steps: (*i*) good lesion preparation; (*ii*) correct stent size selection and positioning; and (*iii*) optimal stent expansion.

Lesion preparation

Direct stenting has a very limited role in the treatment of diffusely diseased arteries requiring long or overlapped stents. Balloon predilatation is recommended in the vast majority of cases. Conventional predilatation with low profile, compliant balloons may be adequate to allow the transit of the stents through the lesion and to guarantee its complete expansion. However, in case of calcified or fibrotic lesions, these kinds of balloons are not able to reach their nominal diameter even when inflated over their maximal burst pressure. If lesion preparation is performed only with compliant balloons, the operator may experience two different errors:

(*1*) The operator does not recognize with angiography the incomplete balloon expansion and places a stent over an unbreakable plaque. The presence of an incompletely expanded stent is one of the most unwelcome and frustrating conditions the operator may encounter. The use of debulking devices (rotational atherectomy, cutting balloon, FX-miniRAIL balloon) is banned by the presence of the stent and the only possible action is limited to high-pressure stent postdilatation with short noncompliant balloons.

(*2*) The operator recognizes the incomplete balloon expansion at the maximal balloon pressure (burst pressure or over) and selects a larger balloon to increase the lumen size. Even though this action may improve the lumen area, it inevitably carries a consistent risk of coronary rupture. This dramatic event is more likely to occur when using a compliant balloon. When inflated at high pressure in a diseased coronary artery, the compliant balloon does not expand homogeneously and may reach a diameter much larger than its nominal one in some spots. The use of a low-compliant balloon should be preferred in the phase of lesion preparation. The new generation of low profile, high-pressure resistant balloons (Quantum Maverick®, Boston Scientific; Sprinter®, Medtronic; Jocath Mercury®, Abbott) may access the target lesion even in the presence of vessel tortuosity or calcifications.

Our suggestion is to perform multiple balloon inflations with relatively short balloons (better trackability), starting from the distal part of the lesion and moving backward to cross the entire lesion with the balloon uninflated and to ensure a preserved profile. The inflations can be performed at high pressure (rated burst pressure or above), but with the precaution of selecting a slightly undersized balloon diameter (for instance 2.5 mm diameter balloon for predilatation if it is anticipated to use a 3.0 diameter stent). The routine use of noncompliant balloons before stenting in our practice has largely reduced the use of rotational atherectomy (rotablator) or cutting balloon angioplasty. Nevertheless, the role of these debulking devices still has a pivotal role in the treatment of long lesions. Rotablator is used in a minority of cases even in centers with large experience with its use. The reason for such limited use is probably due to a concern of complications. The two most frequent complications associated with the use of rotablator are vessel perforation and onset of slow flow for distal embolization. These adverse events may occur even when the device is properly used. However, in order to minimize the incidence and clinical consequences of adverse events, operators should keep in mind the following: (*i*) Select small burrs (1.25 or 1.5 mm); (*ii*) avoid long runs without a proper interval between; (*iii*) avoid the rotablator in tortuous vessels or in bend lesions; (*iv*) electively place an intraaortic balloon pump in patients with low left ventricular ejection fraction or high jeopardy score.

In our practice currently, the use of a rotablator is limited to the following conditions: (*i*) lesions that can be crossed by the coronary wire but not by the smallest balloon available (1.25 mm or 1.5 mm in diameter); (*ii*) evidence of incomplete balloon expansion (during high-pressure inflation of noncompliant balloons); (*iii*) inability to cross the lesion with the stent despite multiple predilatations; (*iv*) IVUS evidence of extensive calcifications (>180°).

Stent size selection and correct positioning

When dealing with very long lesions involving the distal portion of coronary vessels, the correct choice of stent diameter and stent length might create some difficulties. Several studies have reported a significant discrepancy between angiographic and IVUS measurement of vessel size. Due to the presence of a large plaque burden that involves, in most cases, the coronary vessel for its entire length, the quantification of vessel diameter based on angiography may be significantly smaller than the true vessel size. This discrepancy can reach 1 mm or more and is more relevant in small vessels, in diabetic patients, and in the presence of diffuse disease (11). Besides the correct stent sizing, stent positioning also might present some technical problems. Despite good lesion preparation, it can be difficult to advance the stent to the target lesion. A deep catheterization with the guiding catheter will increase catheter back up and can be helpful for lesions located in right coronary artery (especially when using 6 French catheters). However, if the lesion is located in the left anterior descending artery or in the left circumflex artery, deep catheterization through the left main and the proximal portion of the target artery is not recommended. In these cases, stent advance can be facilitated by positioning parallel wires in the same artery ("buddy wire") in order to straighten the vessel and reduce stent friction against the vessel wall. The operator can use a second standard floppy wire as a buddy wire or, as an alternative, a heavy support wire (Ironman®, Balance Heavyweight®, Universal®, Guidant®). In the latter situation, the stent shall not necessarily be advanced on the stiff wire. In actuality, we have often found it easier to advance the stent on the standard floppy wire while keeping a stiff parallel wire in place.

Optimal stent expansion

A recent insight in morphological characteristics of in-stent restenosis following DES implantation has shown that the two most frequent conditions contributing to the restenostic process were incomplete lesion coverage and stent under expansion (12,13). These findings provided useful insights on the best implantation strategy for DES. One important point is to fully cover with stents the vessel area that underwent balloon predilatation. This precaution avoids leaving injured areas outside the stent. Similarly, operators should avoid injuring the areas at stent edges during stent implantation. This phenomenon is usually caused by the delivery balloon that protrudes outside the stent edges during its deployment. It is more likely to occur distally to the stent due to the smaller vessel diameter and is dependent on the maximal balloon pressure reached during stent expansion. All DES are crimped on compliant or semicompliant balloons and if high pressures are used for stent implantation, the balloon will significantly increase both its diameter and its length, damaging the artery outside the intended treatment area. Low-compliant balloons are stiffer, thicker, and less susceptible to growth outside of the stent. When used to post dilate a stent, low-compliant balloons hold their shape despite added pressure. This results in the balloon's ability to exert more force against a stent or a hard lesion, potentially increasing dilatation success (Fig. 1).

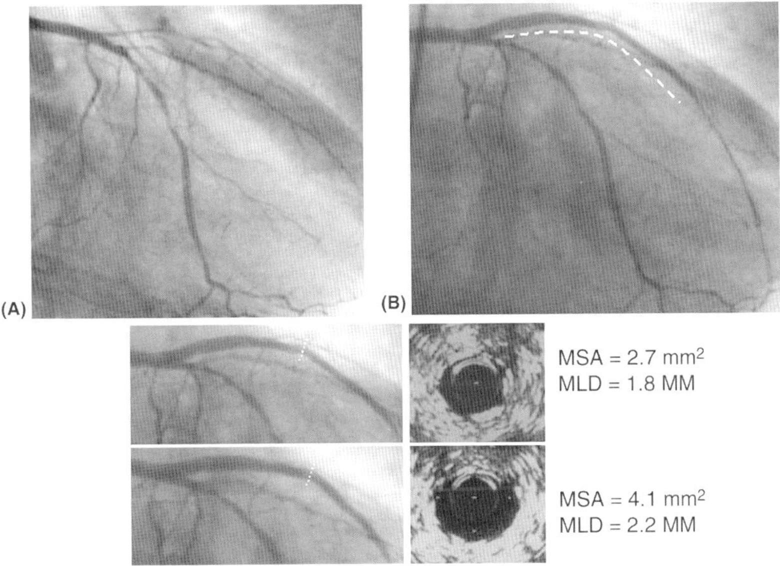

Figure 1 (**A**) Long lesion in the proximal segment of the left anterior descending artery. (**B**) Final result after stent implantation (Costar® 2.5 × 33 mm, 3.0 × 33 mm, and 3.5 × 16 mm). The lower panel shows the intravascular ultrasound (IVUS) examination of the treated segment indicating the smallest cross sectional area of the stented segment at two different times: (*1*) after stent deployment with the delivery balloon (2.5 mm at 16 atm); (*2*) after postdilatation with a low-compliant balloon having the same diameter, but inflated at higher pressure (Quantum Maverick® 2.5 × 15 mm at 30 atm).

SIDE BRANCH PROTECTION

The problem of side branch compromise has received attention following the increased use of long and multiple stents. The closure of side branches when stenting the parent vessel is more likely to occur in the left anterior descending (LAD) artery than in other coronary arteries due to the large numbers of septal and diagonal branches originating from the LAD (Fig. 2). The TAXUS-V trial has been the first large-scale study stressing the problem of side branch closure during the implantation of long stents. The 8.3% incidence of myocardial infarction in patients treated with multiple overlapping Taxus stents represents an unacceptable incidence of adverse event (5). Transient or definitive closure of side branches appears to be the most likely explanation of the phenomenon. Whatever the difference between one DES versus another, we are now treating long segments of vessels with multiple overlapping stents, and the risk to occlude small side branches leading to myocardial infarction becomes a real issue. In our experience with stenting lesions longer than 60 mm on the LAD, the incidence of periprocedural myocardial infarction is 16% (8).

This concern has led us to significantly change our strategy when implanting long stents. Currently, we routinely protect most of the side branches by positioning and jailing coronary wires underneath stent struts during stent implantation. The wires are removed following the documentation that the side branch has maintained patency with at least TIMI three-flow grade. In a few rare occasions, wire recrossing and balloon dilatation on the side branch becomes necessary. This strategy has been applied to most of the side branches involved in the stented segment, regardless of their diameter. Therefore, not only relevant side branches, with reference to diameter suitable for balloon angioplasty or stent implantation, but also branches of 1 mm diameter are protected by wire positioning and jailing. This strategy contributed to a marked reduction in the incidence of non-Q-wave myocardial infarctions in our clinical practice. It may require placing two or three wires in side branches while stenting the LAD. The presence of this relatively large number of wires in a 6 French guiding catheter does not interfere with the transit of any type of coronary stent to be placed on the main vessel. As already recommended for any bifurcational lesions, wire jailing can be safely performed with standard wires (Hi-torque Balance Middleweight®, Universal®, Guidant®; Rinato Asahi Intecc Co.),

(A)

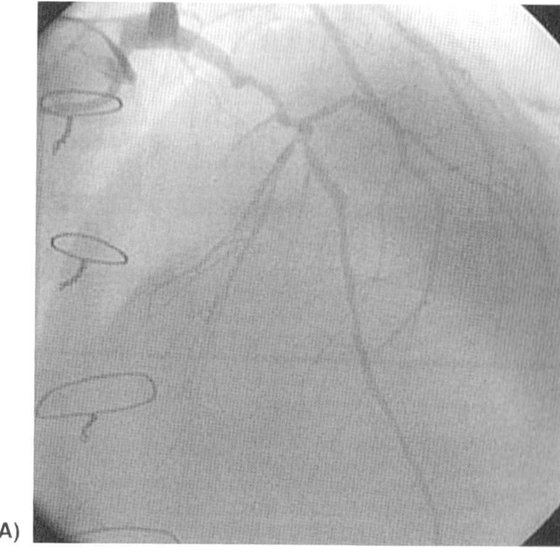

(B)

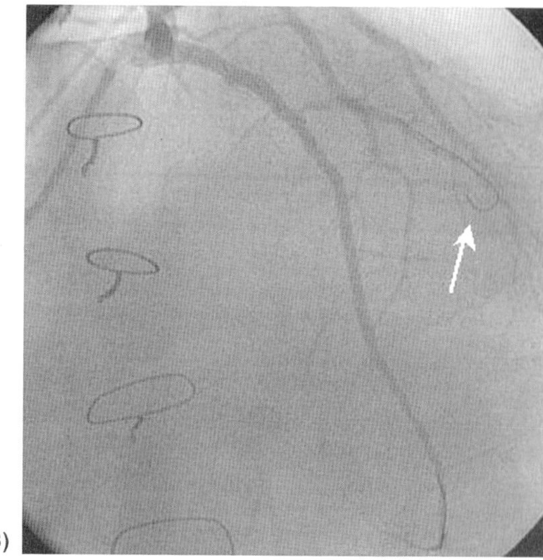

Figure 2 (**A**) Long lesion on the mid portion of the left anterior descending artery. (**B**) Final result after stent implantation (Costar®, 30 × 33 mm at 18 atm and Costar®, 2.5 × 33 m at 18 atm). Note the patency of the diagonal branch protected by jailing a standard floppy wire underneath the stents (*white arrow*) and the abrupt of a large septal branch originating at the same site, but not protected by the jailed wire.

while the use of hydrophilic wire should be strongly discouraged because of the risk of wire entrapment or peeling of the hydrophilic coating during wire removal after stent implantation.

USE OF GLYCOPROTEIN IIb-IIIa INHIBITORS

The treatment of long lesions with DES is associated with prolonged intracoronary manipulation and great metal and polymer density. This feature may correspond to a more pronounced vascular injury. Consequently, it may trigger platelet activation and increase the risk of periprocedural cardiac events. Glycoprotein IIb-IIIa inhibitors should be considered when dealing with lesions requiring long or multiple stents. Their use in this setting may have a double target: (*i*) decrease the incidence of intraprocedural stent thrombosis (IPST); (*ii*) reduce in-hospital myocardial infarction.

IPST is a rare event defined as thrombus formation during stent implantation in the absence of acute myocardial infarction (AMI) thrombus containing lesions, and residual peri-stent dissections. In our experience it has been reported to occur in 0.7% of patients treated with DES implantation. Even if rare, operators should be alert for this potential complication. In this setting, it is worthwhile to note that IPST occurred only in patients who did not receive glycoprotein IIb-IIIa inhibitors and was more likely to happen when long or multiple stents were implanted in the same artery (14). When using DES, the incidence of periprocedural myocardial infarction, revealed by CK rise, increases progressively with stent length (15). In long lesions the occurrence of in-hospital myocardial infarction is remarkable and varies from 16% to 18% (Table 1). The administration of glycoprotein IIb-IIIa inhibitors has been reported to reduce the frequency of periprocedural myocardial infarction in unselected lesions (15). Even in the absence of evidence from prospective dedicated trials, when using multiple, long stents, platelet inhibition with glycoprotein IIb-IIIa blockade should be performed in all cases if not contraindicated.

LONG-TERM THERAPY

Optimal long-term care after coronary stent implantation in the presence of diffuse disease requires aggressive systemic pharmacotherapy (antiplatelet agents and statins) in conjunction with therapeutic lifestyle changes (smoking cessation, weight reduction, dietary adjustment and exercise). In this context, dual antiplatelet therapy (aspirin plus clopidogrel) is recommended for at least 12 months after stenting for prophylaxis of future antithrombotic events. Stent length has been reported to be a predictor of late thrombosis occurring during the first nine months following stent implantation

Table 1 Clinical and angiographic outcome following DES implantation in long lesions

No. of patients	*Lesion length (mm)*	*Stent type*	*GP IIb-IIIa inhibitors (%)*	*In-hospital MI (%)*	*TLR (%)*	*Restenosis (%)*	*Thrombosis (%)*	*Reference*
577	29 ± 13	PES	42	4.9	8.6	18.9	0	5
99	63 ± 13	PES and SES	11	18.6	6.7	NA	0	6
96	61 ± 21	SES	31	NA	4.2	11.9	0	7
66	84 ± 22	PES and SES	47	16.6	15[a]	19.6	1.5[b]	8

[a]TVR, target vessel revascularization.
[b]All in-hospital.
Abbreviations: PES, paclitaxel eluting stent; SES, sirolimus eluting stent; TLR, target lesion revascularization; MI, myocardial infarction.

nevertheless (16). At present, no information is available regarding the potential benefit of maintenance of dual antiplatelet therapy over one year.

REFERENCES

1. Kobayashi Y, De Gregorio J, Kobayashi N, et al. Stented segment length as an independent predictor of restenosis. J Am Coll Cardiol 1999; 34: 651–659.
2. Serruys PW, Foley DP, Suttorp MJ, et al. A randomized comparison of the value of additional stenting after optimal balloon angioplasty for long coronary lesions: final results of the additional value of NIR stents for treatment of long coronary lesions (ADVANCE) study. J Am Coll Cardiol 2002; 39:393–399.
3. Bauters C, Hubert E, Prat A, et al. Predictors of restenosis after coronary stent implantation. J Am Coll Cardiol 1998; 31:1291–298.
4. Colombo A, De Gregorio J, Mousssa I, et al. Intravascular ultrasound-guided percutaneous transluminal coronary angioplasty with provisional spot stenting for treatment of long coronary lesions. J Am Coll Cardiol 2001; 38:1427–1433.
5. Stone GW, Ellis SG, Cannon L, et al. Comparison of a polymer-based paclitaxel-eluting stent with a bare metal stent in patients with complex coronary artery disease: A randomized controlled trial (TAXUS V). JAMA 2005; 294:1215–1223.
6. Mishra S, Wolfram R, Torguson R, et al. Procedural results and outcomes after extensive stent coverage with drug-eluting stent implantation in single coronary lesions. Am J Cardiol 2006; 98:357–361.
7. Degertekin M, Arampatzis C, Lemos P, et al. Very long sirolimus-eluting stent implantation for de novo coronary lesions. Am J Cardiol 2004; 93: 826–829.
8. Tsagalou E, Stankovic G, Iakovou I, et al. Early outcome of treatment of ostial de novo left anterior descending coronary artery lesions with drug-eluting stents. Am J Cardiol 2006; 97: 187–191.
9. Corbett SJ, Cosgrave J, Melzi G, et al. Patterns of restenosis after drug-eluting stent implantation: insights from a contemporary and comparative analysis of sirolimus- and paclitaxel-eluting stents. Eur Heart J 2006; 27:2330–2337.
10. Cosgrave J, Melzi G, Biondi-Zoccai G, et al. Drug-eluting stent restenosis: the pattern predicts the outcome. J Am Coll Cardiol 2006; 47:2399–2404.
11. Briguori C, Tobis J, Nishida T, et al. Discrepancy between angiography and intravascular ultrasound when analysing small coronary arteries. Eur Heart J 2002; 23:247–254.
12. Lemos PA, Saia F, Ligthart JM, et al. Coronary restenosis after sirolimus-eluting stent implantation. Morphological description and mechanistic analysis from a consecutive series of cases. Circulation 2003; 108:257–260.
13. Sonoda S, Morino Y, Ako J, et al. Impact of final stent dimension on long-term results following sirolimus-eluting stent implantation. J Am Coll Cardiol 2004; 43:195.
14. Chieffo A, Bonizzoni E, Orlic D, et al. Stankovic G et al. Intraprocedural stent thrombosis during implantation of sirolimus-eluting stents. Circulation 2004; 109:2732–2736.
15. Stankovic G, Chieffo A, Iakovou I. Creatine kinase-myocardial band isoenzyme elevation after percutaneous coronary interventions using sirolimus-eluting stents. Am J Cardiol 2004; 93: 1397–1401.
16. Iakorou I, Schmidt T, Bonizzoni E, et al. Incidence, predictors, and outcome of thrombosis after successful implantation of drug-eluting stents. JAMA 2005; 293:2123–2130.

7

Calcified and undilatable lesions

Paul S. Teirstein, Raghava R. Gollapudi, and Matthew J. Price

- **Background** • **Initial evaluation** • **Angioplasty techniques** • **Rotational artherectomy**
- **Other devices** • **Conclusion**

BACKGROUND

Calcified and undilatable lesions (CULs) remain a technical challenge in interventional cardiology despite novel approaches and devices. When compared to noncalcified lesions, angioplasty of calcified lesions is more often associated with insufficient balloon expansion, dissection, acute closure, and perforation. The geographic distribution of calcification within the vessel wall may impact the dynamics of balloon expansion and stent delivery. Typically, undilatable lesions consist of heavy, circumferential superficial calcification, although occasionally calcification can be limited to a localized region. In cases of localized calcification, balloon angioplasty results in an expansion of the contralateral calcium-free wall with insufficient balloon dilation. Calcification also impairs stent delivery and can lead to stent underexpansion with the attendant risks of subsequent stent thrombosis and restenosis. When contemplating an intervention on CULs, the interventionalist can achieve optimal outcomes and avoid therapeutic misadventures through a stepwise approach.

INITIAL EVALUATION

The initial evaluation involves assessing three key factors: (*i*) lesion location, (*ii*) angiographic characteristics (calcification and vessel tortuosity), and (*iii*) patient characteristics that may influence the risk of adjunctive procedures. With respect to the lesion location, the left main coronary artery is unique in its propensity for calcification, elastic recoil, and large plaque burden. Lesions involving the ostium of major epicardial arteries and large side branches tend to be fibrotic, and the risk of a suboptimal result after balloon angioplasty at these sites is greater. Severe calcification is undoubtedly present when densities can be seen within the plaque when viewing a still-frame fluoroscopic image, especially radio-oapacities noted without cardiac motion prior to contrast injection. In such cases, the operator should have a very high suspicion that the lesion may be difficult to dilate. Vessel tortuosity at the lesion site increases the risk of perforation with atheroablative devices and may warrant reconsideration of such an approach. Finally, patient characteristics, such as hemodynamic instability, reduced ejection fraction, and recent myocardial infarction, are relative contraindications to rotational atherectomy and argue against this technique as an initial approach. After taking into account these variables, we typically approach a calcified lesion with balloon-based devices initially, and then proceed with rotational atherectomy only if there is insufficient balloon inexpansion (Fig. 1).

Some investigators advocate the use of intravascular ultrasound (IVUS) to further

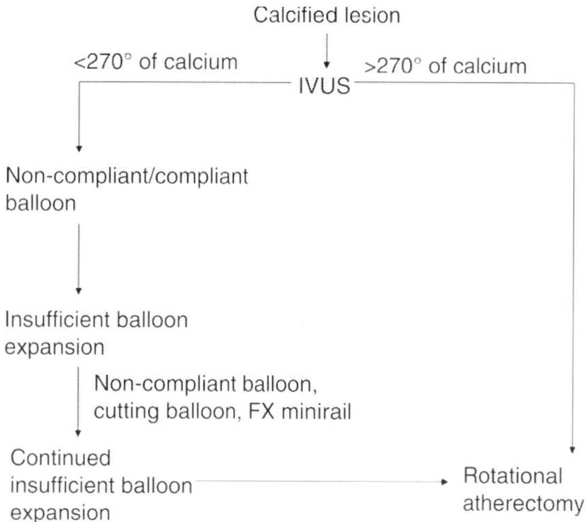

Figure 1 Algorithm for management of calcified and undilatable lesions.

evaluate a lesion prior to intervention as well. IVUS can help identify circumferential, deep, and superficial plaque. In the setting of calcium arcs of <270°, an initial balloon-based strategy is often successful with rotational atherectomy reserved for insufficient balloon inexpansion. In the setting of circumferential calcification (>270°), an initial strategy of rotational atherectomy may be beneficial to facilitate debulking prior to stenting.

ANGIOPLASTY TECHNIQUES

Generally, we perform a trial of balloon angioplasty to ascertain the potential for poor lesion expansion, and proceed to rotational atherectomy if the balloon angioplasty is unsuccessful. Although prior balloon angioplasty is traditionally considered a relative contraindication to rotational atherectomy, in our experience, such a "bailout" approach to rotational atherectomy appears safe. In a group of 20 patients undergoing unplanned rotational atherectomy at Scripps Clinic for suboptimal balloon angioplasty (nine of whom had angiographic evidence of dissection postangioplasty), technical success was 100% and there were no angiographic complications.

In the setting of a potentially undilatable lesion, the choices for balloon-based devices include noncompliant balloons, the cutting balloon, and FX minirail balloon (Table 1).

Table 1 Noncompliant balloons

Balloon name	*Device manufacturer*	*Delivery system*	*Available sizes (mm)*	*Nominal pressure (atm)*	*Rated burst pressure*
Quantum Maverick	Boston Scientific	Monorail, OTW	2.0, 2.25, 2.5, 2.75, 3.0, 3.25, 3.5, 3.75, 4.0, 4.5, 5.0	8	16–20
Ranger	Boston Scientific	Monorail, OTW	2.5, 2.75, 3.25, 3.5, 3.75, 4.0, 4.5	8	20
Cutting balloon	Boston Scientific	Monorail, OTW	2.0, 2.25, 2.5, 2.75, 3.0, 3.25, 3.5, 3.75, 4.0	6	10
FX miniRAIL	Guidant	Monorail	2.0, 2.5, 3.0, 3.5, 4.0	6–8	12–14
Highsail	Guidant	OTW	1.5, 2.0, 2.25, 2.5, 2.75, 3.0, 3.25, 3.5, 3.75, 4.0, 4.5, 5.0	10	18
Powersail	Guidant	Monorail	2.0, 2.25, 2.5, 2.75, 3.0, 3.25, 3.5, 3.75, 4.0, 4.5, 5.0	10	18

Abbreviation: OTW, over the wire.

Noncompliant balloons

As the name implies, noncompliant balloons exert a high-pressure localized force without overexpansion of the balloon, and thus can lead to controlled localized plaque fissuring and dissection. Initial high-pressure inflation of a noncompliant balloon can still result in under-expansion; in such a case, inflation for a prolonged duration (as tolerated by the patient) and at pressures equal to the rated burst pressure can lead to full balloon expansion. During this technique, the operator must be aware that balloon inflation at pressures higher than the rated burst pressure, although sometimes successful, can result in balloon rupture and subsequent dissection, perforation, and the introduction of air into the coronaries from poor balloon preparation. "Watermelon seeding" of the balloon is a frequent phenomenon when performing angioplasty of undilatable lesions; in this situation, gentle traction of the balloon during inflation or the use of a longer length balloon is helpful.

The nondilatable lesion will sometimes respond to a short, noncompliant balloon (i.e., an 8-mm balloon in length) that exerts focal forces on the calcified segment. Care should be taken not to use a balloon larger in diameter than the reference vessel as the risk of perforation is increased, particularly if an oversized balloon "cracks" the plaque and overexpands the vessel at high pressures.

The Cutting® balloon

The Cutting balloon (Boston Scientific, Natick, MA) contains three microsurgical blades that results in scoring of the plaque by severing the elastic and fibrotic continuity of the vessel wall. In our experience, the cutting balloon is helpful in in-stent restenosis lesions as well as calcified ostial lesions. The first generation cutting balloon was a stiff high-profile device that was difficult to deliver across severe lesions and tortuous vessels. However, the newer flexotome cutting balloon is a lower profile, more flexible balloon that is easier to deliver. Importantly, the cutting balloon does not reduce the rate of restenosis compared to standard balloon angioplasty, but is associated with less watermelon seeding and less dissections, requiring additional stent placement when treating in-stent restenosis.

FX MiniRAIL® balloon

The FX MiniRAIL (Guidant Corporation, Santa Clara, CA) is a forced-focus angioplasty device similar to the cutting balloon but, instead of cutting blades, uses a dual-wire dilatation balloon catheter that exerts its force on the two wires alongside the balloon, which can lead to expansion of the plaque along these two planes. This balloon can be used in a manner similar to the cutting balloon.

ROTATIONAL ATHERECTOMY

Basic principles

In cases of persistent balloon inexpansion, rotational atherectomy is used to facilitate plaque modification and subsequent stent delivery (Fig. 2). High-speed rotational atherectomy enables luminal enlargement by differential cutting and orthogonal displacement of friction. Differential cutting is defined by preferential ablation of inelastic tissue (calcium, stents) with deflection away from normal elastic tissue. Similarly, at burr speeds of greater than 60,000 rpm, orthogonal displacement of friction describes elimination of the longitudinal friction vector, resulting in unimpeded forward movement of the burr through tortuous coronary arteries. Data from experimental studies suggest that particulate debris from rotational atherectomy is generally under 5 to 15 μ and is small enough to be cleared by the reticuloendothelial system.

Rotablator® setup

The Rotablator system uses a 0.009-in stainless steel guidewire with varying support strengths (floppy, extra support) with a 0.014-in. distal spring tip to prevent burr advancement off the end of the wire (Fig. 3). The Rotablator catheter is composed of the advancer body, control knob, connector tubing, and burr. The burr is diamond coated on its distal half so that ablation only occurs with forward movement (Fig. 4). The burr is available in different sizes that require different size guiding catheters (Table 2).

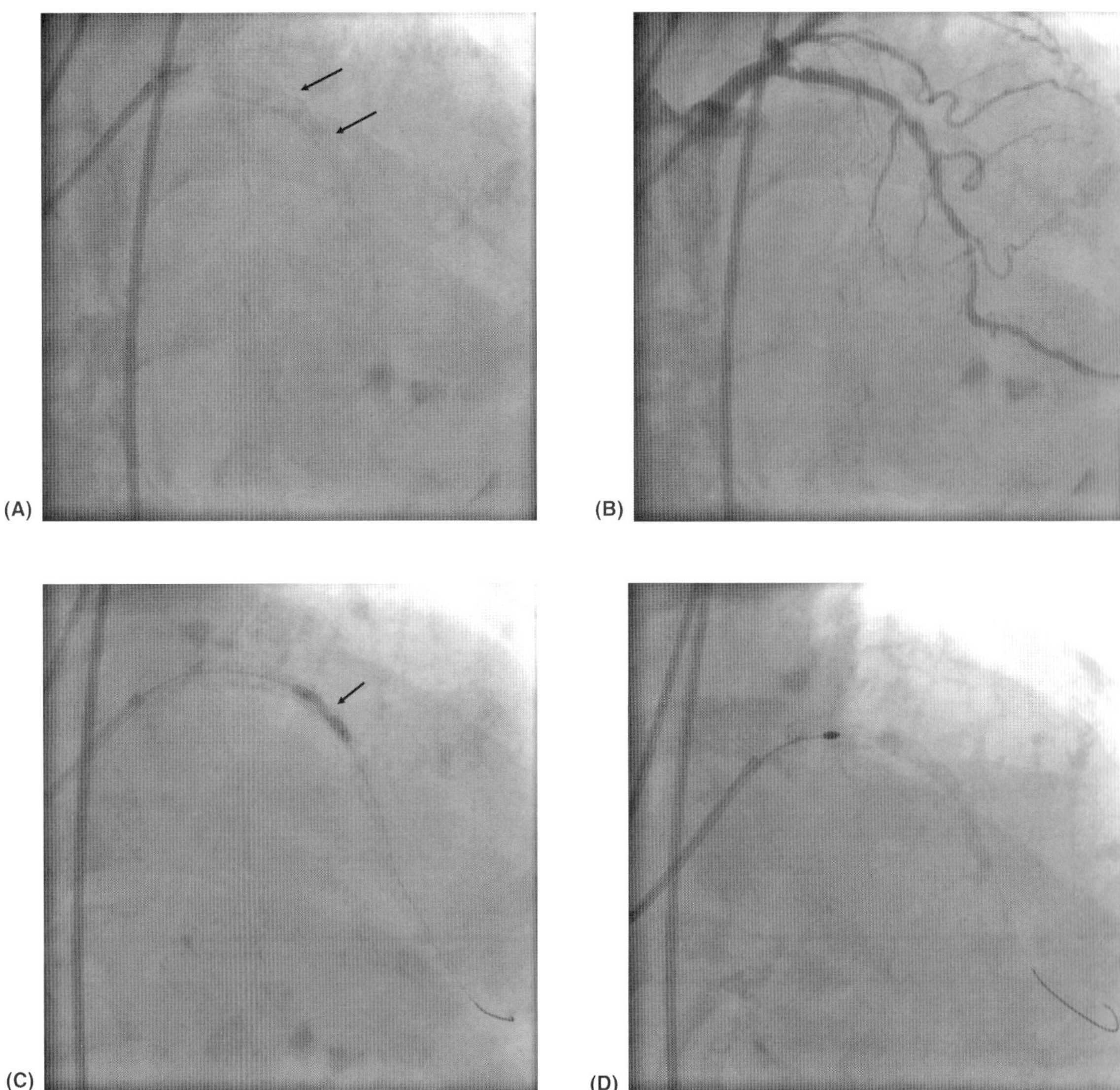

Figure 2 Calcified and undilatable lesion with excellent response to rotational atherectomy prior to stenting. A heavily calcified lesion is noted on fluoroscopy and angiography by arrows (**A,B**) that responds poorly to a noncompliant balloon at high pressure, as indicated by the arrow (**C**). Subsequent rotational atherectomy (**D**) and stenting results in excellent stent expansion, as indicated by the arrow (**E,F**). (*E, F on facing page.*)

Medications

Anticoagulation

During the procedure, intravenous heparin is given to maintain an ACT of at least >250 seconds. The use of bivalirudin (Angiomax®) during rotational atherectomy has not been well reported. Bivalirudin should probably be used with some caution in this situation; perforations are more frequent with atheroablation than with other devices, and bivalirudin has a half-life of approximately 25 minutes without a known reversal agent, which makes management of this complication more challenging. Glycoprotein IIb/IIIa inhibitors may be used during rotational atherectomy to help reduce burr-associated platelet aggregation, CK-MB release, and transient hypoperfusion. No specific IIb/IIIa

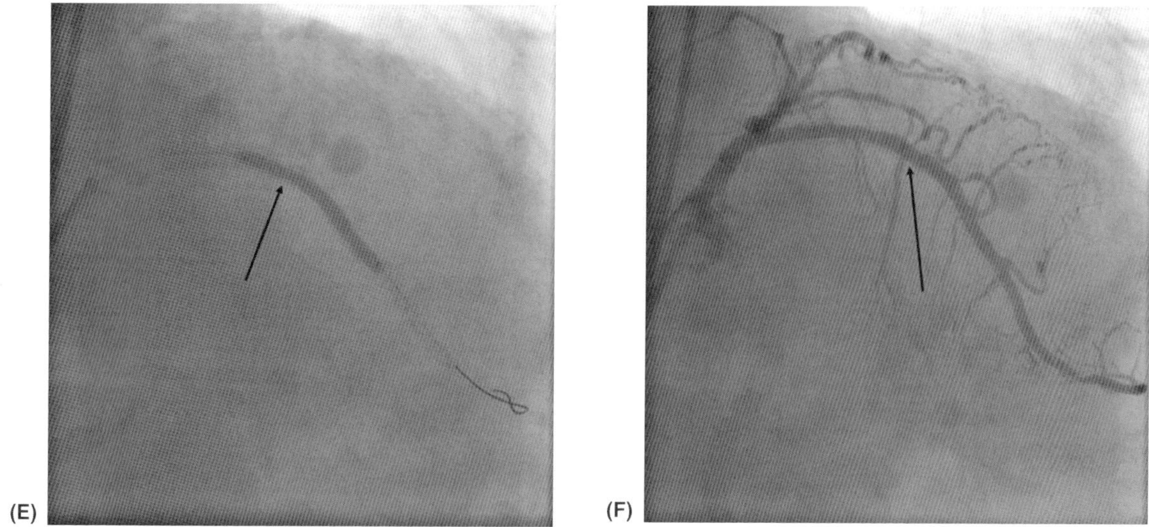

Figure 2 *Continued.*

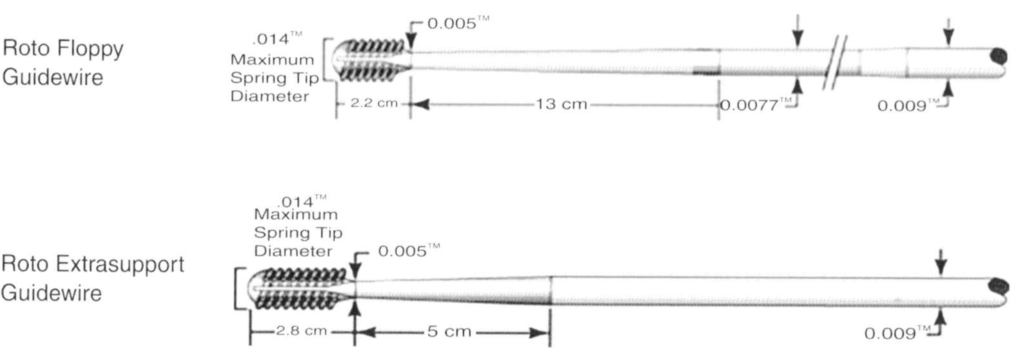

Figure 3 Rotational atherectomy guidewires. The Rotowire floppy wire has a long tapered shaft that minimizes guidewire bias. The extra support guidewire has a short tapered shaft that results in excessive guidewire bias.

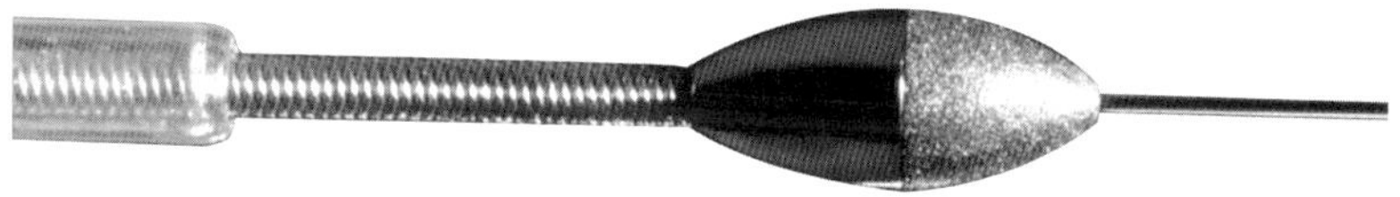

Figure 4 Rotational atherectomy burr. Note that the burr is only diamond coated on its distal half, resulting in ablation during forward advancement only.

inhibitor appears to be better than the others, but the same limitations of bivalirudin hold true with the small molecular IIb/IIIa inhibitors (eptifibatide and tirofiban), which cannot be reversed if a perforation occurs.

Coronary vasospasm related to microparticulate debris, vibration from the burr, the rotowire, and ischemia can be reduced with a cocktail of nitroglycerin, verapamil, and heparin, given via the flush port of the Rotablator system. This also

Table 2 Minimum guide catheter for burr size

Burr size (mm)	*Minimium guide catheter (French)*
1.25	6
1.50	7
1.75	7
2.0	8
2.15	8
2.25	9
2.50	10

has the added benefit of cooling the burr during advancement.

Wire choice

Some operators will cross a lesion with a floppy steerable wire (i.e., Balance Middleweight®, Asahi Prowater®) and then exchange out with an over-the-wire balloon or transit catheter for the Rotowire®; wiring the lesion initially with the Rotowire can be difficult but is sometimes feasible (Fig. 3). Most lesions will only require the use of the Rotowire floppy guidewire. This wire has a long tapered shaft that limits vessel straightening and reduces guidewire bias. In contrast, the Rotowire extra support is short tapered and increases both vessel straightening and guidewire bias. Excessive guidewire bias can direct the burr into the nondiseased arterial wall with subsequent dissection and perforation.

Burr size

Initial recommendations for a burr/artery of >0.7 were found to be associated with increased complications without an increase in lumen area compared to a <0.7 burr/artery ratio. Thus, smaller burrs are recommended with a goal in the drug-eluting stent (DES) era of creating enough plaque modification to facilitate stent delivery that generally limits the need for large burr sizes. We usually begin with a 1.5-mm burr and step up to a 1.75-mm burr, depending on the vessel size and guide catheter (Table 2). Even if this is significantly less than 0.7 times the vessel diameter, such plaque modification through "gentle" rotational atherectomy is often successful in enabling full balloon and DES expansion. Currently, there is no evidence that aggressive plaque debulking can reduce the need for revascularization in the DES era.

Burr technique

Rotational atherectomy is performed using a pecking motion while at all times monitoring the burr RPM. Atherectomy is usually started at a platform speed of 150,000 rpm for 15 to 20 seconds runs with at all times monitoring for excessive burr deceleration (>10,000 rpm). Significant decelerations can signify complications, including dissection, perforation, and burr entrapment.

Temporary pacemaker

A temporary pacemaker is indicated during rotational atherectomy on a dominant right coronary artery, a dominant left circumflex, or in the setting of significant bradycardia (<45 bpm). A temporary pacemaker is occasionally needed when using a large diameter burr (i.e., >2.0 mm).

Intra-aortic balloon pump

An intra-aortic balloon pump (IABP) is indicated in the setting of severe left ventricular dysfunction, especially when intervening on a left main lesion.

Complications

Perforation

Perforations are rare, but can be a potentially catastrophic complication that is more frequent with rotational atherectomy than balloon angioplasty. Angulated lesions (>45) and the use of an extra support guidewire are associated with an increased risk of perforation. Management of a perforation includes: (*i*) rapid reversal of heparin anticoagulation with protamine and platelet administration if abciximab has been given, (*ii*) prolonged balloon inflation at low atmospheric pressure (just enough to occlude flow) and use of a perfusion balloon if needed, (*iii*) placement of an IABP in the contralateral groin if prolonged balloon inflation is not tolerated, and (*iv*) placement of a polytetrafluoroethylene covered stent (JoMed®, Abbott Vascular, Abbott Park, IL) if balloon tamponade is unsuccessful. Recently, a new pericardium covered stent has become available in Europe (Calidad Humana®, Desarrollo Mexicano, Mexico). This stent is more flexible and easier to negotiate in difficult anatomies.

No flow/slow flow

Slow flow during rotational atherectomy may be due to distal embolization, coronary spasm, or dissection. Retraction of the burr usually resolves the slow flow; however, supplemental intracoronary calcium channel blockers or nitroglycerin can help relieve vessel spasm and distal ischemia. Multiple low-pressure balloon inflations can be used to relieve dissection.

Stuck burr

A stalled/entrapped burr occurs rarely and is an extremely disconcerting event for the operator. It is frequently related to the burr being entrapped in the lesion itself or stuck just distal to a lesion through the kokesi effect (Fig. 5). The kokesi is a Japanese wooden doll whose head is bulb-shaped and is larger than the hole on the body to which it is attached. The head is attached to the body by rotating the head and forcing it through the hole, and is thus prevented from coming back through the hole given its bulb shape. Similarly, the rotating burr slips pass a lesion without forward ablation, but cannot be withdrawn because the burr is larger than the hole. Tips on removing an entrapped burr are as follows:

- Gentle manual traction should be done with care to prevent vessel laceration and "sucking" in of the guide, but can be successful occasionally.
- Place and inflate a PTCA balloon and wire (or an Ace® Balloon, Boston Scientific, Natick, MA) along the side of the burr to create a "space" between the lesion and the burr, allowing for retraction of the burr.

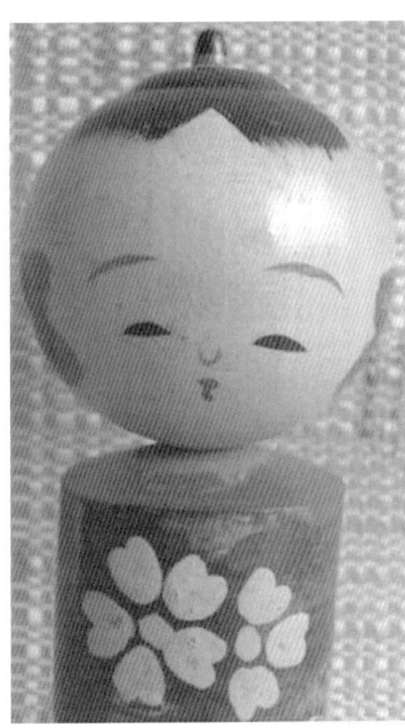

Figure 5 The kokesi effect. The doll has a head that is bulb-shaped and larger than entrance hole on the body. The head is attached onto the body by forcefully rotating and pushing the head into the body. After the head is pushed into the body, the head cannot be retracted from the body given it shape. Similarly, the rotablator burr can be entrapped past a lesion and prevented from being withdrawn by the lesion itself.

- Retract the distal wire against the burr. The diameter of the distal Rotowire is 0.014 in. while that of the burr's wire shaft is only 0.009 in. The operator can now use the wire to gain additional traction on the burr. Withdraw both the burr and the wire together during this maneuver.
- Disassemble the rotablator apparatus to expose the burr shaft. Over the burr shaft, advance a percutaneous snare just proximal to the burr. This snare can provide direct traction on the burr during withdrawal.
- Prepare for the worst after burr withdrawal. An entrapped burr can be associated with vessel laceration and perforation, and the operator should be ready to institute the measures described earlier for perforations.

OTHER DEVICES

Laser atherectomy has been used in the past when treating CULs; however, its use is rare in today's practice.

CONCLUSION

The undilatable, calcified lesion is amongst the most difficult challenges faced by the interventional cardiologist. Proper understanding of potential remedies will often turn an unsuccessful procedure into an excellent final result without complication.

8

Management of coronary thrombotic lesions

Issam D. Moussa and Neil Goyal

INTRODUCTION

In clinical practice, appropriate management of thrombotic coronary lesions can play a major role in procedural success, potentially leading to better patient outcomes. Although current evidence-based medicine suggests that mechanical thrombectomy and embolic protection devices do not improve clinical outcomes when applied to large numbers of patients with varying clinical and angiographic presentation, it should be recognized that these devices might be of benefit in specific patient subsets, particularly in those with large thrombus burden (1–3).

The purpose of this chapter is to describe differing clinical and angiographic case scenarios of coronary thrombotic lesions managed with and without thrombectomy and embolic protection devices.

CLASSIFICATION OF CORONARY THROMBUS BURDEN

The most commonly used classification scheme for thrombus burden is the TIMI thrombus grade scale as outlined in Table 1 (4). Although this classification facilitates thrombus definition for the purpose of conducting clinical trials, it

Table 1 TIMI Thrombus Grade Scale

Grade	Description
Grade 0	no cineangiographic characteristics of thrombus are present
Grade 1	possible thrombus is present, with reduced contrast density, haziness, irregular lesion contour, or a smooth convex "meniscus" at the site of total occlusion suggestive but not diagnostic of thrombus
Grade 2	definite thrombus, with greatest dimensions half of the vessel diameter
Grade 3	definite thrombus but with greatest linear dimension >0.5 but <2 vessel diameters
Grade 4	definite thrombus, with the largest dimension >2 vessel diameters
Grade 5	total occlusion

Table 2 Thrombus Burden Classification II

Incomplete obstruction with an angiographic thrombus with the greatest linear dimension more than three times the RLD (Type II lesion)
Cutoff pattern (i.e., lesion morphology with an abrupt cutoff at the obstructive level)
Presence of accumulated thrombus (i.e., 5 mm of linear dimension) proximal to the occlusion
Presence of floating thrombus proximal to the occlusion
Persistent dye stasis distal to the occlusion
Reference lumen diameter of the IRA of 4.0 mm

lacks the qualitative elements of thrombus description, which is also important in determining potential for embolization during percutaneous coronary intervention (PCI). In particular, grade 5 of this classification (total occlusion) has no value in quantifying the underlying thrombus burden, because a total occlusion can be caused by either a small or large thrombus burden. Yip et al. (5) proposed an alternative classification scheme that may be clinically useful to estimate the potential for embolization during PCI (Table 2). Figures 1 to 4 show angiographic case examples of this classification (5). Indicators of large thrombus

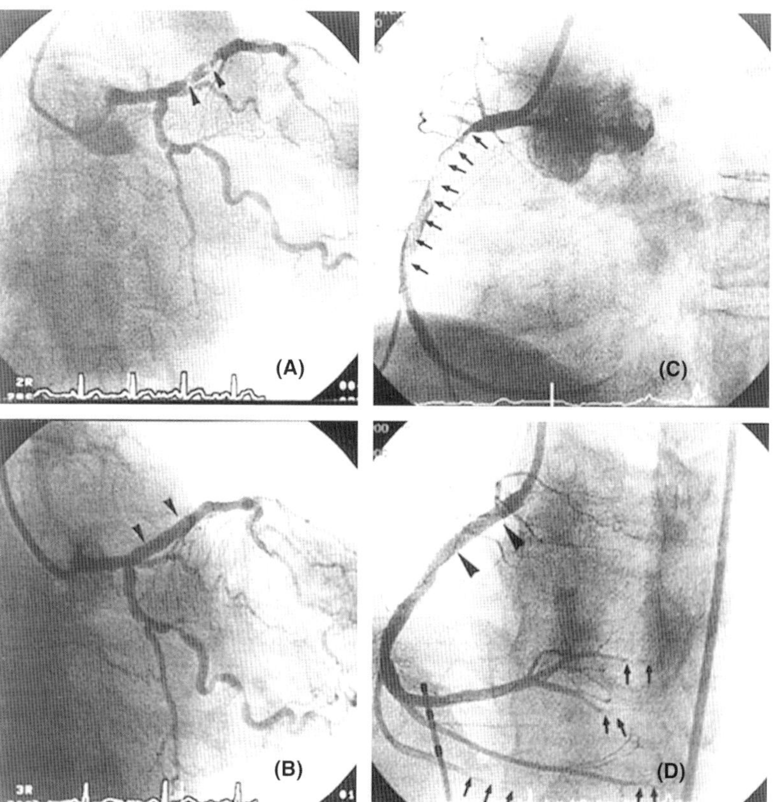

Figure 1 Types I and II lesions. (**A**) Type I lesion. Anteroposterior caudal view demonstrated small amount of intracoronary thrombus (*black arrowheads*) in the proximal left anterior descending artery. (**B**) Anteroposterior caudal view demonstrated that TIMI 3 flow was achieved after coronary stenting (*black arrowheads*). (**C**) Type II lesion. Left anterior oblique view of the RCA demonstrated much intracoronary thrombus (*black arrows*). (**D**) Left anterior oblique cranial view showed that only TIMI 2 flow was achieved after stenting (*black arrow heads*), and distal vessels were embolized (*black arrows*). *Source*: From Ref. 5.

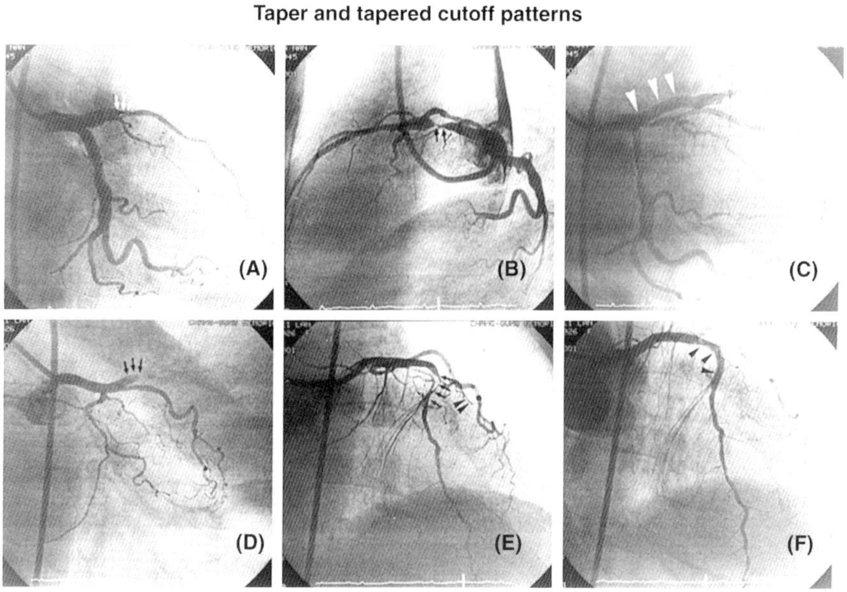

Taper and tapered cutoff patterns

(A) (B) (C) (D) (E) (F)

Figure 2 Taper and tapered cutoff patterns. (**A**) Taper pattern: anteroposterior caudal view demonstrated total occlusion of the proximal left anterior descending artery (LAD) with a tapered end (*white arrows*). (**B**) After the occlusion was opened by wiring, the most stenotic lesion was observed adjacent to the occluded site (*black arrows*), with no obvious thrombus distal to the obstructive site. (**C**) Anteroposterior caudal view demonstrated that TIMI 3 flow was achieved after stenting (*white arrowheads*). (**D**) Tapered cutoff pattern. Anteroposterior caudal view demonstrated total occlusion of the proximal LAD with tapered cutoff end and some thrombus accumulated (*black arrows*). (**E**) After the occlusion was opened by wiring (*black arrowheads*), the most stenotic lesion was observed adjacent to the occluded site (*black arrows*) with some thrombus distal to the obstructive site. (**F**) Right anterior oblique cranial view showed that TIMI 3 flow was achieved after stenting (*black arrowheads*). *Source*: From Ref. 5.

burden according to this classification have been shown to be independent predictors of slow flow during PCI (Fig. 5) (5).

GENERAL APPROACH TO CORONARY THROMBOTIC LESIONS DURING PERCUTANEOUS CORONARY INTERVENTION

Although the majority of patients with coronary thrombotic lesions can be safely managed with a combination of standard pharmacological regimen and percutaneous transluminal coronary angioplasty (PTCA) and/or coronary stent implantation, some of these patients will certainly fail this approach. This would typically manifest by distal embolization and slow flow that may or may not respond to pharmacological and mechanical approaches (intracoronary Nipride infusion, rescue IIb-IIIa receptor antagonists, rescue thrombectomy). Although some may argue that preventing distal embolization and slow flow is not worth the effort because population-based studies have not proven that this would lead to a reduction in infarct size and mortality, this argument is counterintuitive. Distal embolization and slow flow can lead to intraprocedural myocardial ischemia, hemodynamic compromise, and periprocedural myocardial infarction in select cases. Although we cannot reliably predict which lesions are at highest risk for complications from distal embolization, most data suggest that thrombus burden plays a significant role.

Case 1

The clinical presentation was a 63-year-old with acute onset chest pain, pronounced ST segment

Cutoff and presence of accumulated thrombus patterns

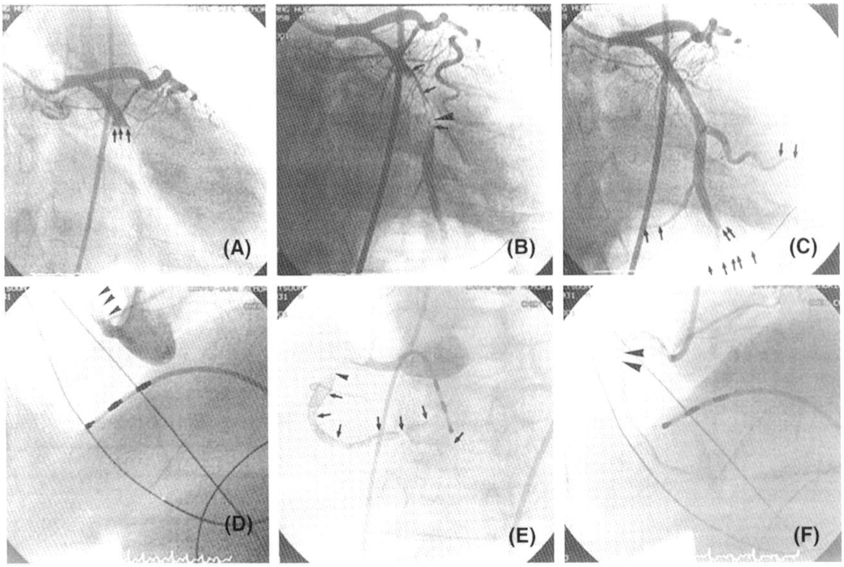

Figure 3 Cutoff and presence of accumulated thrombus patterns. (**A**) Cutoff pattern. Anteroposterior caudal view demonstrated total occlusion of the proximal left circumflex (*black arrows*). (**B**) After the occlusion was opened by wiring, much intracoronary thrombus distal to the occluded level (*black arrows*) and a distance between the occluded level and the most stenotic site (*black arrowshead*) were observed. (**C**) Anteroposterior caudal view showed that only TIMI 1 flow was achieved after stenting (*black arrowheads*), and distal vasculature was embolized (*black arrows*). (**D**) Presence of accumulated thrombus proximal to occluded level pattern. Lateral view demonstrated total occlusion of proximal RCA with presence of accumulated thrombus (*black arrowheads*). (**E**) After the wire crossed the occlusion, repeated angiography demonstrated much intracoronary thrombus distal to the occlusion (*black arrows*), and a distance between the occluded level and the most stenotic site (*black arrowhead*) was observed. (**F**) Lateral view demonstrated that only TIMI 1 flow was achieved after balloon angioplasty, and much intracoronary thrombus was observed (*black arrows*). *Source*: From Ref. 5.

depression in the lateral leads, and positive cardiac troponin. The patient was premedicated with 324 mg of chewed aspirin, 600 mg of clopidogrel, and intravenous (IV) heparin. Diagnostic coronary angiography with 5 French catheters revealed a proximal left circumflex (LCX) artery thrombotic lesion after which IV eptifibatide was begun (Fig. 6). A 6-French extra back-up (EBU) 3.5 guide and BMW wire were used in preparation for PCI. The lesion was predilated with a Maverick 2® (2.5 × 15 mm) balloon inflated at 8 atm. Coronary angiography after predilatation demonstrated delayed flow and a new angiographic cutoff (embolus) of the distal LCX artery with concomitant chest pain (Fig. 7). A Cypher® stent (3.0 × 13 mm) was then deployed at 16 atm. Final coronary angiography demonstrated good stent deployment, but persistent delayed coronary flow and a distal LCX embolus, and the patient did not have ischemic electrocardiographic changes or hemodynamic compromise probably due to the small territory at jeopardy (Fig. 8).

This case illustrates that despite optimal antithrombotic and antiplatelet therapy, even a small thrombus can lead to distal embolization and slow flow.

Case 2

The clinical presentation was a 42-year-old man with diabetes mellitus and hypertension who

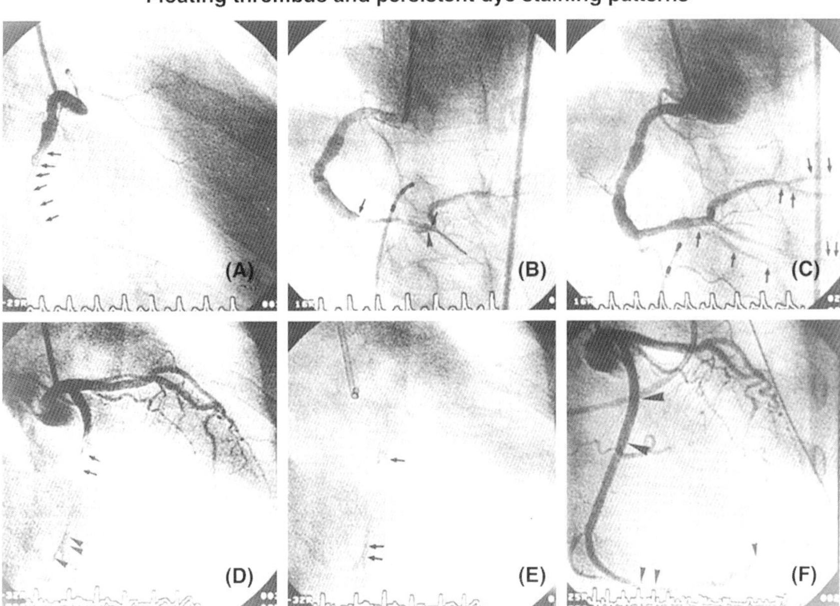

Figure 4 Floating thrombus and persistent dye staining patterns. (**A**) Presence of intracoronary floating thrombus. Right anterior oblique view demonstrated total occlusion of mid RCA with intracoronary floating thrombus (*black arrows*). (**B**) After the wire and balloon were advanced through the occlusion, much intracoronary thrombus distal to the occlusion (*black arrows*) and a distance between the occluded level and the most stenotic site (*black arrowhead*) were observed. (**C**) Left anterior oblique cranial view showed that only TIMI 2 flow was achieved after balloon angioplasty, and distal vasculature were embolized (*black arrows*). (**D**) Persistent dye staining pattern. Right anterior oblique caudal view demonstrated total occlusion of proximal left circumflex (LCX) with much intracoronary thrombus formation (*black arrows*) and distal dye staining (*black arrowheads*). (**E**) Persistent dye staining of proximal and distal LCX (*black arrows*) was still observed after stopping the dye injection. (**F**) Right anterior oblique caudal view demonstrated that only TIMI 2 flow was achieved after stenting (*large black arrowheads*) and distal vasculature was embolized (*small black arrowheads*). *Source*: From Ref. 5.

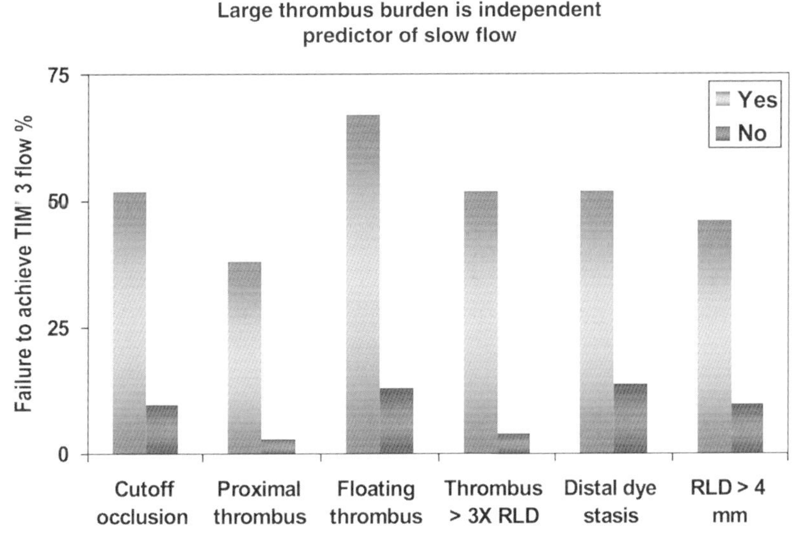

Figure 5 Univariate analysis of angiographic features of IRAs in predicting slow-flow or no-reflow reperfusion after coronary angioplasty in 794 consecutive patients with acute myocardial infarction. *Source*: From Ref. 5.

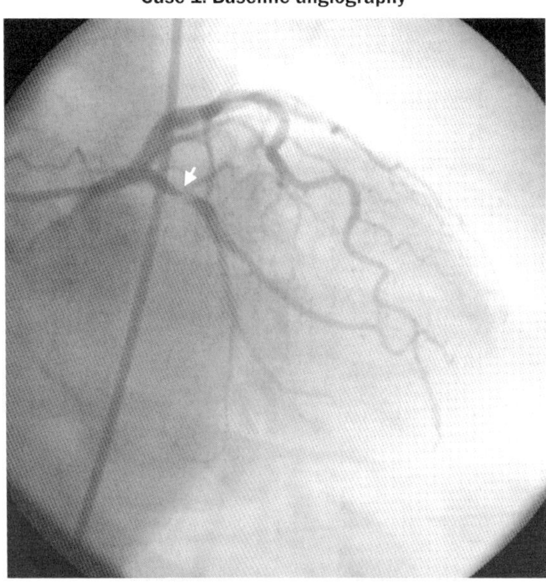

Figure 6 Diagnostic coronary angiography reveals a proximal left circumflex artery thrombotic lesion (*arrow*) in Case 1.

presented with an inferior wall ST segment elevation myocardial infarction (STEMI). He received 324 mg chewable aspirin, clopidogrel 600 mg, and heparin, and was taken to the catheterization laboratory. Diagnostic angiography revealed an occluded ectatic right coronary artery (RCA) with large thrombus burden (Fig. 9). ReoPro was started, and a 7-French hockey-stick guide was advanced into the RCA. A bare-metal wire (BMW) was passed into the RPDA. Aspiration thrombectomy with a Pronto catheter was performed, however, with minimal thrombus removed (Fig. 10). The operator proceeded with balloon angioplasty of the RPLS and RPDA with 3.0- × 15-mm Maverick 2 balloon, resulting in slow flow (TIMI 1 flow). An Ultrafuse-X catheter

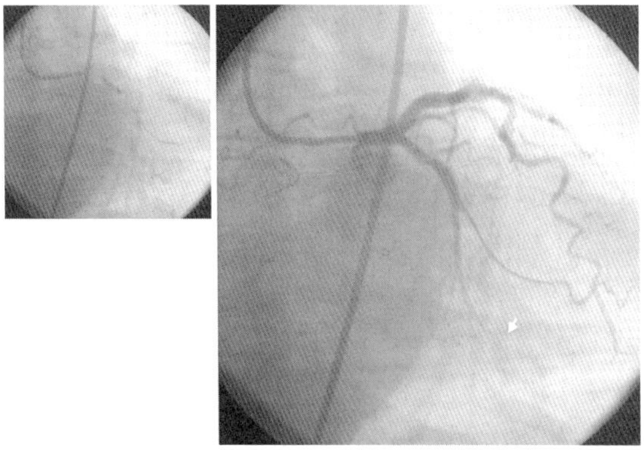

Case 1: After predilatation

Figure 7 Coronary angiography after predilatation of the proximal left circumflex (LCX) lesion with a Maverick 2® (2.5 × 15 mm) balloon inflated at 8 atm demonstrates delayed flow and a new angiographic cutoff (embolus) of the distal LCX artery (*arrow*) in Case 1.

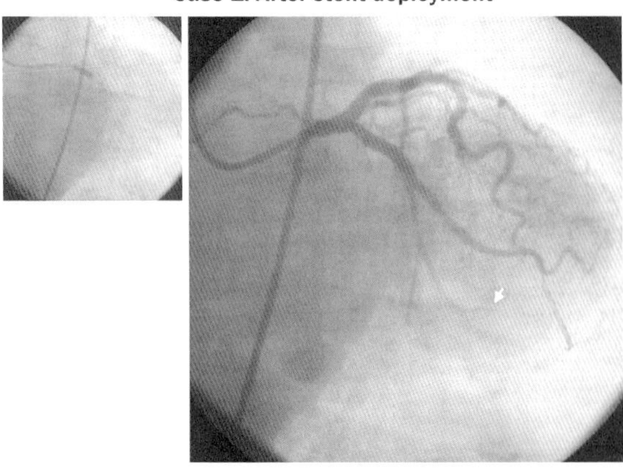

Figure 8 Final coronary angiography for Case 1 shows persistent delayed coronary flow and a distal left circumflex embolus (*arrow*).

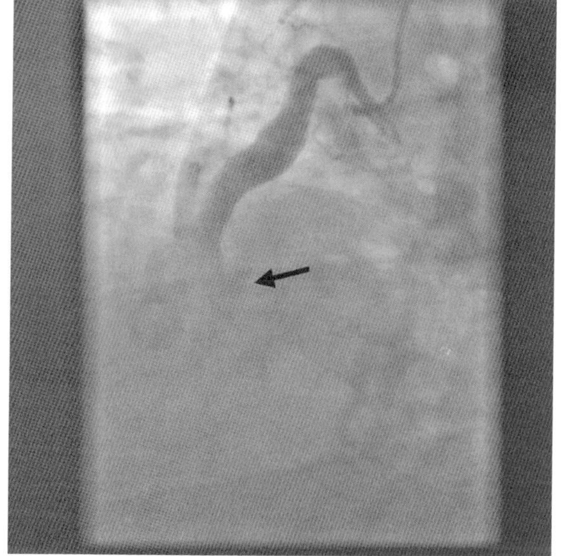

Figure 9 Diagnostic angiography in Case 2 reveals an occluded ectatic RCA with large thrombus burden (*arrow*).

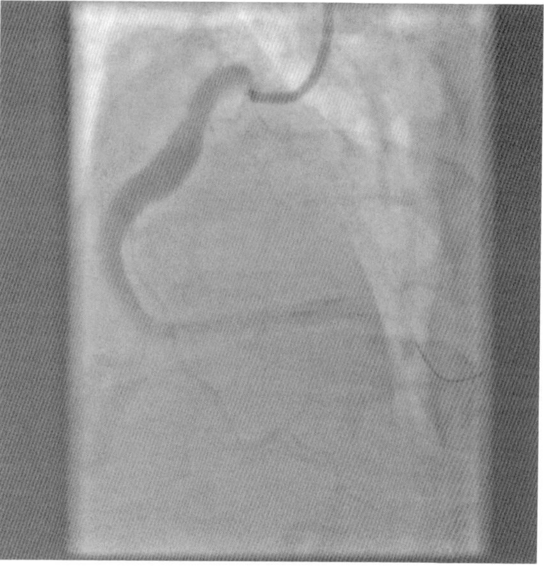

Figure 10 Case 2 angiogram after Pronto aspiration thrombectomy was performed. Note persistent thrombus in distal vessel.

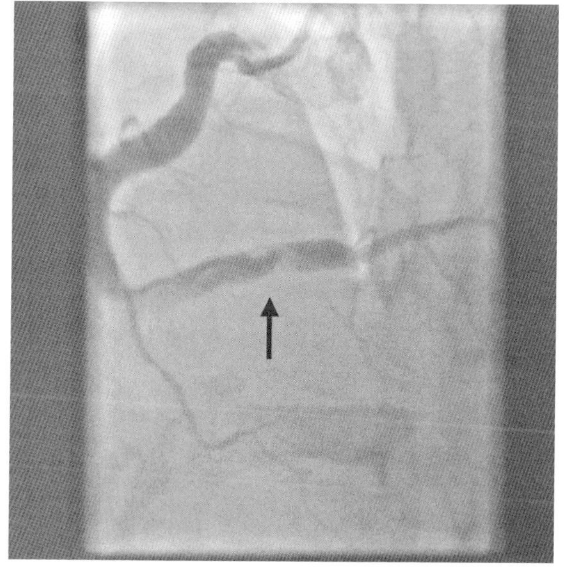

Figure 11 Angiogram in Case 2 after distal infusion of nipride and deployment of two stents in the dRCA. Note persistent thrombus in the dRCA (*arrow*).

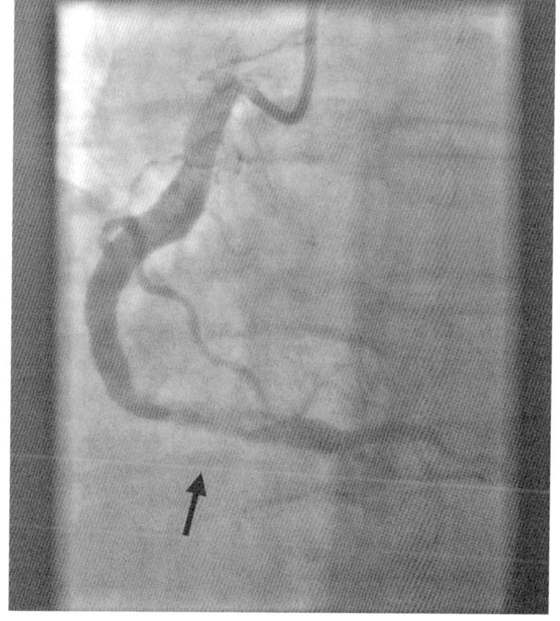

Figure 12 Final angiogram in Case 2 after deployment of a final stent in the distal RCA with persistent thrombus in dRCA (*arrow*).

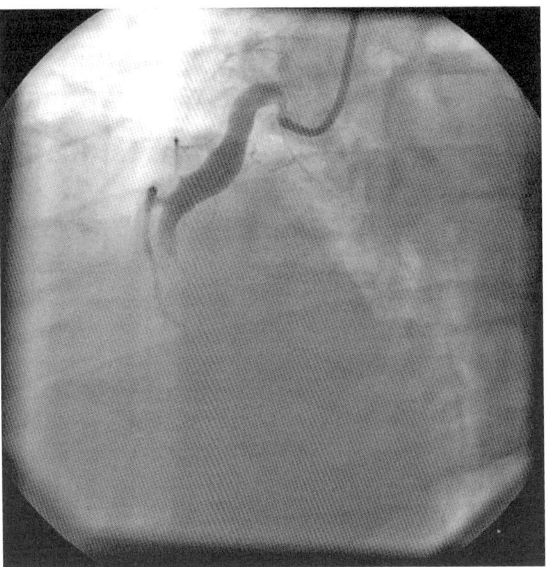

Figure 13 Diagnostic angiogram in Case 2 after cardiac arrest demonstrates stent thrombosis.

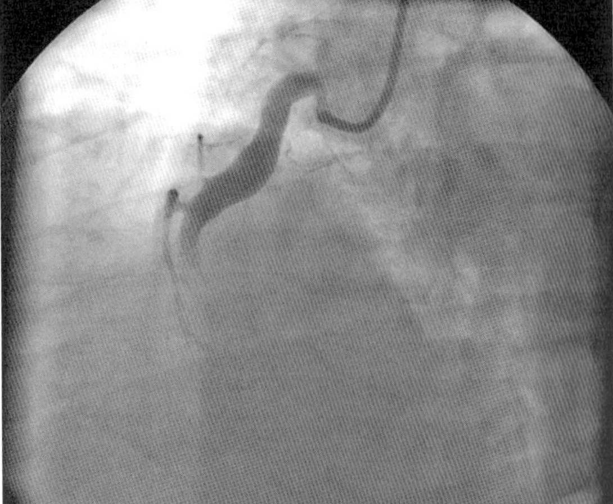

Figure 14 Final result in Case 2 after further stenting of pRCA without the use of thrombectomy.

was placed in the distal coronary, and nipride was administered without noticeable improvement. A 3.5- × 28-mm Cypher stent was deployed at 18 atm in the distal RCA, and a 5.5- × 28-mm Multilink Ultra stent was deployed in the mid RCA at 10 atm (Fig. 11). Final flow in the RCA remained TIMI 1–2 and the patient was transferred to the critical care unit for monitoring (Fig. 12).

The patient had a cardiac arrest with complete heart block 8 hours after the procedure. Coronary angiography revealed stent thrombosis of the mid RCA stent (Fig. 13). The physician managed this situation with PTCA and proximal stent placement without thrombectomy. At the conclusion of the case, the patient had persistent chest pain and ST elevations with angiography showing TIMI 0 flow (Fig. 14).

Several lessons can be learned from this case: (*i*) the presence of large thrombus burden in an ectatic artery is a high risk scenario for distal embolization and slow flow; (*ii*) platelet IIb-IIIa receptor antagonists are often insufficient to prevent slow flow when massive thrombus burden is present; (*iii*) a simple aspiration catheter, such as the Pronto® or Export® catheter, is often ineffective in removing large thrombus burden (hydrolytic thrombectomy or other equivalent devices may be required in these patients); (*iv*) nipride therapy may be ineffective in the face of massive embolization; and (*v*) thrombectomy and/or distal protection should be considered for treatment of acute stent thrombosis.

Case 3

The clinical presentation was a 45-year-old man who presented with an inferior wall STEMI. The patient was treated with chewable aspirin 324 mg, clopidogrel 600 mg, and IV heparin prior to catheterization. Diagnostic angiography revealed extensive thrombus in the RCA with TIMI 1 flow (Fig. 15). A 7 French hockey-stick guide and BMW wires were used for intervention. Eptifibatide infusion was begun together with bivalirudin. A wire was placed in the RPDA after which distal thrombus was seen in the RPLS (Fig. 16). A second BMW was placed

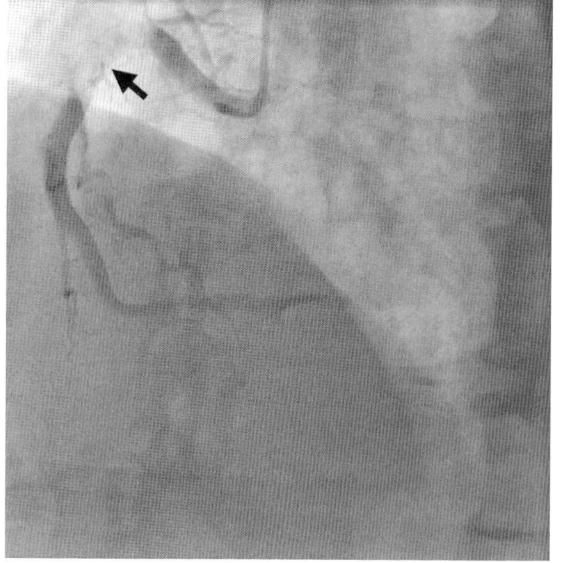

Figure 15 Diagnostic angiography in Case 3 reveals extensive thrombus in the RCA (*arrow*) with TIMI 1 flow.

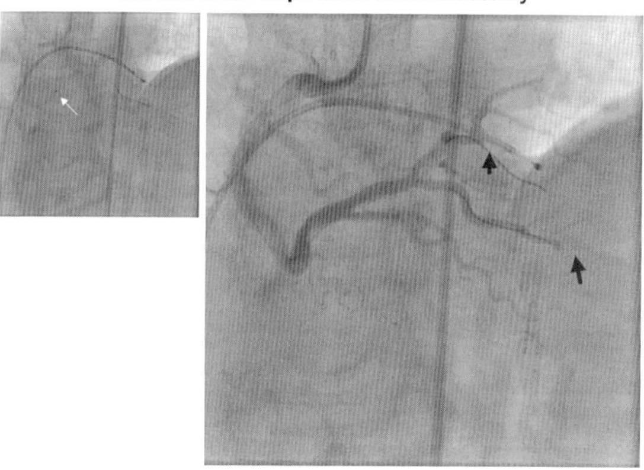

Figure 17 In Case 3, a second wire is placed in the RPLS, and Pronto® extraction (*white arrow*) is performed in the direction over the RPDA wire. Angiography after aspiration atherectomy demonstrates distal embolization of thrombus (*black arrows*) with vessel cutoff.

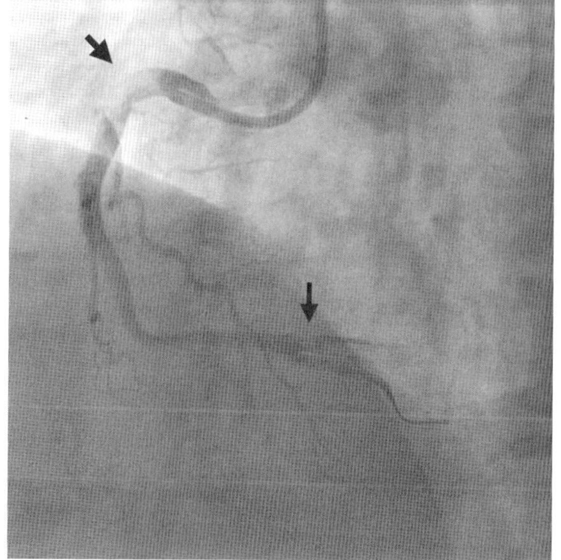

Figure 16 After a wire is placed in the RPDA of Case 3, thrombus is now seen in the RPLS as well as the pRCA (*arrows*), indicating distal embolization.

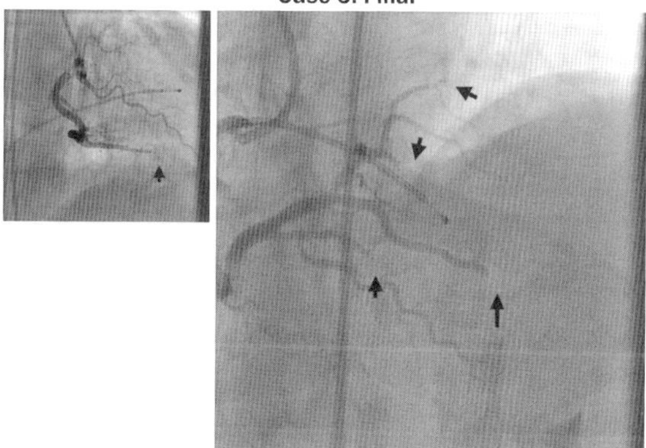

Figure 18 Case 3 final angiography after multiple aspiration attempts and infusion of nipride demonstrated multiple areas of vessel cutoff, secondary to distal embolization (*arrows*).

in the RPLS and Pronto extraction was performed into the RPDA. After aspiration thrombectomy, thrombus with vessel cutoff was seen in the RPLS and RPDA (Fig. 17). The Pronto was then passed into the RPLS and RPDA. Atropine and neosynephrine were used for supportive measures, and a temporary pacing wire was placed in the right ventricle. Despite multiple passes with the Pronto catheter and delivery of nipride, persistent vessel cutoff was seen in the RPDA and RPLS. Final angiography revealed persistent distal thrombus burden in multiple vessels (Fig. 18). The final intravascular ultrasound (IVUS) revealed no plaque burden in the culprit coronary artery. Further workup revealed a PFO, which was subsequently closed percutaneously.

This case is an example of primary thrombus burden from an embolic source. Because of the large thrombus burden, aspiration thrombectomy insufficiently removed thrombus and may have led to distal vessel embolization. Use of hydrolytic thrombectomy with distal protection in this case may have prevented this complication.

Case 4

The clinical presentation was a 58-year-old man with an anterior STEMI and underwent successful thrombolysis. The stress test prior to discharge was remarkable for VT and severe ischemia. Prior to diagnostic catheterization, the patient was premedicated with clopidogrel 600 mg. Angiography revealed a severe proximal left anterior descending artery (LAD) lesion with irregular lesion contour, suggestive of thrombus (Fig. 19). A 7 EBU 3.5 guide was used with a BMW in anticipation of thrombectomy. The lesion was predilated with a Maverick 2 balloon (3.0 × 20 mm) (Fig. 20). The lesion was then stented with a 4.0- × 23-mm Vision to 10 atm. After stent deployment TIMI 1 flow was noted with anterior ST elevations. Distal vessel cutoff consistent with thrombus embolization was seen (Fig. 21). Thrombus was extracted with a Pronto extraction catheter. About 200 ug of nipride was infused distally using the Ultrafuse X catheter. TIMI 3 flow was restored with these maneuvers (Fig. 22). Two Vision stents were placed in the mLAD (3.5 × 15 mm and

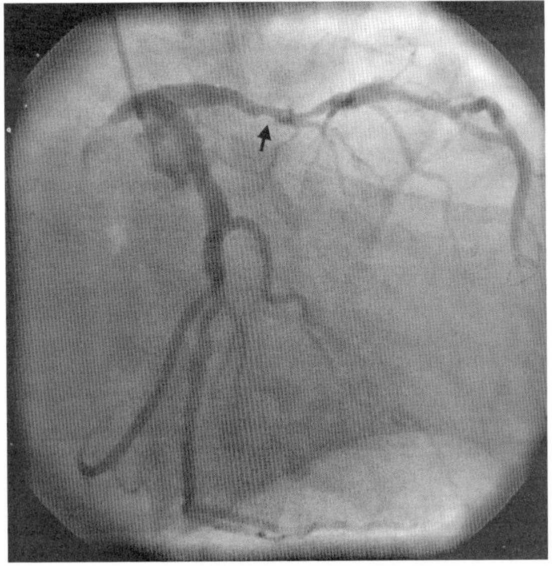

Figure 19 Baseline angiography in Case 4 reveals a severe proximal left anterior descending artery lesion with irregular lesion contour suggestive of thrombus (*arrow*).

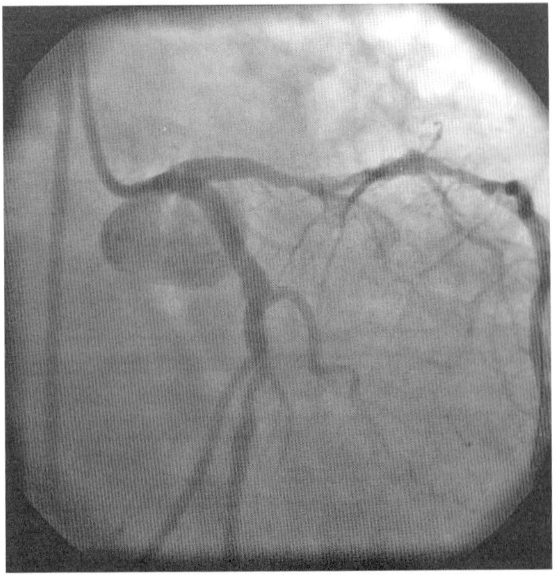

Figure 20 Case 4 after PTCA.

Case 4: After stent

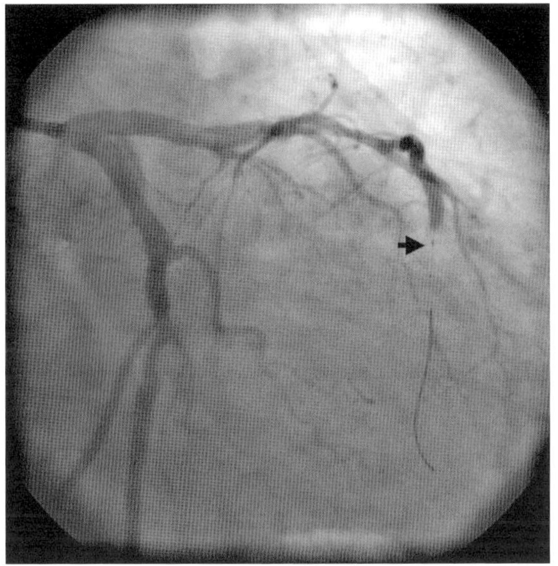

Figure 21 After stenting of the proximal left anterior descending artery in Case 4, distal vessel cutoff consistent with thrombus embolization is seen (*arrow*).

3.0 × 18 mm). Final angiogram revealed widely patent stents with TIMI 3 flow (Fig. 23). From this case, we see that despite thrombolysis therapy, thrombus burden may be large and under appreciated in large coronaries with heavy plaque burden. Once distal embolization is recognized, use of the Pronto extraction catheter and nipride infusion through the Ultrafuse X restore TIMI flow in the distal vessel. The Pronto catheter is best used through a 7 guide in order to monitor pressure. Prevention of distal embolization with use of a distal protection device would have been useful had the thrombus burden been appreciated prior to PCI.

Case 5

The clinical presentation was a 74-year-old male presenting within 24 hours of onset of chest pain with inferior ST elevations. The patient was premedicated with 324 mg of chewable ASA, 600 mg of clopidogrel, and IV heparin, and taken to the catheterization laboratory. Diagnostic angiography showed a proximal thrombotic

Case 4: After thrombectomy

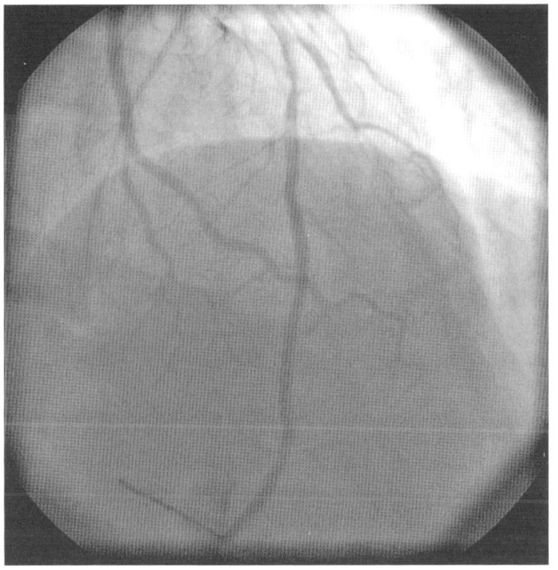

Figure 22 After aspiration thrombectomy and infusion of nipride distally in Case 4, TIMI flow is restored with improved distal flow.

Case 4: Final

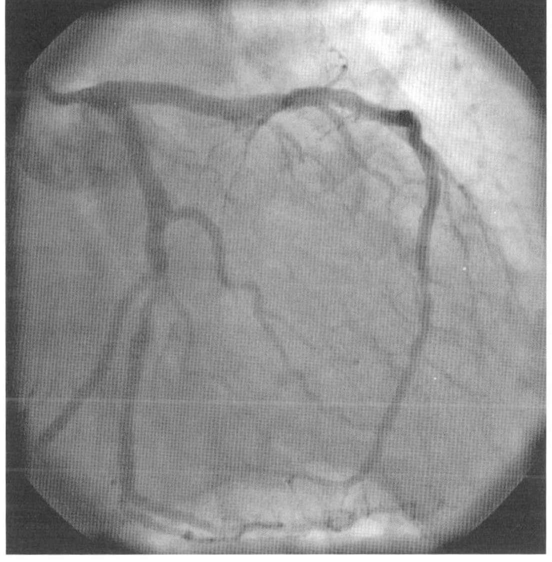

Figure 23 Final angiogram in Case 4 with TIMI 3 flow.

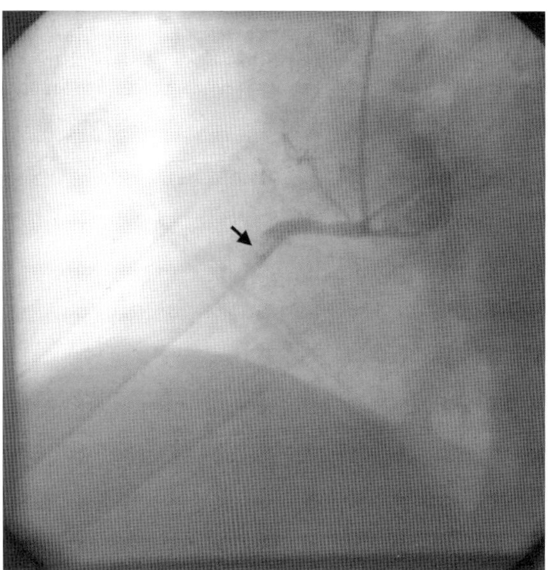

Figure 24 Diagnostic angiography in Case 5 shows a proximal thrombotic RCA lesion (*arrow*).

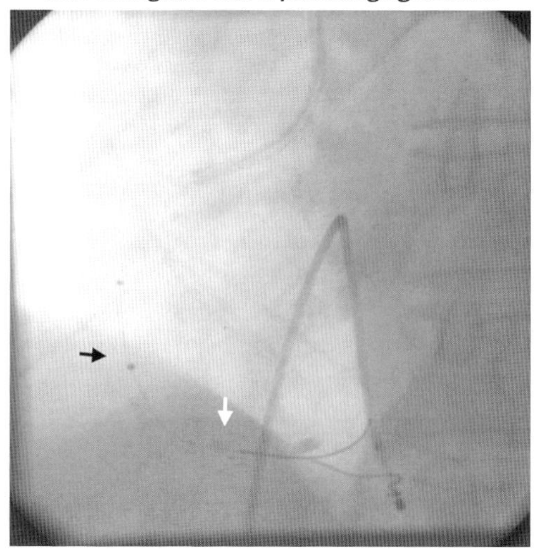

Figure 26 Hydrolytic thrombectomy with the POSSIS AngioJet® device (*black arrow*) is performed in conjunction with distal protection using the PercuSurge® Guardwire (*white arrow*) in Case 5.

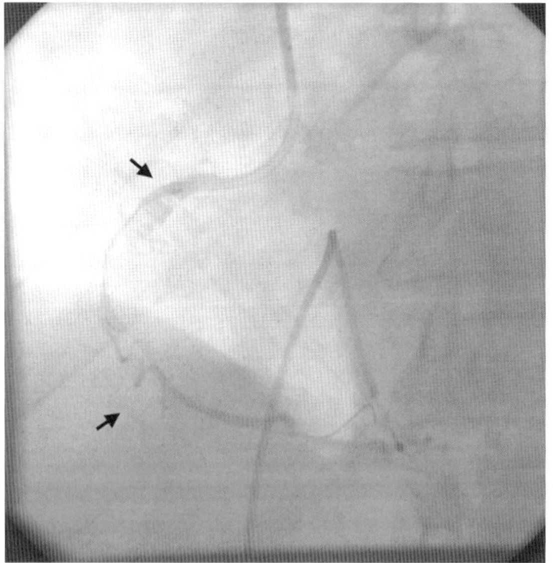

Figure 25 Coronary angiography after wire introduction in Case 5 illustrates a very large thrombus extending from proximal to distal RCA (*arrows*).

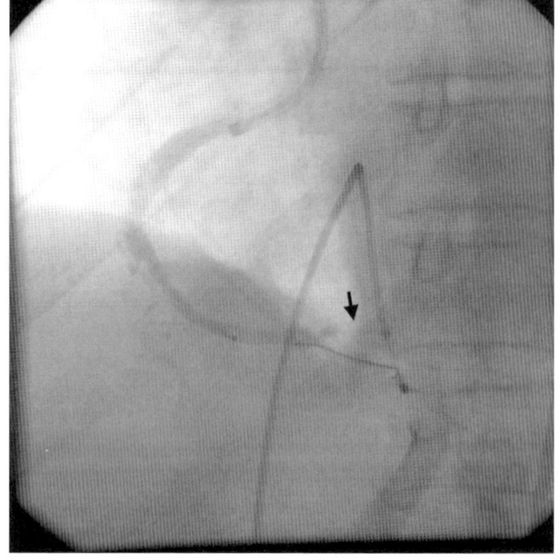

Figure 27 Coronary angiography in Case 5 demonstrates abrupt angiographic cutoff of the posterolateral branch (*arrow*).

RCA lesion (Fig. 24). IV abciximab and bivalirudin were initiated. A 7 hockey-stick guide with sideholes and BMW wire were prepared for PCI. A 5 balloon tip pacing wire was placed in the right ventricle in preparation for possible hydrolytic thrombectomy. Coronary angiography after wire introduction illustrated a very large thrombus, extending from proximal to distal RCA with aneurysmal dilatation (Fig. 25). Hydrolytic thrombectomy with the Possis AngioJet® device was performed in conjunction with distal protection using the PercuSurge® Guardwire (Fig. 26). Coronary angiography after hydrolytic thrombectomy demonstrated significant reduction in thrombus burden, but with abrupt angiographic cutoff of the posterolateral (PLS) branch (Fig. 27). An Ultra Fuse X® catheter was placed into the PLS branch and 200 μg of nipride was infused (Fig. 28). Final coronary angiography demonstrates a patent RCA with TIMI 3 flow (Fig. 29).

Lessons from this case include: (*i*) the presence of very large subacute thrombus burden, such as in this case, makes it extremely unlikely that balloon angioplasty and stenting alone can achieve acceptable arterial patency with TIMI 3 flow; (*ii*) the use of thrombectomy alone is plausible, but still carries the risk of distal embolization. The use of large profile filter-based distal protection devices may cause distal embolization during the delivery stage. The use of balloon-based distal protection may be effective; however, the export catheter tip may get occluded when such a large thrombus burden is present. When distal embolization is present, use of a distal delivery system such as the Ultrafuse X catheter will allow delivery of nipride into the vessel, distal to the occlusion, thereby improving TIMI flow.

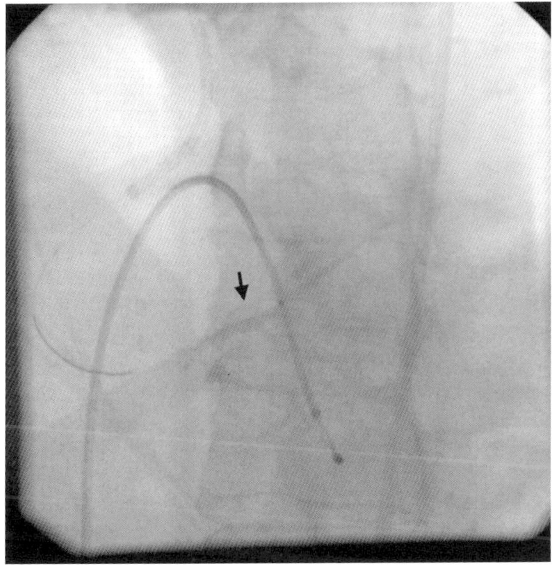

Figure 28 Angiogram after distal Nipride infusion with an Ultrafuse X® catheter shows improved RPLS flow (*arrow*) in Case 5.

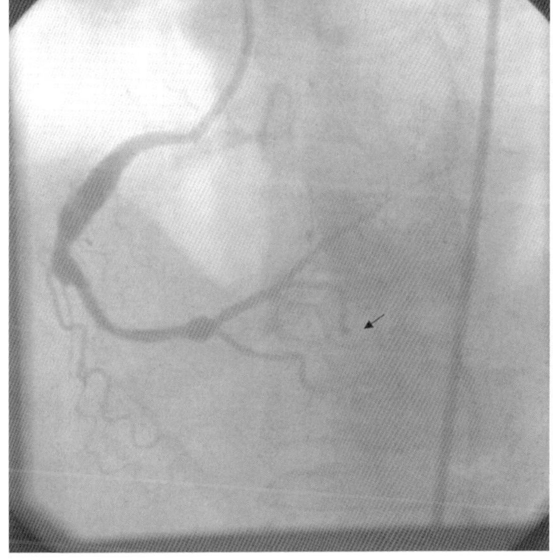

Figure 29 Final angiogram in Case 5 with improved flow and a small vessel cutoff from distal embolization (*arrow*).

Case 6

The clinical presentation was a 78-year-old male with ST elevations anteriorly. The patient underwent thrombolysis with tPA without resolution of symptoms or EKG changes. The patient was also initially treated with aspirin 324 mg chewed and IV heparin. Because of failed thrombolysis, the patient was brought to the catheterization lab. The patient was loaded with clopidogrel 600 mg, and IV heparin was used to maintain a therapeutic ACT. A baseline RAO cranial angiographic view illustrated a proximal LAD thrombotic subocclusion (TIMI 1 flow), involving the ostium of the 1st diagonal branch (TIMI 1 flow) (Fig. 30). Preparation for PCI included an 8-Fr EBU 3.5 guide in anticipation of the need for thrombectomy as well as bifurcation stent techniques. A BMW wire was placed in the diagonal. A decision was made to use hydrolytic thrombectomy with the POSSIS AngioJet and distal protection. The PercuSurge Guardwire was passed through the LAD and then thrombectomy was performed (Fig. 31). Coronary angiography after hydrolytic thrombectomy demonstrated significantly reduced thrombus burden and TIMI 3 flow in the LAD and diagonal branch (Fig. 32). The ostium of the first diagonal branch was dilated with a Maverick 2 balloon (2.5 × 15 mm) (Fig. 33). Two Cypher stents were deployed in the LAD (3.0 × 23 mm) and diagonal branch (3.0 × 18 mm) using the crush technique. Post dilatation was performed with a Quantum Maverick balloon (3.5 × 15 mm) in the LAD and a Quantum Maverick balloon (2.5 × 15 mm) in the diagonal branch using kissing inflation (Fig. 34). Final coronary angiography demonstrated widely patent stents with TIMI 3 flow without any evidence of distal embolization (Fig. 35).

The approach to thrombus-laden bifurcation lesions presents several challenges:

1. A simple approach using balloon dilatation to both the LAD and diagonal branch increases the likelihood of distal embolization to one or both territories.

Case 6: Baseline

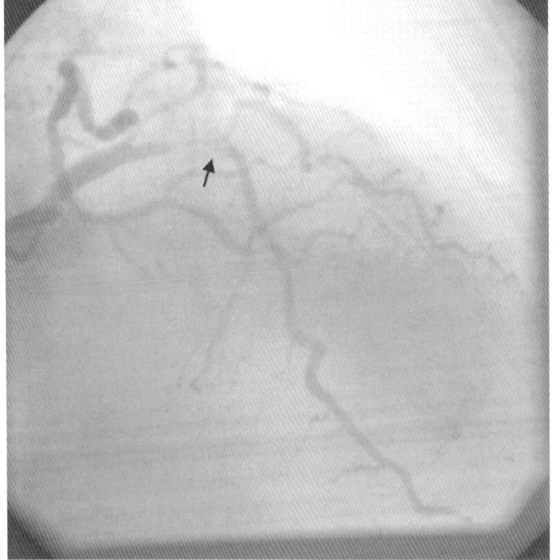

Figure 30 Baseline angiogram in Case 6 shows a proximal left anterior descending artery thrombotic subocclusion (*arrow*), involving the ostium of the first diagonal branch.

Case 6: AngioJet over PercuSurge

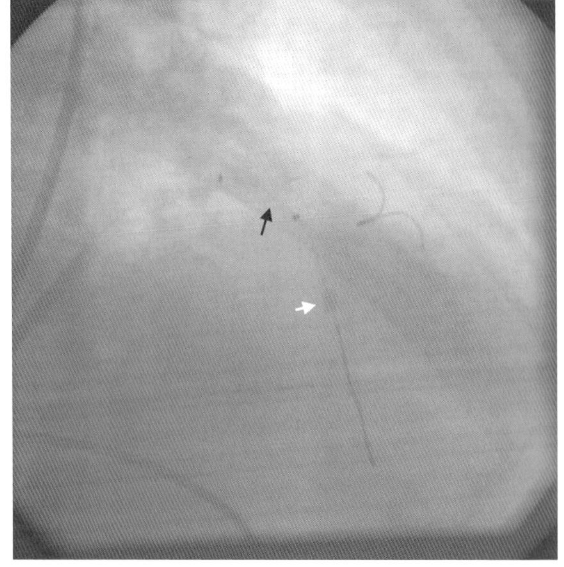

Figure 31 Wires are placed into the left anterior descending artery and diagonal. Hydrolytic thrombectomy (*black arrow*) with Percusurge distal protection (*white arrow*) is performed in Case 6.

Case 6: After AngioJet

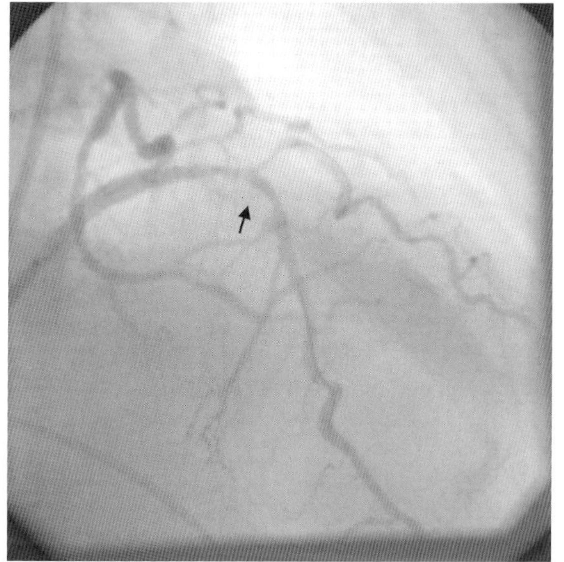

Figure 32 Coronary angiography after hydrolytic thrombectomy demonstrates significantly reduced thrombus burden (*arrow*) and TIMI 3 flow in the left anterior descending artery and diagonal branch in Case 6.

Case 6: After PTCA to diag oral

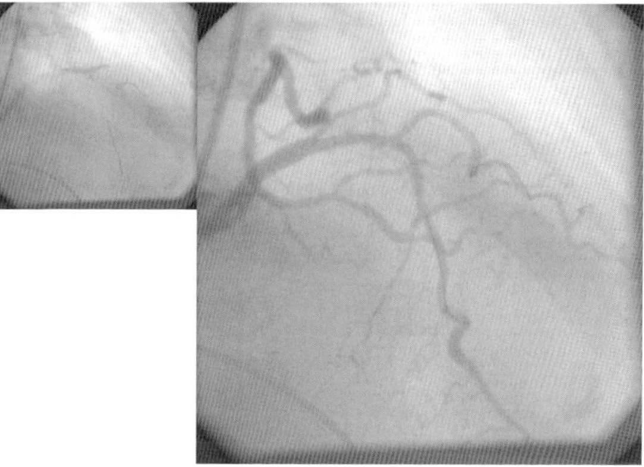

Figure 33 After PTCA of the diagonal in Case 6, a dissection is seen in the diagonal branch.

Case 6: Bifurcation stent deployment: Crush technique

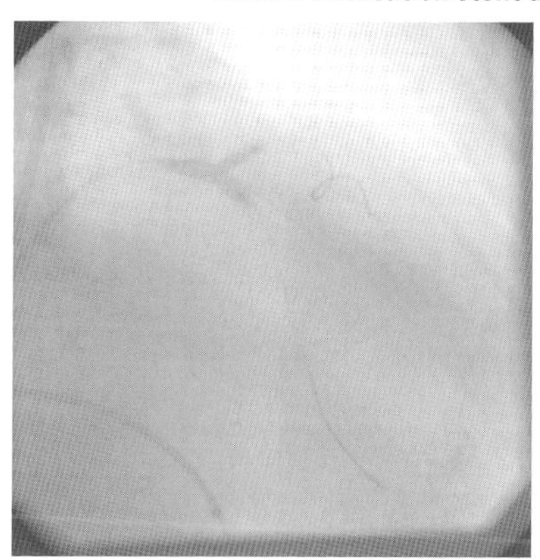

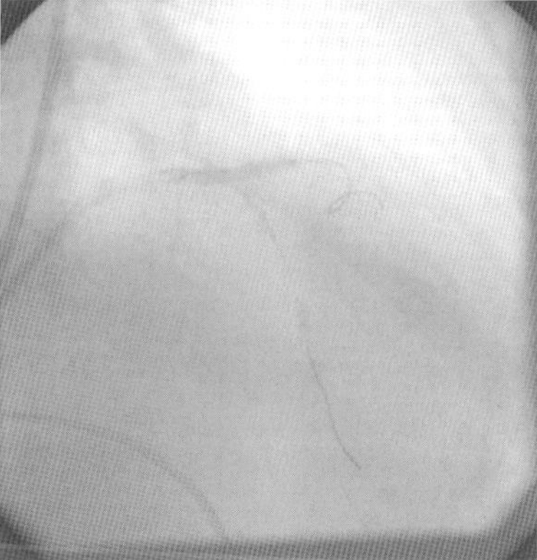

Figure 34 Bifurcation stenting using the crush technique is demonstrated in Case 6.

2. An attempt to use balloon dilatation with distal protection in only one territory does not eliminate the risk of embolization to the other unprotected territory.

One could employ simultaneous distal protection in both branches. We chose to perform thrombectomy with distal protection in the main vessel to remove the thrombus from the bifurcation area. This reduces the risk of embolization to the side branch during balloon angioplasty. After thrombus removal, we proceeded with bifurcation stenting using the crush

Case 6: Final

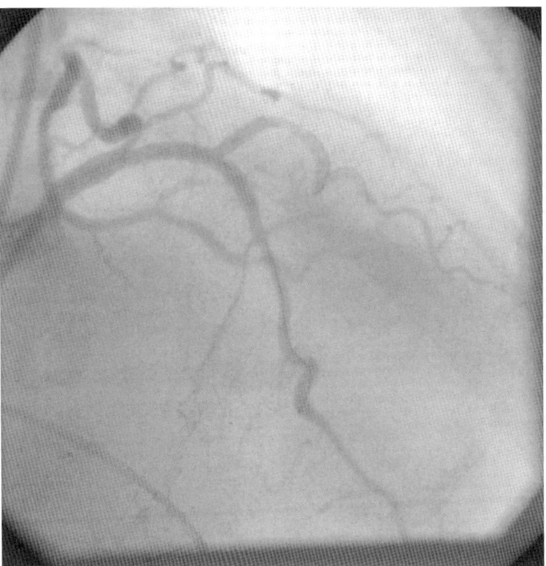

Figure 35 Final angiogram in Case 6 with excellent TIMI 3 flow.

technique. Provisional stenting was not attempted due to severe ostial branch disease, which reduces the chances of success with balloon angioplasty alone.

REFERENCES

1. Stone GW, Webb J, Cox DA, et al. Enhanced Myocardial Efficacy and Recovery by Aspiration of Liberated Debris (EMERALD) Investigators. Distal microcirculatory protection during percutaneous coronary intervention in acute ST-segment elevation myocardial infarction: a randomized controlled trial. JAMA 2005; 293: 1063–1072.
2. Gick M, Jander N, Bestehorn HP, et al. Randomized evaluation of the effects of filter-based distal protection on myocardial perfusion and infarct size after primary percutaneous catheter intervention in myocardial infarction with and without ST-segment elevation. Circulation 2005; 112: 1462–1469.
3. Ali A. AngioJet rheolytic thrombectomy in patients undergoing primary angioplasty for acute myocardial infarction. TCT abstract presentation, 2004. Information available at tctmd.com.
4. Gibson MC, de Lemos JA, Murphy SA, et al. Combination therapy with abciximab reduces angiographically evident thrombus in acute myocardial infarction. A TIMI 14 substudy. Circulation 2001; 103:2550–2554.
5. Yip HK, Chen MC, Ghang HW, et al. Angiographic morphologic features of infarct-related arteries and timely reperfusion in acute myocardial infarction. Chest 2002; 122:1322–1332.

9

Tips and tricks in acute myocardial infarction

Susheel Kodali and Gregg W. Stone

Acute ST segment elevation myocardial infarction (STEMI) most commonly results from occlusive thrombus formation after rupture of a previously undetected vulnerable plaque in a native coronary artery. As thrombus formation and endogenous thrombolysis is a dynamic process, intermittent coronary occlusion presenting as stuttering chest pain is common, especially in patients with a functioning collateral circulation. For patients presenting with ongoing chest pain and electrocardiographic changes consistent with STEMI, percutaneous coronary intervention (PCI) is emergently performed to re-establish normal antegrade blood flow and myocardial perfusion. Primary angioplasty refers to the strategy of immediate cardiac catheterization during evolving acute myocardial infarction (AMI), followed by patient triage to either angioplasty (usually in ~90% of patients), surgery (~5%, rarely emergent), or medical therapy (~5%) as dictated by the coronary anatomy, left ventricular function, and patient clinical status.

ANGIOPLASTY TREATMENT ALGORITHMS (WITH AND WITHOUT THROMBOLYTIC THERAPY)

Primary PCI in STEMI (without preceding fibrinolytic therapy) has been shown to result in lower rates of death, reinfarction, stroke, and intracranial bleeding compared to thrombolytic therapy (1). The results are optimized when performed by an experienced team of interventional cardiologists, nurses, and technicians, and as expeditiously as possible. Delays to reperfusion beyond 90 to 120 minutes have been associated with increased mortality (2,3), and a median door to balloon time of 90 minutes or less has become widely accepted as the optimal quality initiative target.

If a patient presents to a hospital where primary PCI is not rapidly available, immediate transfer to a PCI center should be initiated for all patients with contraindications to thrombolysis or patients in cardiogenic shock. In all other patients, withholding of thrombolysis for preferential interhospital transfer for PCI should be considered, if it can be done with a total door to balloon time of <120 minutes. Recent studies have shown that transfer for PCI rather than administering thrombolytic therapy is associated with better clinical outcomes, especially for the patient presenting after three hours (4,5). Transfer delays are also of less relevance for low risk patients, such as those with non-anterior MI (6). However, it is important to remember that in these studies the incremental transfer related delays were less than 45 minutes; longer transfer times have not been formally studied.

For the patient who received thrombolytic therapy, a routine strategy of early angiography and PCI should be considered. The large-scale, multicenter REACT trial has shown that rescue PCI after failed thrombolytic therapy saves lives, prevents reinfarction, and markedly enhances event-free survival (7). Moreover, in several moderate sized recent randomized trials, early angiography and PCI, even after successful thrombolysis, reduces recurrent ischemia and promotes myocardial recovery (8–10). Recommendations for patient triage stratified by use of thrombolytic therapy, time to presentation, and expected delays appear in Figure 1.

EMERGENCY ROOM MANAGEMENT AND MEDICATIONS

All patients presenting to the emergency department with ongoing ischemic symptoms, even if atypical, should have a 12 lead electrocardiogram (ECG) performed within 10 (preferably five) minutes of arrival, and read by a physician within five minutes. If abnormal, the decision to bring the patient to the cardiac catheterization laboratory should be reached and a coordinated beeper system activated to immediately notify all necessary personnel (including the attending interventional cardiologist, cardiology fellow if applicable, two nurses, and an angioplasty technician). All such persons should be on site or live within 30 minutes of the hospital to minimize delays. ECG may be performed in the field and transmitted to an interventional hospital, allowing earlier mobilization of the catheterization laboratory and personnel, avoiding many of the emergency room delays. Bedside, two-dimensional ECG may be useful in borderline cases to identify regional wall motion abnormalities consistent with STEMI, or other causes of chest pain such as pericarditis or aortic dissection.

While the cath lab is being mobilized, the patient should undergo an abbreviated history and physical examination, and blood drawn for chemistry and hematologic panels, as well as cardiac biomarkers (CKMB, troponins). A portable chest X-ray may be obtained, but

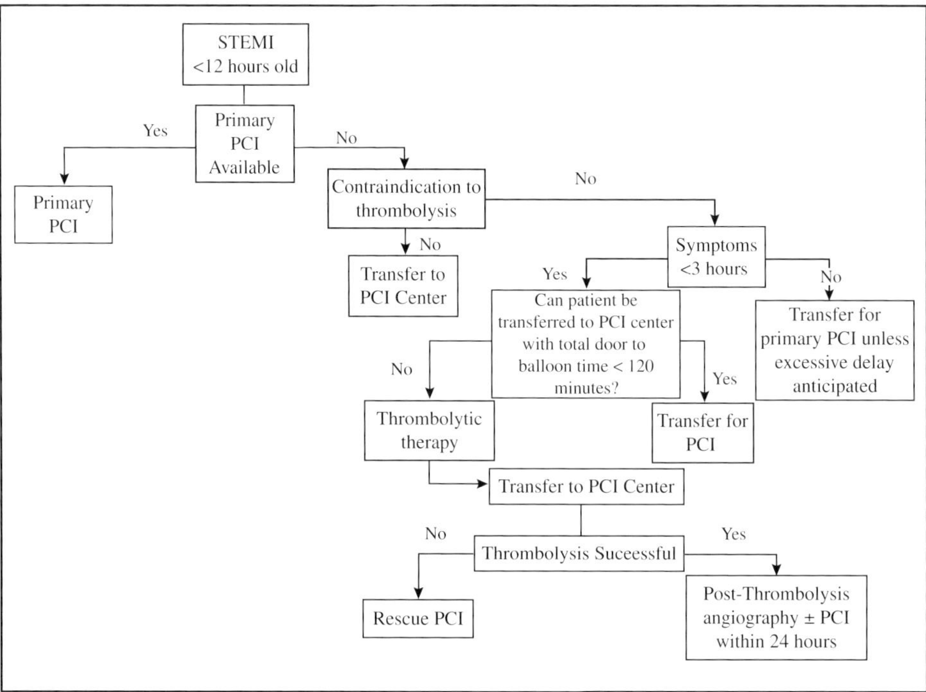

Figure 1 Algorithm for triaging patients presenting with ST-segment elevation myocardial infarction.

transfer to the cath lab should not be delayed for the performance of radiography. Pharmacologic treatment should be initiated in the emergency room with chewable (325 mg) or intravenous (250–500 mg) aspirin on arrival. Patients should also be loaded with 600 mg of clopidogrel in the emergency room. Recent data from the COMMIT trial have shown that clopidogrel, as adjunctive therapy in STEMI patients undergoing thrombolysis improves survival (11). A subset of the CLARITY trial that looked at patients, who underwent PCI following fibrinolytic therapy, showed a marked benefit of clopidogrel preloading in STEMI patients undergoing rescue PCI within six hours (12). Concerns about postoperative bleeding after a clopidogrel load are usually not warranted in the STEMI setting as <5% of patients undergoing an emergent primary PCI strategy require bypass graft surgery within three to five days.

In addition to antiplatelet agents, patients should receive an intravenous bolus of heparin (60 u/kg). A glycoprotein IIb/IIIa inhibitor (preferably abciximab, as eptifibatide has not been extensively studied in primary PCI) may be started in the emergency room or deferred for use during primary PCI in the cath lab. A recent meta-analysis of six trials found no benefit to early initiation of IIb/IIIa inhibitors (13). IIb/IIIa inhibitors should in most cases be withheld if the patient had recently received thrombolytic therapy. To minimize bleeding, some operators are currently using the direct antithrombin bivalirudin. This has not yet been extensively studied during primary PCI, however, and thus cannot currently be recommended. A large-scale study of 3400 patients [Harmonizing Outcomes with Revascularization and Stents in Acute Myocardial Infarction (HORIZIONS)] is underway to examine this issue. Patients should also receive intravenous beta blockers in the absence of contraindications (14).

THE ANGIOPLASTY PROCEDURE

After consent, the patient should be brought to the cardiac catheterization laboratory as quickly as possible. ECG leads and oximetry provide for continuous monitoring. The presence of two working intravenous lines is verified. Radiolucent defibrillation pads are attached to the patient. The patient is then prepped and draped quickly, and access is obtained via the right femoral artery (though some operators prefer the radial artery approach). Although primary PCI can usually be safely performed through a 6 French sheath, a 7 French sheath is recommended in most cases to provide more backup for crossing difficult lesions, facilitate treatment of bifurcations (which may not be initially be evident due to a proximal occlusion), and to accommodate thrombectomy and aspiration devices, if needed. Femoral vein access is not routinely required (and in fact should not be obtained to minimize bleeding and other vascular complications), but should be considered for patients who are hemodynamically or electrically unstable to allow for temporary pacemaker insertion, pulmonary artery catheterization, or administration of pressor agents.

If the patient is in cardiogenic shock (systolic blood pressure <80 mmHg for >30 minutes, unresponsive to fluids or requiring pressors, with no secondary causes of shock), an intra-aortic balloon pump should be placed and counterpulsation obtained before any contrast material is injected. A low threshold for intra-aortic counterpulsation should also be applied for patients in borderline shock (systolic blood pressure persistently <100 mmHg, pulmonary edema, or large anterior MI). However, the routine use of intra-aortic balloon pumps in all high-risk non shock patients following AMI was not shown to be of benefit in the randomized PAMI-2 trial (15). Similarly, routine right heart catheterization is not necessary, but may be useful in certain cohorts, including hemodynamically unstable patients, those in shock, and patients with right ventricular infarction. In such patients the right heart catheter is usually placed after the PCI procedure has restored coronary flow.

Prior to angioplasty, bilateral coronary arteriography and left ventriculography are performed. Left ventriculography prior to angioplasty is essential as it provides useful information about left ventricular and valvular function, as well as left ventricular filling pressures. The knowledge of which is useful if hypotension develops. More importantly, occasionally an unexpected major mechanical complication of

STEMI will be revealed, such as papillary muscle rupture with severe mitral regurgitation, ventricular septal defect, or left ventricular freewall rupture with pseudoaneurysm formation (Fig. 2). Aortic dissection will also occasionally be seen, which may involve a coronary artery presenting as STEMI (Fig. 2). In such cases, angioplasty should not be performed, heparin should be reversed with protamine, and a surgeon immediately consulted. Left ventriculography may be performed safely in almost all patients with 35 cc of low or iso-osmolar contrast, and is especially important to perform prior to angioplasty in patients with cardiogenic shock, to rule out mechanical complications, though not until after a balloon pump is placed.

The choice of guide catheter will be determined by the patient's anatomy. In general, a moderately supportive guide, such as an EBU 3.5 or XB 3.5 without sideholes, is recommended for the left coronary system. For the right coronary artery (RCA), either a JR4 or hockey stick guide will typically provide the necessary support if the artery is courses inferior or horizontal, respectively. If there is a prominent shepard's crook in the proximal vessel or significant calcification, an Amplatz left guide may be needed. For the right coronary artery (RCA), a guide with sideholes is recommended.

Once the decision is made to proceed with angioplasty, additional heparin is given if necessary to ensure an activated clotting time of >300 seconds (200–250 seconds if a IIb/IIIa inhibitor is used). Abciximab is recommended in most patients without excessive bleeding risk, given evidence from a meta-analysis of randomized studies showing reduced rates of mortality and reinfarction (16). An intravenous beta blocker should be administered if not administered earlier. Low or iso-osmolar contrast should be used in all patients.

The thrombotic acute infarct lesion typically can be crossed with a nonhydrophilic, medium support coronary guide wire, such as the BMW Universal (Guidant) or Forte (Boston Scientific), and most interventions performed using a

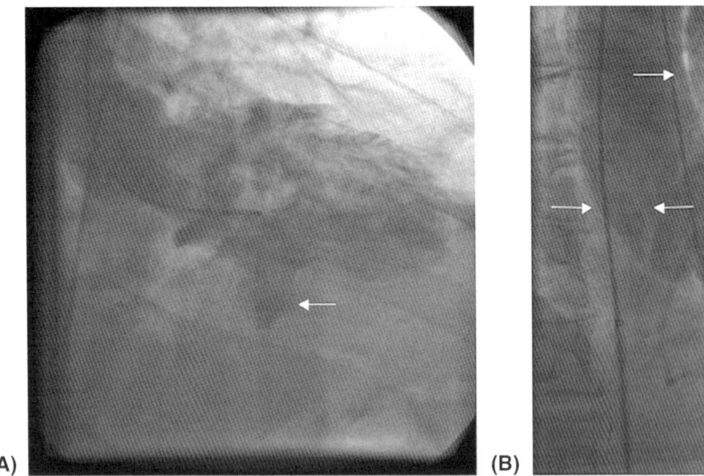

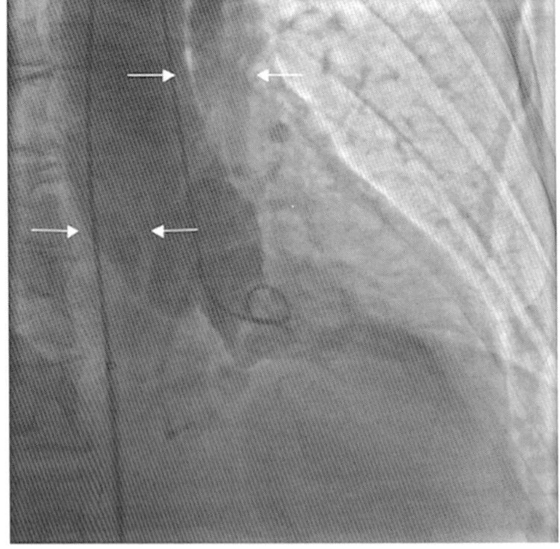

Figure 2 The left ventriculogram performed during an acute myocardial infarction prior to primary angioplasty may occasionally reveal unexpected findings that alter the treatment plan. (**A**) In a patient with a left circumflex artery occlusion, rupture of the lateral wall of the left ventricle with pseudoaneurysm formation is seen (*arrow*). Had angioplasty been performed before the left ventriculogram, the circumflex artery would have been needlessly stented and the patient exposed to dangerous additional anticoagulation, as the appropriate therapy is an urgent surgery. (**B**) In a patient with crushing chest pain and precordial ST-segment elevation, an ascending aortic dissection is seen with normal left ventricular function (*arrows*). The patient also had an 80% stenosis of the left anterior descending artery, which may have been erroneously stented had the left ventriculogram not been performed first.

180 cm guidewire. If there is significant difficulty in crossing the lesion, it is important to reassess whether or not the lesion is an acute or chronic occlusion. Most acute occlusions can be crossed easily with the guidewire and balloon angioplasty catheter, due to the fresh nature of the thrombus. Whenever possible, coronary stents should be implanted as they markedly reduce the rate of clinical and angiographic restenosis (17,18). If the vessel is patent such that the extent of the lesion can be seen, direct stenting may be attempted, which may result in less distal embolization and improved myocardial perfusion than predilatation (19). When selecting a stent diameter, it should be recognized that there often is marked myogenic vasospasm in the infarct-related vessel. If the blood pressure is sufficient (>100 mmHg), liberal 50 to 200 mcg boluses of intracoronary nitroglycerin should be administered to reduce vascular tone.

The safety of drug-eluting stents in STEMI has not yet been firmly established, and concerns about the thrombogenicity of these devices persist, especially in the thrombotic AMI milieu. Several registries and a small single center randomized trial have suggested that the use of drug-eluting stents during AMI is safe and decreases target vessel revascularization (20–22). In contrast, in the multicenter PREMIER registry, the use of drug-eluting rather than bare metal stents resulted in a three-fold increase in mortality (23). The excess deaths in this study with drug-eluting stents occurred between two and four weeks, a period during which stent thrombosis might be expected. The ongoing HORIZONS trial will determine the safety and efficacy of drug-eluting stents in STEMI.

Primary angioplasty is considered successful when normal antegrade epicardial TIMI-3 flow is restored, and all lesions >50% in the infarct vessel have been reduced to <30% (to avoid inflow or outflow stenoses). In general, high-grade lesions in the non infarct vessel should not be treated during the index procedure, as embolization or a complication in a second territory may put an undue amount of myocardium at risk. There are two exceptions to this rule: first, a significant minority of patients present with rupture of multiple coronary plaques in different epicardial vessels, in which case both vessels should be stabilized with angioplasty (24); second, angioplasty of the nonculprit vessel may be considered for the patient in cardiogenic shock who remains hypotensive despite successful PCI of the culprit vessel, if left ventriculography shows hypokinesis (or lack of compensatory hyperkinesis) in the noninfarct myocardial zones.

PREVENTION OF DISTAL EMBOLIZATION

One of the major complications, which can occur during primary PCI is distal embolization (Fig. 3). Macroscopic distal embolization occurs in 10% to 20% of patients, and markedly increases infarct size and mortality (25). Microscopic embolization is even more frequent, and may contribute to suboptimal restoration of myocardial perfusion in more than one-third of patients after primary PCI, despite restoration of TIMI-3 epicardial flow (26,27). Abnormal myocardial perfusion may readily be recognized after primary PCI either by absent myocardial blush (27) or incomplete ST-segment resolution (26).

Thrombectomy and distal protection devices effectively remove thrombus in the majority of patients undergoing primary PCI for STEMI, but have not been shown to be of clinical benefit in

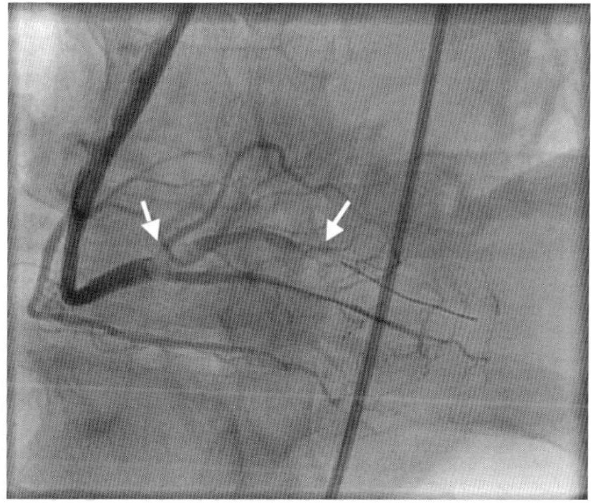

Figure 3 Distal embolization during primary angioplasty. A large filling defect is seen at the distal bifurcation of the right coronary artery and in the posterolateral branch following primary angioplasty of a mid right coronary artery lesion.

multicenter randomized trials, to date. In the randomized EMERALD trial, use of the GuardWire Plus for distal protection during AMI did not improve microvascular blood flow, ST-segment resolution, infarct size, or clinical events compared to primary PCI without distal protection (28). Similarly, disappointing results were found with the FilterWire in the randomized PROMISE trial (29). As presented by Arshad Ali at the TCT 2004 scientific sessions, thrombectomy with the Possis AngioJet during acute MI in the multicenter, AngioJet Rheolytic Thrombectomy in Patients Undergoing Primary Angioplasty for Acute Myocardial Infarction (AIMI) trial resulted in increased infarct size and mortality. A variety of manual thrombus aspiration catheters have been developed, such as the Pronto, Diver CE, and Export catheters, which are able to extract thrombus in AMI patients. Small registries have shown feasibility but the only large trial performed to date (as presented by Anna Kaltoft at TCT 2005) showed an increase in infarct size with the Rescue catheter compared to control.

Thus, to date, no mechanical strategy to prevent distal embolization has proven successful in reducing infarct size or enhancing event-free survival. Most cases of primary PCI may thus be performed without the use of complex thrombectomy or distal protection devices. The AngioJet, X-Sizer, or aspiration catheters may empirically be used for the occasional patient with stuttering infarcts and a massive thrombus burden. Early registry studies have also reported favorable results with proximal microcirculatory protection using the Proxis catheter, though randomized trials with this device have not been performed. If microscopic distal embolization occurs or ST-segment elevation persists after an otherwise successful angioplasty, intracoronary vasodilators may be administered (e.g., diltiazem, nicardipine, nitroprusside, adenosine, or epinephrine, the latter if hypotension is present). For true no reflow, these agents must be given to the distal coronary bed through an infusion catheter. However, the efficacy of these agents in this setting has not been demonstrated, so their excessive use should be avoided to minimize the occurrence of hypotension or arrhythmias.

SPECIAL SITUATIONS

Management of saphenous vein graft occlusion

Though mechanical reperfusion is preferred over intravenous thrombolytic therapy for acute saphenous vein graft occlusion, PCI in this setting is technically challenging, and is associated with lower success rates than primary angioplasty in native coronary vessels (30). These lesions typically have a large atherosclerotic and thrombus burden, and intervention is often complicated by no-reflow secondary to distal embolization. Saphenous vein graft PCI is one situation in which distal protection devices can be used once reperfusion is restored with an undersized balloon, if the anatomy is appropriate. Proximal protection may be considered for distal vein graft occlusions. In cases where the operator feels the likelihood of distal embolization is high, intervention of the native vessel supplied by the graft should be strongly considered if technically possible.

Cardiogenic shock

Cardiogenic shock due to left ventricular failure is the most common cause of death in patients presenting with AMI, with mortality in as many as 50% of patients despite primary PCI. The SHOCK trial demonstrated a clear mortality benefit at six months and one year with emergency percutaneous or surgical revascularization compared to initial medical stabilization (despite the frequent administration of thrombolytic therapy and intra-aortic balloon counterpulsation) in patients younger than 75 years presenting with cardiogenic shock (31). As previously discussed, an intra-aortic balloon pump should be inserted prior to any other diagnostic or therapeutic maneuver in all patients with cardiogenic shock. Left ventriculography is then mandatory prior to PCI to exclude mechanical complications of AMI. If the intra-aortic balloon pump provides inadequate hemodynamic support, a percutaneous left ventricular assist device, such as the Tandem Heart or Impella, may be used to mechanically unload the heart and restore normal cardiac output. However, these devices are complex and large, and have significant associated risk, especially in critically ill patients. In one small randomized study, percutaneous left ventricular assist with the Tandem Heart device improved hemodynamic variables but did not reduce mortality, and resulted in a higher rate of serious complications such as bleeding and limb ischemia (32). Finally, surgical left and/or right ventricular assist devices may be considered as a final resort, usually as a bridge to transplantation, though right ventricular recovery may frequently occur after successful reperfusion.

Management of left main occlusion

Presentation with acute left main occlusion and STEMI is rare in patients without prior bypass graft surgery as most such patients die prior to hospital arrival. Those who do survive to reach the cardiac catheterization laboratory almost always present in cardiogenic shock. An intra-aortic balloon should be placed immediately, and PCI rapidly performed to restore flow. In such cases the motto "the simpler the better" should be remembered. The main goal should be to restore TIMI-3 flow in all major branches. Striving for a perfect result will often result in distal embolization and no reflow. Complex bifurcation stenting during primary PCI for left main occlusion is typically not advisable. If the distal bifurcation is involved, a simple "crossover" strategy (stenting across the left circumflex artery into the left anterior descending artery) is recommended in most cases, with a final kissing inflation to obtain a reasonable lumen in the circumflex. Depending on the extent of disease, bypass graft surgery or a second more definitive PCI can then be performed days later, once myocardial recovery has begun and the patient is more hemodynamically stable.

Role of coronary artery bypass graft surgery for acute reperfusion

Emergent bypass graft surgery initiated directly from the cardiac catheterization laboratory is rarely required during AMI (33). Emergent surgery for failed angioplasty in the stent era is extremely rare, and as such surgical standby is not generally considered to be necessary. Even with left main occlusion or severe triple vessel disease, in most cases the best immediate course will be PCI, followed by surgical consultation for possible surgery days later, after the patient has stabilized. Early surgery is occasionally required for the patient with a mechanical complication of transmural infarction such as ventricular septal defect, papillary muscle rupture, or a pseudoaneurysm. For less urgent indications, clopidogrel should be discontinued for five to seven days before surgery to reduce the bleeding risk. If the patient is at high risk, a small molecule of IIb/IIIa inhibitor (eptifibatide or tirofiban) can bridge this period, and be discontinued four to six hours prior to surgery.

PRIMARY ANGIOPLASTY COMPLICATIONS

Ventricular arrhythmias

Arrhythmias are common after reperfusion and are most often short-lived and not deleterious. The most common postreperfusion arrhythmia is accelerated idioventricular rhythm (AIVR) with a ventricular rate of 60 to 100 beats per minute. This rhythm is typically benign and resolves within 60 seconds. Other more malignant arrhythmias include polymorphic ventricular tachycardia (VT) and sustained monomorphic VT. Polymorphic VT typically is often related to ongoing ischemia and/or hypokalemia or hypomagnesemia. Polymorphic VT must be treated quickly as it often degenerates into pulseless arrest. In addition to early defibrillation, electrolytes (especially magnesium and potassium) should be repleted aggressively. A bolus of amiodarone should also be given. In addition, a lidocaine infusion may assist in the management of refractory arrhythmia. Defibrillation may be necessary for monomorphic VT, after which amiodarone should be considered. With all arrhythmias, electrolytes should be checked and repleted to normal levels. Ventricular arrhythmias developing after primary PCI period are less common if intravenous beta blockade is administered before reperfusion.

Bradycardia and heart block

Significant bradycardia commonly occurs in the peri infarct period. Sinus bradycardia or type I atrioventricular block is common in inferior MI, and if the patient is symptomatic may be interrupted with intravenous atropine (0.6–1 mg). A temporary pacemaker is usually not required. Bradycardia may also be seen after reperfusion of inferior MI due to the Bezold-Jarisch reflex and is self-limited, typically responding to atropine or vigorous coughing. If severe, reinflation of the angioplasty balloon will typically restore sinus rhythm. Advanced heart block, (Mobitz type II and complete atrioventricular block) secondary to damage to the conduction system, may develop in patients with large anterior infarcts, and typically warrant temporary transvenous pacemaker insertion, and frequently permanent pacing.

Hypotension

Hypotension is common before, during, and after primary PCI, and ascertaining its cause is essential to appropriate care. In this regard the measurement of left ventricular end diastolic pressure with a pigtail catheter prior to angioplasty is helpful. Contrast left ventriculography is also essential to exclude mechanical complications of MI as discussed earlier. Volume depletion with reduced or normal filling pressures responds to intravenous saline. Elevated filling pressures with left ventricular dysfunction often necessitate intravenous pressors, and if severe, intra-aortic balloon pumping. Such patients may empirically benefit by placement of an in-dwelling right heart catheter, following angioplasty to allow ongoing measurement of intravascular fluid status. If hypotension is persistent postprocedure, coronary perforation with tamponade must always be considered, and may be rapidly diagnosed with echocardiography. Delayed tamponade hours to a day or more postprocedure has also been described and warrants repeat catheterization, though the site of perforation may not be readily visualized. Typically, pericardial drainage and reversal of anticoagulation will suffice to restore stability, though occasionally surgical exploration and creation of a pericardial window is required. Occult hemorrhage, especially retroperitoneal bleeding, should also always be considered as a frequent cause of unexpected hypotension.

Large residual thrombus burden

In patients with significant residual thrombus burden after balloon inflation or stent implantation, thrombectomy with an aspiration catheter, such as the Pronto or Export catheter, may be performed. Often it is difficult to fully remove the thrombus, however. Glycoprotein IIb/IIIa inhibitors should be administered as well, if not previously used. In situations where the thrombus has embolized distally and resulted in side branch loss, crossing the branch with the guidewire and performance of low pressure balloon inflations is often sufficient to restore flow. This is another situation where a perfect result may not be in the best interests of the patient. Repeated angioplasty will often just embolize the thrombus further downstream. Rather, restoring antegrade flow and maintaining a IIb/IIIa inhibitor for 12 to 24 hours is usually sufficient to resolve the remaining thrombus.

Coronary vasospasm

Profound vasospasm may occur on a neurohumoral or myogenic basis following infarct artery recanalization, especially in patients with long symptom-to-balloon times. Liberal amounts of intracoronary nitroglycerin and/or arterial vasodilators should be administered prior to stenting to ensure appropriate balloon, and stent sizing decisions should be made. If the vessel "grows" after stent implantation, the stent should be more fully expanded with a larger balloon to avoid malapposition. If spasm is severe, low-pressure balloon inflations may be rarely required and are useful to "break" the spasm.

POSTANGIOPLASTY CARE

Following successful angioplasty, no additional heparin is administered, IIb/IIIa inhibitors are continued for 12 hours in the absence of bleeding, and the sheaths are removed as soon as the activated clotting time falls below 170 seconds (or immediately if a closure device is used). High-risk patients are observed in the coronary care unit for at least 24 hours. Low-risk patients in whom angioplasty is successful, however, may be managed in the usual angioplasty step-down unit (34).

Optimizing the postprocedural medication regimen is critical. Patients should receive aspirin indefinitely (at least 162 mg enteric coated recommended); clopidogrel for at least 1 year; oral beta blockade (highest dose tolerated); angiotensin converting enzyme inhibitors or receptor blockers if the patient has hypertension or left ventricular dysfunction; and a statin to decrease the LDL to <70 mg/dl. The patient may be progressively ambulated, and most patients after successful primary PCI may be discharged on day three to five in the absence of complications.

EDITORS' COMMENTS

PCI in patients with acute MI is most probably one great benefit for our patients. Few points to be kept in mind:

- We are quite liberal in using IIb/IIIa inhibitors (we prefer abciximab) in patients with acute MI. Prior to administration, always check for contraindications including possible wrong diagnosis of MI or any associated problem such as mitral regurgitation or interventricular septal rupture that require surgery.
- If the patient is in shock or with poor hemodynamics insertion of balloon pump (IABP) prior to angiography may be of value. If the surgeon even thinks that the patient may need an IABP, it should be inserted.
- In the era of DES we should be careful to obtain adequate history from patients or family in order to exclude possible contraindications to prolonged double antiplatelet therapy. In any doubtful situation bare-metal stent may be preferable.
- Never overestimate the ability to find the infarct related artery. Look carefully at any old ECG, if available, echo, prior angiograms, and current LV gram.
- Do not forget that a baseline LV gram can give important diagnostic information to radically change the approach to the patient.
- Direct stenting is important but predilatation is not contraindicated and in case of doubts, this approach may give additional information.
- If the hemodynamics permits, always give intracoronary nitroglycerin to obtain maximal vasodilatation and currently evaluate vessel size, especially after predilatation.
- Do not use oversized stents, too long stents, or very high pressures because you may increase myogenic spasm and profoundly impair distal flow. Even if many randomized trials have shown no role for thrombectomy, do not forget that typical cases where careful and well-performed removal of thrombus may have value.
- For intractable slow flow, the combination of nitroprusside intracoronary and adrenaline systemically may be the only way to keep acting on the distal coronary bed.

REFERENCES

1. Keeley EC, Boura JA, and Grines CL. Primary angioplasty versus intravenous thrombolytic therapy for acute myocardial infarction: a quantitative review of 23 randomised trials. Lancet 2003; 361(9351):13–20.
2. Cannon CP, Gibson CM, Lambrew CT, et al. Relationship of symptom-onset-to-balloon time and door-to-balloon time with mortality in patients undergoing angioplasty for acute myocardial infarction. JAMA 2000; 283(22):2941–2947.
3. De Luca G, Suryapranata H, Ottervanger JP, Antman EM. Time delay to treatment and mortality in primary angioplasty for acute myocardial infarction: every minute of delay counts. Circulation 2004; 109(10):1223–1225.
4. Andersen HR, Nielsen TT, Rasmussen K, et al. A comparison of coronary angioplasty with fibrinolytic therapy in acute myocardial infarction. N Engl J Med 2003; 349(8):733–742.
5. Widimsky P, Budesinsky T, Vorac D, et al. Long distance transport for primary angioplasty vs immediate thrombolysis in acute myocardial infarction. Final results of the randomized national multicentre trial–PRAGUE-2. Eur Heart J 2003; 24(1):94–104.
6. Brodie BR, Hansen C, Stuckey TD, et al. Door-to-balloon time with primary percutaneous coronary intervention for acute myocardial infarction impacts late cardiac mortality in high-risk patients and patients presenting early after the onset of symptoms. J Am Coll Cardiol 2006; 47(2):289–295.

7. Gershlick AH, Stephens-Lloyd A, Hughes S, et al. Rescue angioplasty after failed thrombolytic therapy for acute myocardial infarction. N Engl J Med 2005; 353(26):2758–2768.
8. Scheller B, Hennen B, Hammer B, et al. Beneficial effects of immediate stenting after thrombolysis in acute myocardial infarction. J Am Coll Cardiol 2003; 42(4):634–641.
9. Fernandez-Aviles F, Alonso JJ, Castro-Beiras A, et al. Routine invasive strategy within 24 hours of thrombolysis versus ischaemia-guided conservative approach for acute myocardial infarction with ST-segment elevation (GRACIA-1): a randomised controlled trial. Lancet 2004; 364(9439):1045–1053.
10. Le May MR, Wells GA, Labinaz M, et al. Combined angioplasty and pharmacological intervention versus thrombolysis alone in acute myocardial infarction (CAPITAL AMI study). J Am Coll Cardiol 2005; 46(3):417–424.
11. Chen ZM, Jiang LX, Chen YP, et al. Addition of clopidogrel to aspirin in 45,852 patients with acute myocardial infarction: randomised placebo-controlled trial. Lancet 2005; 366(9497):1607–1621.
12. Sabatine MS, Cannon CP, Gibson CM, et al. Effect of clopidogrel pretreatment before percutaneous coronary intervention in patients with ST-elevation myocardial infarction treated with fibrinolytics: the PCI-CLARITY study. JAMA 2005; 294(10): 1224–1232.
13. Keeley EC, Boura JA, and Grines CL. Comparison of primary and facilitated percutaneous coronary interventions for ST-elevation myocardial infarction: quantitative review of randomised trials. Lancet 2006; 367(9510):579–588.
14. Halkin A, Grines CL, Cox DA, et al. Impact of intravenous beta-blockade before primary angioplasty on survival in patients undergoing mechanical reperfusion therapy for acute myocardial infarction. J Am Coll Cardiol 2004; 43(10): 1780–1787.
15. Stone GW, Marsalese D, Brodie BR, et al. A prospective, randomized evaluation of prophylactic intraaortic balloon counterpulsation in high risk patients with acute myocardial infarction treated with primary angioplasty. Second Primary Angioplasty in Myocardial Infarction (PAMI-II) Trial Investigators. J Am Coll Cardiol 1997; 29(7): 1459–1467.
16. De Luca G, Suryapranata H, Stone GW, et al. Abciximab as adjunctive therapy to reperfusion in acute ST-segment elevation myocardial infarction: a meta-analysis of randomized trials. JAMA 2005; 293(14):1759–1765.
17. Stone GW, Grines CL, Cox DA, et al. Comparison of angioplasty with stenting, with or without abciximab, in acute myocardial infarction. N Engl J Med 2002; 346(13):957–966.
18. Grines CL, Cox DA, Stone GW, et al. Coronary angioplasty with or without stent implantation for acute myocardial infarction. Stent Primary Angioplasty in Myocardial Infarction Study Group. N Engl J Med 1999; 341(26):1949–1956.
19. Loubeyre C, Morice MC, Lefevre T, Piechaud JF, Louvard Y, Dumas P. A randomized comparison of direct stenting with conventional stent implantation in selected patients with acute myocardial infarction. J Am Coll Cardiol 2002; 39(1):15–21.
20. Valgimigli M, Percoco G, Malagutti P, et al. Tirofiban and sirolimus-eluting stent vs abciximab and bare-metal stent for acute myocardial infarction: a randomized trial. JAMA 2005; 293(17):2109–2117.
21. Hofma SH, Ong AT, Aoki J, et al. One year clinical follow up of paclitaxel eluting stents for acute myocardial infarction compared with sirolimus eluting stents. Heart 2005; 91(9):1176–1180.
22. Saia F, Lemos PA, Lee CH, et al. Sirolimus-eluting stent implantation in ST-elevation acute myocardial infarction: a clinical and angiographic study. Circulation 2003; 108(16):1927–1929.
23. Kernis SJ, Cohen D, Reid K, et al. Clinical Outcomes Associated with Use of Drug-Eluting Stents Compared with Bare-Metal Stents for Primary Percutaneous Intervention. American Journal of Cardiology 2005; 96(7(1)):47H.
24. Goldstein JA, Demetriou D, Grines CL, Pica M, Shoukfeh M, O'Neill WW. Multiple complex coronary plaques in patients with acute myocardial infarction. N Engl J Med 2000; 343(13): 915–922.
25. Henriques JP, Zijlstra F, Ottervanger JP, et al. Incidence and clinical significance of distal embolization during primary angioplasty for acute myocardial infarction. Eur Heart J 2002; 23(14): 1112–1117.
26. McLaughlin MG, Stone GW, Aymong E, et al. Prognostic utility of comparative methods for assessment of ST-segment resolution after primary angioplasty for acute myocardial infarction: the Controlled Abciximab and Device Investigation to

Lower Late Angioplasty Complications (CADILLAC) trial. J Am Coll Cardiol 2004; 44(6):1215–1223.

27. Henriques JP, Zijlstra F, van 't Hof AW, et al. Angiographic assessment of reperfusion in acute myocardial infarction by myocardial blush grade. Circulation 2003; 107(16):2115–2119.
28. Stone GW, Webb J, Cox DA, et al. Distal microcirculatory protection during percutaneous coronary intervention in acute ST-segment elevation myocardial infarction: a randomized controlled trial. JAMA 2005; 293(9):1063–1072.
29. Gick M, Jander N, Bestehorn HP, et al. Randomized evaluation of the effects of filter-based distal protection on myocardial perfusion and infarct size after primary percutaneous catheter intervention in myocardial infarction with and without ST-segment elevation. Circulation 2005; 112(10):1462–1469.
30. Stone GW, Brodie BR, Griffin JJ, et al. Clinical and angiographic outcomes in patients with previous coronary artery bypass graft surgery treated with primary balloon angioplasty for acute myocardial infarction. Second Primary Angioplasty in Myocardial Infarction Trial (PAMI-2) Investigators. J Am Coll Cardiol 2000; 35(3):605–611.
31. Hochman JS, Sleeper LA, White HD, et al. One-year survival following early revascularization for cardiogenic shock. JAMA 2001; 285(2): 190–192.
32. Thiele H, Sick P, Boudriot E, et al. Randomized comparison of intra-aortic balloon support with a percutaneous left ventricular assist device in patients with revascularized acute myocardial infarction complicated by cardiogenic shock. Eur Heart J 2005; 26(13):1276–1283.
33. Stone GW, Brodie BR, Griffin JJ, et al. Role of cardiac surgery in the hospital phase management of patients treated with primary angioplasty for acute myocardial infarction. Am J Cardiol 2000; 85(11):1292–1296.
34. Grines CL, Marsalese DL, Brodie B, et al. Safety and cost-effectiveness of early discharge after primary angioplasty in low risk patients with acute myocardial infarction. PAMI-II Investigators. Primary Angioplasty in Myocardial Infarction. J Am Coll Cardiol 1998; 31(5):967–972.

10

Saphenous vein grafts and arterial conduits

Eberhard Grube, Swee Guan Teo, and Lutz Buellesfeld

Options for revascularization in cases of saphenous vein graft (SVG) disease include either percutaneous coronary interventions (PCI) or repeat coronary artery bypass graft surgery (CABG). Due to a significantly higher risk of performing a repeat CABG, PCI is the preferred method of treating patients with SVG lesions. Especially in the presence of advanced age and comorbidities such as cerebrovascular, renal, malignancy, or pulmonary disease, the outcome of a second surgical approach is limited. In addition, re-CABG carries the potential for jeopardizing patent bypass vessels, and it is associated with less complete revascularization and control of symptoms when compared to the first procedure. Percutaneous revascularization of bypass grafts or native vessels is, therefore, the preferred treatment option for recurrent ischemia in CABG patients—particularly surgical high-risk candidates—associated with a high procedural success (97%) and an acceptable in-hospital major adverse cardiac event (MACE) rate (6–11%) (1). Furthermore, percutaneous intervention is standard in patients with degenerated grafts who still have patent arterial grafts, or patients with no suitable arterial or venous grafts for re-operation.

TYPES OF CORONARY ARTERY BYPASS GRAFT SURGERY FAILURES

Early failure

Ischemia after CABG can be divided into three groups—early, midterm and late ischemia. Graft failure related to thrombosis, prolonged spasms, or suture problems at the anastomosis site, is often the cause of recurrent ischemia within 30 days of CABG. Other causes include incomplete revascularization, stenoses distal to anastomosis, and bypass of the wrong vessel. Urgent coronary angiography is indicated to determine the cause of ischemia and emergency percutaneous intervention if required, often successfully relieving the ischemia in the majority of patients. Balloon dilatation across suture lines has been performed safely within a few days of surgery. Intracoronary fibrinolytic, in contrast, should be avoided especially within the first week after operation, due to high rate of mediastinal bleeding, often requiring exploration.

Midterm failure

When ischemia occurs within 1 to 12 months after CABG, it is usually due to perianastomotic graft stenosis from intimal hyperplasia. Both arterial and venous graft disease at distal anastomotic sites have been treated successfully with balloon dilatation alone, and have better long-term prognosis than midshaft or proximal vein graft anastomotic stenoses. Based on a retrospective study of 252 patients who had percutaneous revascularization to SVG at distal anastomotic site, stenting deployment compared to balloon angioplasty may further improve the long-term outcome of these patients by reducing the need for repeat revascularization (14% versus 25%, $P = 0.058$) (2).

Late failure

In late ischemia (more than one year) after CABG, the cause is usually new stenoses in graft conduits and/or native vessels. Accelerated atherosclerotic disease predominates in SVG, with plaque being friable and often thrombus-laden. This typical morphology contributes to the high occurrence of slow flow, distal embolization, and periprocedural myocardial infarction (MI), after percutaneous intervention of SVG lesions.

SAPHENOUS VEIN GRAFTS—CHARACTERISTICS AND TECHNICAL APPROACH

SVGs begin to deteriorate within five to seven years due to accelerated atherosclerosis. Only about 80% of SVGs remain patent five years after surgery and about 60% at 7 to 10 years. Long-term patency rates are much higher (about 85–90%) with internal mammary artery grafts. From three years after CABG, SVGs particularly degenerate quickly with the formation of large, friable, lipid-rich atherosclerotic plaque. The most common presentation is recurrent angina and less often acute MI. It is especially important that graft problems be investigated earlier, since stenoses in these vessels can progress rapidly to total occlusion.

Due to the typical plaque composition of SVG lesions, distal embolization resulting in elevated cardiac enzymes is more common after percutaneous intervention in SVG. Angiographic predictors of MACE in percutaneous intervention of SVG are thrombus, diffuse disease, and impaired flow at baseline. In a report of 1056 consecutive patients who had SVG intervention, 15% of patients had CK-MB > 5 times normal. This carried higher one-year mortality compared to normal CK-MB (11.7% versus 4.8%) and was the strongest predictor of late mortality (3). Overall, the outcome of PCI in SVG stenoses is worse than in native vessels with higher mortality rates at 30 days (2.1% versus 1%, $P = 0.006$) and six months followup (4.7% versus 2%, $P < 0.001$) (4).

Distal embolization

Distal embolization, being the main complication of PCI with stenting of degenerated SVGs, results in "slow flow"/"no reflow," secondary to diffuse microvascular occlusion, mainly caused by debris arising from manipulation of the friable lesion within a diseased vein graft. Although the use of glycoprotein (GP) IIb/IIIa inhibitors have enhanced the safety of PCI, these drugs have no significant impact on patient outcome after distal embolization in interventions of diseased SVGs, due to the specific composition of vein graft emboli, which are primarily based on atherofibrotic particles. Pooled data of 627 patients (32% abciximab and 31% eptifibatide) from five trials involving SVG treatment failed to show clinical efficacy of IIb/IIIa inhibitors in this lesion subset (5); therefore, SVG lesion patients remain at high risk for peri-procedural embolization with consecutive development of non-Q-wave/Q-wave MIs. In the past decade, several techniques and devices have been developed to limit distal embolization (intracoronary administration of urokinase, directional coronary atherectomy, laser angioplasty, or ultrasound thrombolysis), but failed to prove efficacy. Studies on thrombectomy devices revealed controversial results. In the VEGAS II trial, 349 patients undergoing percutaneous intervention for a coronary artery or SVG lesion with angiographically evident thrombus were randomized to urokinase versus rheolytic thrombectomy device (AngioJet, Possis Medical Inc., Minneapolis, MN). AngioJet is a catheter-based system that uses high-velocity water jets to produce a vacuum for thrombus aspiration and extraction. The treated vessel was an SVG in 53% in the AngioJet group and 54% in the urokinase group. The results showed that AngioJet is superior to urokinase with higher procedural success (86% versus 72%, $P < 0.002$), lower periprocedural MI (14% versus 31%, $P < 0.001$) and fewer major hemorrhagic complications (5% versus 12%, $P = 0.03$) (5).

The X-Sizer thrombectomy device, which uses spinning blades to macerate thrombus and allows its extraction into a vacuum bottle, was studied in the X-TRACT trial (6). A total of 797 patients with diseased SVGs or thrombus-containing coronary arteries were randomized to X-Sizer followed by stenting versus stenting alone. There were no differences in periprocedural MI, and MACE at 30 days and at one year. However, large MI at 30 days occurred less often in the X-Sizer group (5.5% versus 9.6%, $P = 0.03$). In those patients with identifiable thrombus on angiography, the rate of death or large MI at 30 days was lower in X-Sizer group (4.7% versus 9.9%, $P = 0.04$). It appears that X-Sizer device is most effective when the target lesion contains thrombus.

Direct stenting without prior balloon inflation is believed to be beneficial in order to minimize peri-interventional complications, but it is still not sufficient to lower complication rates substantially.

Covered stents

Polytetrafluoroethylene (PTFE)-covered stents were designed to trap friable degenerated material and thus prevent protrusion of proliferating tissue, resulting in reduced microembolization and restenosis. However, trials of covered stents have been disappointing with higher rates of target vessel revascularization (SYMBIOT III) and of nonfatal MI (RECOVERS). There was no difference in angiographic restenosis (STING, SYMBIOT III, RECOVERS)(7–9).

However, in lesions with a large plaque load prone to embolize, the use of a covered stent might still be considered.

Distal protection devices

The most successful approach to reduce distal embolization is the use of distal protection devices that capture the embolic debris or thrombus released during intervention, using either a balloon occlusive or a filter-based system (Figs. 1 and 2). In the SAFER trial, 801 patients with SVG intervention were randomized to have usual PCI with or without the PercuSurge GuardWire System (PercuSurge, Medtronic AVE, Sunnyvale, CA). This device uses an inflated balloon placed distally from lesion, to stop distal embolization during intervention. An export catheter was used to aspirate the debris before deflating the occlusive balloon. In the PercuSurge group, there was a 42% relative reduction in the 30-day MACE (9.6% versus 16.5%, $P = 0.004$) (10). This was, predominantly the result of a reduction in myocardial infarctions. In addition, rates of TIMI grade 3 flow were higher for the PercuSurge arm (98%) compared with the control arm (95%; $P = 0.04$), and the incidence of clinically evident no-reflow was reduced (3% versus 9%; $P = 0.001$).

A filter-based system was studied in the FIRE trial (11). A total of 650 patients undergoing percutaneous intervention of SVG were randomized to the EPI FilterWire EX (Boston Scientific, Santa Clara, CA) versus the PercuSurge GuardWire (Medtronic). Device success was high (> 95%) for both systems. Postprocedural epicardial flow and angiographic complications were similar between the two groups. The primary end point, the composite incidence of death, myocardial infarction, or target vessel revascularization at 30 days, occurred in 9.9% of FilterWire EX patients and 11.6% of PercuSurge patients (P for superiority = 0.53).

Another filter-based system (Spider Embolic Protection Device, eV3) was compared to with distal protection using either the FilterWire or GuardWire device among patients (n = 732) undergoing percutaneous intervention for de novo SVG lesions (SPIDER) (12). MACE at 30

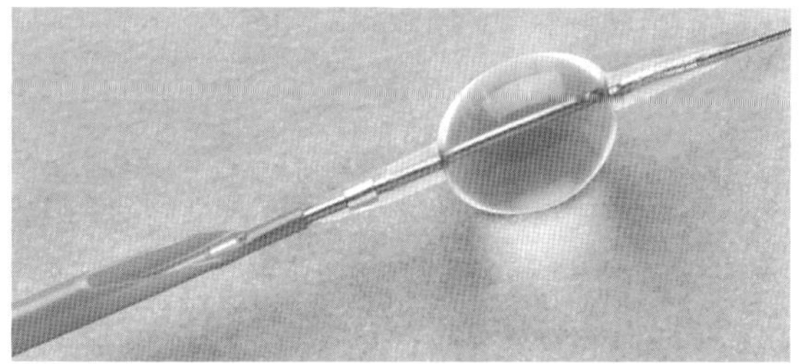

Figure 1 Example of balloon occlusion device: GuardWire with export catheter.

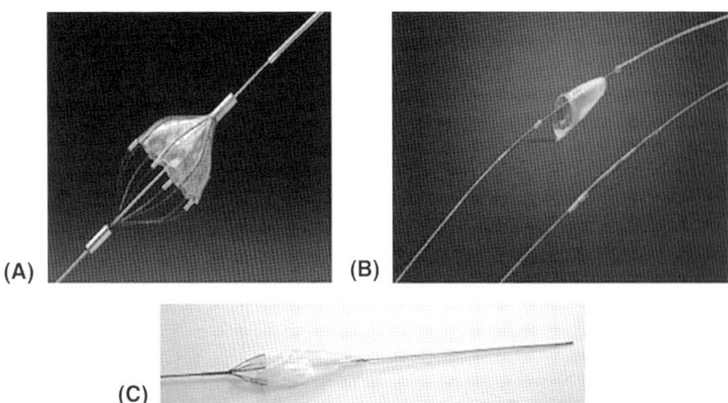

Figure 2 **A–C** Examples of filter protection devices. AngioGuard (**A**), EPI EZ (**B**) and Rubicon (**C**).

days (primary endpoint) was noninferior, and there was no difference in device or procedure success between the two groups. Today, comparable study results are available for various protection devices (Fig. 3).

More recently, a proximal embolic protection device (Proxis System, St Jude Medical, Inc) was developed and studied in a randomized SVG intervention trial (PROXIMAL). The Proxis system is designed to be placed before the lesion and works by briefly stopping and then reversing flow in the treated vessel to remove debris that may be dislodged during stent placement. In an intention-to-treat analysis of 30-day major adverse events, patients in the Proxis arm (Proxis system whenever possible and a FilterWire or GuardWire when use of Proxis was not possible for proximal lesions) and control arms (FilterWire or GuardWire whenever possible and no protection when use of either wire was not possible) had statistically similar incidence rates of 9.2% versus 10% (13).

Drug-eluting stents

Beside safety issues, restenosis after PCI of SVG lesions is another important problem, occurring in 46% of treated patients (1). Risk predictors are lesion location (ostial > mid-shaft), lesion morphology (length, diameter), and individual risk factors (diabetes, etc.). Drug-eluting stents (DES) have been proven safe and highly effective in treatment of coronary artery lesions. However, up to now, there are not much data available on DES in SVG lesions. Nevertheless, early reports suggest that DES is superior to bare-metal stents (BMS) in saphenous vein graft (SVG) stenosis. Ge et al. (14) conducted a study comparing 61 DES patients with 89 bare metal stent patients. DES were associated with significantly lower rates of in-segment restenosis (10% versus 27%, $P = 0.03$) and target lesion revascularization (3% versus 20%, $P = 0.003$) at six-month follow-up. There was no difference in in-hospital outcomes, mortality, or MI. With treatment effects of 50% to 90%

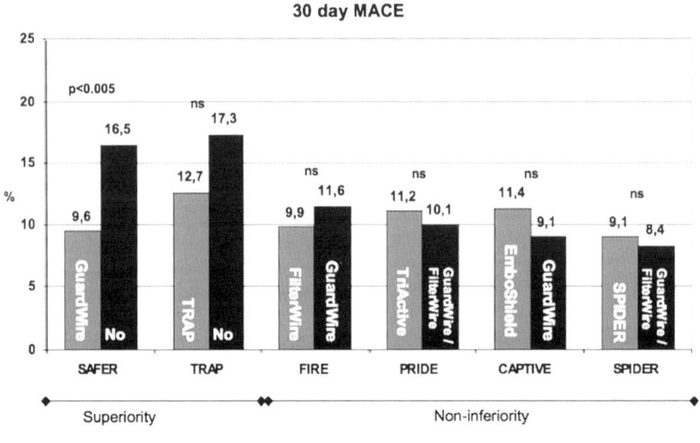

Figure 3 Clinical trial results of various protection devices for treatment of saphenous vein graft lesions.

in various lesion subsets, DES are likely to reduce the incidence of restenosis in SVG interventions as well. Further studies are ongoing to evaluate both safety and efficacy of DES for SVG failures.

SPECIFIC TECHNICAL CONSIDERATIONS

Left-sided SVGs with more posterior destination are usually placed higher in the aorta. Generally, the top graft goes to the distal LCX and the lower graft goes to the LAD. The right Judkins and left venous bypass catheters are suitable guides for left-sided grafts. However, the Amplatz left guiding catheter often provides the best support. For right bypass grafts, a Multipurpose guide provides the best coaxial alignment, while an Amplatz Left may be needed for a posteriorly located RCA graft.

In balloon angioplasty for vein grafts, balloons are generally sized in the ratio of 1:1 to venous grafts. Lesions with high elastic recoil respond well to stenting. Stenting (or directional atherectomy) is often used in aorto-ostial vein graft intervention, although the result remains disappointing. Overdilatation with balloons should be avoided as this may squeeze soft atheromatous plaque, increasing the risk of distal embolization. In the placement of multiple stents, distal stent should be deployed before proximal, if possible. This is to avoid recrossing the proximal stent with the increased risk of distal embolization.

Today, distal embolization protection should be the standard of care in bypass graft interventions and must be routine in the treatment of degenerative vein grafts with de novo lesions. Case examples are shown in Figures 4 and 5. Both filter and balloon-occlusive devices have similar efficacy. Filter-based devices preserve antegrade flow and allow contrast imaging throughout the procedure. However, the filter may clog with large amounts of embolic debris and the emboli cannot be removed intermittently to relieve the overload. Balloon-occlusive devices trap large and small debris reliably. However, there is no antegrade flow during balloon inflation, making contrast imaging difficult and prolonging the ischemia time. Intermittent occlusion and aspiration partially alleviates these problems.

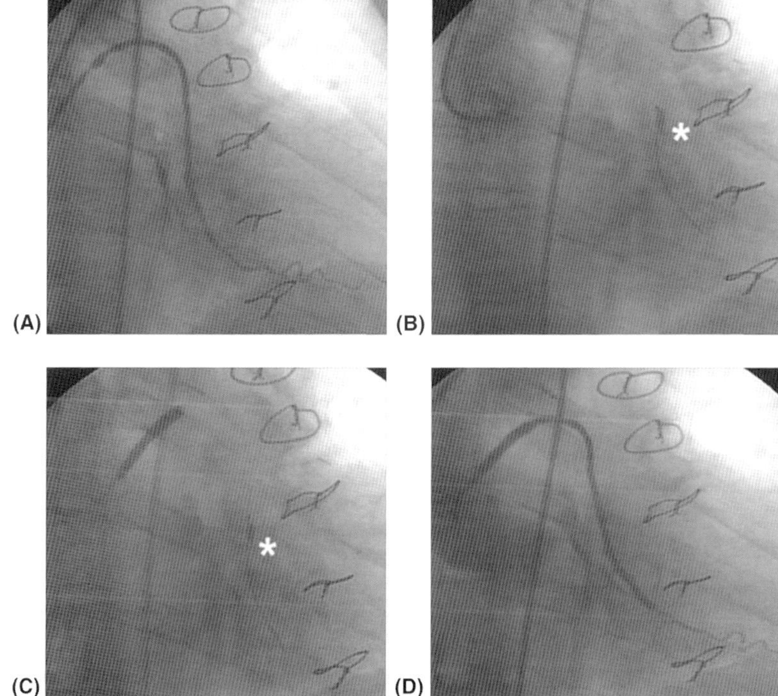

Figure 4 A–D: Case example with balloon occlusion device. (**A**) Proximal saphenous vein graft lesion. (**B**) Placement of distal occlusion balloon (*). (**C**) TCA/stenting of proximal lesion, balloon still inflated. (**D**) Final result after balloon deflation.

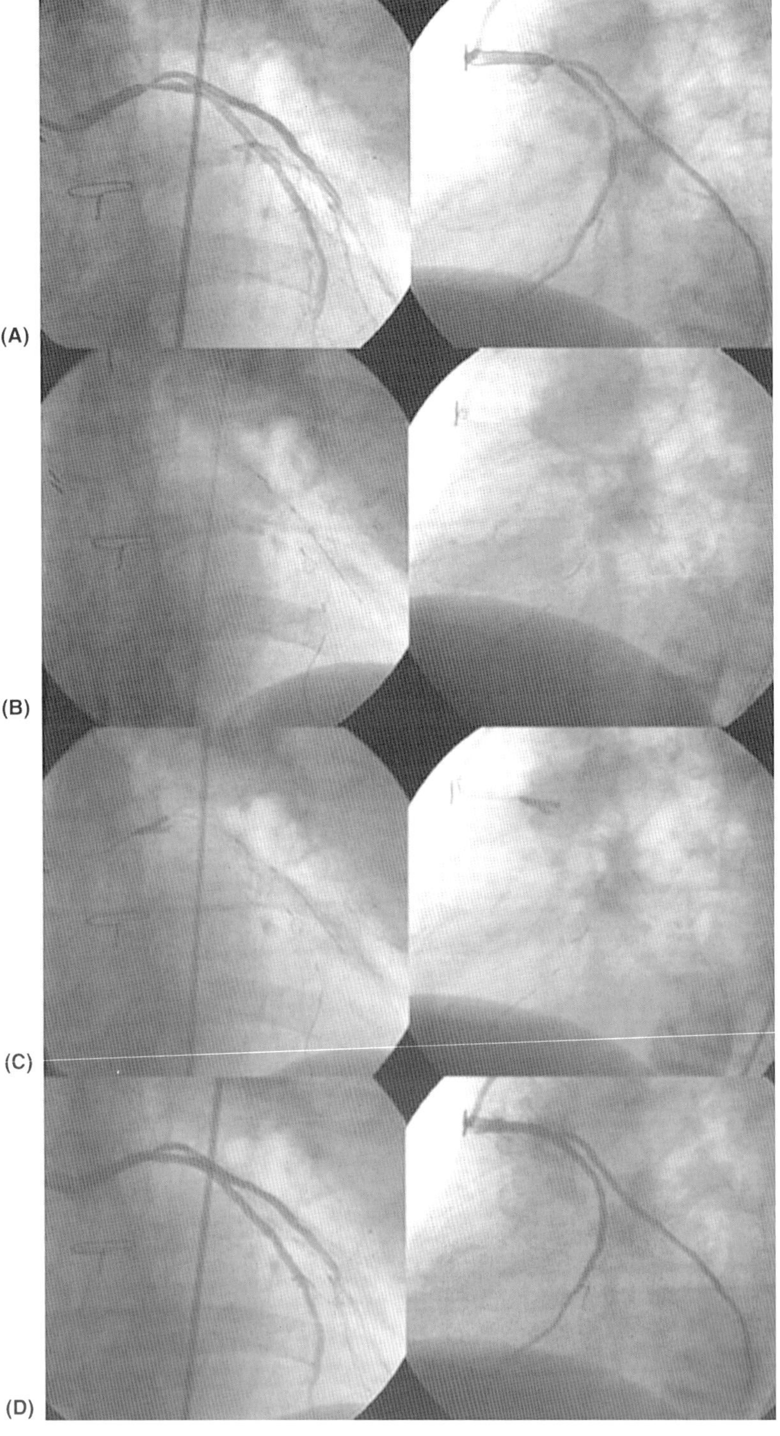

Figure 5 **A–D**: Case example with simultaneous use of two filter devices (biplane) for treatment of bifurcation stenosis in a sequential vein graft. (**A**) Pre-angio. (**B**) Placement of two filter wires to protect each arm. (**C**) Kissing balloon/stent. (**D**) Final result.

PROXIMAL PROTECTION DEVICES

The Proxis system overcomes the shortcomings of filter and balloon-occlusive devices when there is no landing zone distal to the SVG lesion, or when there is complete occlusion where a safe landing zone cannot be visualized. It also theoretically reduces the risk of distal embolization associated with the passage of filter or balloon-occlusive devices. Operators are also free to use guidewires of their choice, as the device is not fixed to a guidewire. The system is however not suitable for proximal lesion and there is no antegrade flow during proximal balloon inflation.

In case of in-stent restenosis of graft lesions, the value of distal protection is not yet determined. The more stable morphology of ISR lesions might decrease the likelihood of distal embolization, which theoretically reduces the benefit of distal protection devices. Further studies are needed to evaluate this issue.

ARTERIAL CONDUITS—CHARACTERISTICS AND TECHNICAL APPROACH

The internal mammary artery (IMA) is now considered the bypass conduit of choice for left anterior descending artery in patients undergoing elective CABG. Furthermore, complete arterial revascularizations have been proven superior to combined arterial and venous graft implantations. IMA grafts, when compared to SVG grafts, showed superior long-term patency rates, lower frequency of reoperation, lower long-term MI, and mortality. However, the IMA remains susceptible to atherosclerotic disease and damage to the vessel during harvest procedure. The results of IMA graft intervention have been favorable with high procedural success and low clinical restenosis. However, the available data on interventions for failed IMA grafts are limited due the beneficial long-term outcome of arterial conduits as well as the current dominance of vein grafts.

Prior to the use of stent, early case reports have shown that percutaneous balloon angioplasty of arterial grafts achieved high procedural success and low restenosis rate. In general, distal anastomotic stenoses respond well to balloon dilation alone and have a more favorable long-term prognosis than stenoses, involving the midshaft or ostial IMA graft lesions. There have been no randomized trials comparing balloon angioplasty and stenting in IMA grafts. Gruberg et al. reported in-hospital and one-year clinical outcomes of 174 consecutive patients who had percutaneous revascularization of 202 lesions in IMA grafts (15). The choice between angioplasty and stenting was decided by operators. Ostial lesions, due to their accessibility and larger vessel diameter, were usually opted for stenting. Anastomotic lesions were more often treated with angioplasty, due to tortuosity and smaller vessel size. Procedural success was 97% with favorable in-hospital outcome: 0.6% mortality rate, 0.6% rate of urgent bypass surgery, and no Q-wave MI. Cumulative one-year rates were: mortality 4.4%, MI 2.9%, and target lesion revascularization 7.4%. Although this study was not intended to compare PTCA and stenting strategies, the overall TLR in angioplasty group was low (5.4% versus 15.4%). Therefore, percutaneous revascularization of IMA grafts by balloon or stenting can be performed with high procedural success and excellent long-term outcome. Balloon angioplasty of anastomotic lesions without stenting was not associated with worse outcomes, and avoids the possibility of compromising the retrograde flow in the native vessel proximal to the anastomosis.

Due to the increasing use of IMA grafts in CABG, there will be a growing need for percutaneous revascularization in this special lesion subset.

SPECIFIC TECHNICAL CONSIDERATIONS

The Judkins right catheter can often engage subclavian artery more easily due to less acute primary curve. This can then be exchanged for the LIMA guide over a 0.035 in. guidewire. The LIMA is then advanced over the wire beyond the origin of IMA and is gently withdrawn. The origin of LIMA is inferior to thyrocervical trunk and distal to the vertebral artery. Gentle counterclockwise rotation of the catheter tip directs it anteriorly, and enables it to engage the IMA selectively. The usual engagement view for LIMA is the anteroposterior view, although a 60° LAO projection is sometimes helpful (as it elongates the arch).

For IMAs that are difficult to engage, there are several alternative techniques. With the LIMA guide in the vicinity of IMA ostium, a slippery hydrophilic or a steerable soft wire can be used to superselect the IMA. It can then be used as guide rail for a LIMA guide. For IMA that descends medially, ipsilateral brachial or radial approach will aid in engagement of LIMA guide and provide better support. If a 5 French or 6 French LIMA catheter is not able to select the ostium, a 4 French LIMA catheter might be used. Its distal bend is sometimes more suitable to reach the ostium than one of larger catheters. Whatever the technique used, every maneuver must be carried out gently as the IMA is particularly prone to spasm and dissection. Intracoronary nitroglycerin or verapamil can be used generously preintervention, and when spasm is suspected. Contrast must not be injected if the position of the guidewire is uncertain or the pressure is dampened.

Beside obstruction in IMA graft and anastomotic site, the obstruction of subclavian artery proximal to the origin to IMA can cause ischemia, rarely. This is suspected if there is a more than 20 mmHg difference between the two-arm pressures. This can be confirmed on angiography and dealt with by percutaneous intervention.

REFERENCES

1. Savage MP, Douglas JS Jr, Fischman DL, et al. Stent placement compared with balloon angioplasty for obstructed coronary bypass grafts. Saphenous Vein De Novo Trial Investigators. N Engl J Med 1997; 337(11):740–747.
2. Gruberg L, Hong MK, Mehran R, et al. In-hospital and long-term results of stent deployment compared with balloon angioplasty for treatment of narrowing at the saphenous vein graft distal anastomosis site. Am J Cardiol 1999; 84(12): 1381–1384.
3. Hong MK, Mehran R, Dangas G, et al. Creatine kinase-MB enzyme elevation following successful saphenous vein graft intervention is associated with late mortality. Circulation 1999; 100(24):2400–2405.
4. Roffi M, Mukherjee D, Chew DP, et al. Lack of benefit from intravenous platelet glycoprotein IIb/IIIa receptor inhibition as adjunctive treatment for percutaneous interventions of aorto-coronary bypass grafts: a pooled analysis of five randomized clinical trials. Circulation 2002; 106(24):3063–3067.
5. Kuntz R, Baim DS, Cohen DJ, et al. for the VeGAS 2 Investigators. A Trial Comparing Rheolytic Thrombectomy With Intracoronary Urokinase for Coronary and Vein Graft. Thrombus (The Vein Graft AngioJet Study [VeGAS 2]). Am J Cardiol 2002; 89:326–330.
6. Stone GW, Cox DA, Babb J, et al. Prospective, randomized evaluation of thrombectomy prior to percutaneous intervention in diseased saphenous vein grafts and thrombus-containing coronary arteries. J Am Coll Cardiol 2003; 42(11): 2007–2013.
7. Maurice Buchbinder. Symbiot III: A prospective randomized trial of a PTFE self-expanding stent graft during SVG intervention. Presentation at Transcatheter Cardiovascular Therapeutics, October 2004.
8. Stankovic G, Colombo A, Presbitero P, et al, for the RECOVERS Investigators. Randomized Evaluation of polytetrafluoroethylene-covered stent in saphenous vein grafts. Circulation 2003; 108: 37–42.
9. Schächinger V, Hamm CW, Münzel T, et al. STING (STents IN Grafts) Investigators. A randomized trial of polytetrafluoroethylene-membrane-covered stents compared with conventional stents in aorto-coronary saphenous vein grafts. J Am Coll Cardiol 2003; 42:1360–1369.
10. Baim DS, Wahr D, George B, et al. Saphenous vein graft Angioplasty Free of Emboli Randomized (SAFER) trial investigators. Randomized trial of a distal embolic protection device during percutaneous intervention of saphenous vein aorto-coronary bypass grafts. Circulation 2002; 105(11):1285–1290.
11. Stone GW, Rogers C, Hermiller J, et al. FilterWire EX Randomized Evaluation Investigators. Randomized comparison of distal protection with a filter-based catheter and a balloon occlusion and aspiration system during percutaneous intervention of diseased saphenous vein aorto-coronary bypass grafts. Circulation 2003; 108(5):548–553.
12. Dixon SD. Presentation at Transcatheter Cardiovascular Therapeutics, October 2005.
13. Campbell R. Proximal protection during saphenous vein graft intervention (PROXIMAL). Presentation at Transcatheter Cardiovascular Therapeutics, October 2005.
14. Ge L, Iakovou I, Sangiorgi GM, et al. Treatment of saphenous vein graft lesions with drug-eluting stents: immediate and midterm outcome. J Am Coll Cardiol 2005; 45(7):989–994.
15. Gruberg L, Dangas G, Mehran R, et al. Percutaneous revascularization of the internal mammary artery graft: short- and long-term outcomes. J Am Coll Cardiol 2000; 35:944–948.

11

Approach to intermediate lesions

Konstantinos Dimopoulos, Liviu Ghilencea, Alessio La Manna, and Carlo Di Mario

INTRODUCTION

Interventional cardiologists often have to decide whether to treat a moderately stenotic lesion or not, and they often miss an objective confirmation of its potential to induce ischemia. Deferral of treatment for performing noninvasive stress imaging investigations can be costly, time consuming, and is accompanied by additional discomfort and risks for patients who will need to undergo a second catheterization for treatment. On the other hand, patients with intermediate but hemodynamically nonsignificant lesions that undergo percutaneous coronary intervention (PCI) have no direct benefit from this procedure while facing peri-procedural risks and the risk of restenosis—the use of angioplasty for "plaque sealing" or to prevent disease progression in critical segments is still an unproven controversial approach. Means for assessing the hemodynamic significance of intermediate lesions in the catheter lab is thus essential (Table 1).

Table 1 Factors limiting angiographic assessment of intermediate coronary lesions
Diffuse atherosclerotic disease
Pre- and poststenotic ectasias
Eccentric lesions
Ostial lesions
Bifurcation lesions
Long lesions
Reduced distal flow
Suboptimal visualization (vessel overlap, obesity)

CORONARY ANGIOGRAPHY

The most frequently used definition of an intermediate (IL) or borderline lesion is that of a lesion causing a 40% to 60% diameter stenosis on angiography. This definition stems from experimental models showing that a 75% lumen area stenosis corresponding to a 50% lumen diameter stenosis significantly impairs maximal hyperemic flow. Nevertheless, visual estimation, which is most often used to evaluate stenosis severity with angiography, is beset by a high inter-observer variability and inaccuracy when compared to physiologic assessment. In one study, only half of the physiologically nonsignificant lesions were characterized as such by three independent operators. Presumably for this reason, the most recent

American College of Cardiology (ACC) and European Society of Cardiology (ESC) guidelines have broadened the angiographic definition of intermediate coronary stenoses up to 70% luminal narrowing (1,2).

These angiographic definitions, however, are plagued by the inherent limitations of angiography that requires a normal reference segment for comparison in the calculation of percent diameter stenosis (3). Pathology, intravascular ultrasound, and other tomographic imaging techniques such as angio-CT and CMR indicate that atherosclerosis is often a diffuse process and long hemodynamically significant lesions in diffusely diseased vessels may be underestimated on angiography. Automated measurement of minimal luminal diameter (MLD) with quantitative angiography is a possible solution (cutoff 1.5 mm), but lesion eccentricity, diffuse disease, limitations in calibration, and suboptimal visualization lead to inaccuracy.

To overcome the limits of angiography, functional (physiologic) and morphologic techniques have been developed and validated for the assessment of IL (Table 2):

- Flow-derived measurement of coronary flow reserve;
- Pressure-derived fractional flow reserve;
- Intravascular ultrasound.

Table 2 Rationale for invasive physiological evaluation of angiographically intermediate coronary lesions

Angiography alone is unreliable for assessing the severity of intermediate lesions
A large proportion of patients undergo angiography without previous provocative tests
Referral to noninvasive testing after angiography is time consuming and costly, induces unnecessary delays in the procedure, and increases the patient's anxiety and discomfort
Physiologic assessment of intermediate stenoses in the catheter lab is:
Safe
Reliable
Fast and straightforward
Cost effective
Helpful in assessing treatment results

PHYSIOLOGIC ASSESSMENT OF CORONARY STENOSES IN THE CATHETER LABORATORY

Coronary flow reserve

Myocardial oxygen consumption at rest is relatively high compared to skeletal muscle. For this reason, oxygen extraction in the myocardium is maximal at rest, and changes in oxygen demand are met mainly through increases in myocardial blood flow (4). Various mechanisms are activated synergistically to increase myocardial perfusion and meet the oxygen demand, mainly through regulation of resistance in the microcirculatory bed. The maximum achievable increase in coronary flow is called coronary flow reserve (CFR) and is the ratio of coronary flow during maximal hyperemia ($F_{hyperemia}$) to coronary flow at rest (F_{rest}) (5).

$$CFR = \frac{F_{hyperemia}}{F_{rest}}$$

CFR is used to assess the degree of flow impediment caused by stenotic lesions. Resting coronary flow is unaffected by lesions with a diameter stenosis of <80% to 85% (6). With intermediate lesions, flow impediment appears only during physiologic (postexercise) or pharmacologically induced hyperemia. Achievement of maximal hyperemia through maximal vasodilatation of the coronary micro-vessels is mandatory for accurate determination of CFR.

CFR can be measured using a 0.014 in. Doppler wire connected to a stationary flow module (FloWire, Volcano Therapeutics). The Doppler transducer is positioned at the tip and the sample volume is approximately 0.5 cm in front of the tip. The Doppler transducer is advanced distally (>2 cm) to the stenosis after the patient is heparinized, and flow velocity is recorded at rest and during pharmacologically induced hyperemia.

In the catheterization lab, maximal hyperemia can be achieved pharmacologically either by intracoronary administration of adenosine, ATP,

Table 3 Vasodilator agents used for inducing myocardial hyperemia

Route of administration	*Agent*	*Doses*
Intracoronary bolus injection	Adenosine	30 μg RCA; 40–80 μg LCA
	ATP	30–80 μg
	Papaverine	10 mg RCA; 15–20 mg LCA
	Nitroprusside	0.3–0.9 μg/kg
Intravenous infusion	Papaverine	20 mg
	Adenosine	140–180 μg/kg/min
	ATP	140–180 μg/kg/min

Abbreviations: RCA, right coronary artery; LCA, left coronary artery

or papaverine, or by intravenous infusion of adenosine or ATP (Table 3) (7). More recently, intracoronary injection of sodium nitroprusside (0.3–0.9 μg/kg) has been shown to produce equivalent coronary hyperemia with a longer duration compared with intracoronary adenosine (8). Even though intracoronary injection has the advantage of a quick response to the medication, it has certain limitations (Table 4):

- Medication could leak into the aorta if the catheter is not selectively engaged into the coronary artery or if a catheter with side-holes is being used.
- The injection produces a significant artefact in the tracings that could take a few seconds to clear.
- Adenosine and ATP, given through the intracoronary path, have very short effects and do not permit pullback studies.

Table 4 Pitfalls in inducing maximal hyperemia

Inadequate dosage:
- Error in the drug preparation (dosage, dilution)
- Blood pressure below the autoregulatory range
- Nonresponders

Intracoronary administration:
- Inadequate drug delivery secondary to:
  - Inadequate flush with normal saline after injection
  - Leakage into the aorta through sideholes
  - Spill into the aorta due to nonselective catheter engagement
  - Leakage through stopcocks or valves
- Slow restoration of tracings after injection (missing maximal hyperemia by intracoronary ATP and adenosine)

Intravenous administration:
- Inadequate drug delivery due to:
  - Pooling in the peripheral vein (kinking of the arm, inappropriate vein incannulation)
  - Valsalva or other maneuvers that decrease venous return

Adenosine is probably the most frequently used agent for inducing maximal hyperemia. Adenosine induces hyperemia by stimulating specific receptors, mainly A2 arteriolar receptors. Therefore, hyperemia is not affected by medication such as nitrates, beta blockers, or calcium channel blockers. Nevertheless, intravenous adenosine has side effects, (chest tightness, flushing, bradyarrhythmias), and requires one to three minutes to achieve maximal vasodilation. For the right coronary artery, it might be wise to start with an initial smaller test bolus to assess patient tolerability. An approach commonly used is the injection of a high-dose intracoronary bolus of adenosine (>36 and up to 72 μg for the left coronary artery and 24 to 36 μg for the right coronary artery) to induce hyperemia. This dose is enough to achieve in most patients a hyperemia sufficiently prolonged enabling the catheter to be withdrawn outside the ostium, should damping develop.

Multiple comparative studies with scintigraphy and other noninvasive methods demonstrated that the cutoff value for a "normal" CFR ranges between 1.7 and 2.0 (9,10,11). A CFR < 2.0 correlates well with abnormal noninvasive stress perfusion imaging and indicates that the lesion should be treated unless there is evidence or suspicion of an impaired microcirculatory response to vasodilatation (12). CFR above 2.5 to 3.0 virtually excludes the need for angioplasty.

CFR takes into account both the epicardial vessels and the microcirculation. An abnormal CFR in the absence of epicardial vessel disease can be related to microvascular dysfunction due to left ventricular hypertrophy, previous myocardial infarction, and diabetes mellitus. The microcirculation plays a dominant role in the regulation of coronary resistance and flow, especially in the presence of intermediate lesions. The correlation between degree of epicardial stenosis and CFR is, in fact, best in high-grade stenoses when the effect of the microcirculation becomes obscured by the severity of the epicardial disease. CFR becomes less accurate when assessing intermediate lesions. CFR is also influenced by central hemodynamic parameters that affect resting coronary flow such as heart rate and blood pressure.

To obviate this, Gould et al. developed the concept of relative coronary flow reserve (rCFR), defined as the ratio between the CFR in the target vessel and the CFR in a reference vessel.

$$rCFR = \frac{CFR_{\text{target vessel}}}{CFR_{\text{reference vessel}}}$$

Gould et al. demonstrated that rCFR is independent of aortic pressure and rate-pressure product. A rCFR value of above 0.8 excludes significant epicardial stenosis, assuming that microvascular disease, if present, is distributed homogenously throughout the myocardium (13,14). Unfortunately, rCFR requires additional recordings in a healthy artery and cannot be used in 3-vessel disease.

Fractional flow reserve

To overcome the limitations of CFR (Table 5), Pijls et al. developed an index reflecting myocardial perfusion unaffected by blood pressure, heart rate, and contractility, relatively independent of

Table 5 Limitations of coronary flow reserve and relative coronary flow reserve for the assessment of intermediate lesions

CFR does not have a clearcut threshold of normal/abnormal values
CFR depends on basal flow and changes in heart rate and blood pressure
CFR is not specific for epicardial lesion and is affected by the response of the microvascular coronary circulation
rCFR requires additional recording in a healthy artery
rCFR is not feasible in 3-vessel disease
A clear Doppler signal can at times be challenging to acquire
Automatic tracking of the peak Doppler velocity trace can occasionally be unreliable

Table 6 Advantages of fractional flow reserve compared to coronary flow reserve

	FFR	*CFR*	*rCFR*
Assesses epicardial disease only	+ + +	−	+ + [a]
Assesses microvascular disease	−	+ + +	−
Independent of central hemodynamics	+ +	−	+
Well-defined cutoff value for ischemia	+ +	−	+
Collateral flow taken into account	+ + +	+	−
Reproducible	+ + +	+	+
Easy and fast to perform	+ +	+	−
Feasible in multivessel disease	+ +	+ +	−

[a] If homogeneously distributed microvascular disease

the state of the microcirculation (15) and which takes into account the contribution of collaterals to maximal myocardial perfusion (Table 6) (16). Fractional flow reserve (FFR) is defined as the ratio of hyperemic flow in a coronary artery in the presence of a stenotic lesion to the theoretical hyperemic flow in the same artery in the absence of the stenosis. It is, in fact, the peak flow in the diseased artery expressed as a fraction of its theoretical normal value. FFR can be calculated as the ratio of the coronary pressure distal to the stenosis by the coronary pressure in the absence of the stenosis (which is equal to the pressure proximal to the lesion and within the aorta):

$$\mathrm{FFR} = \frac{P_{\mathrm{distal}}}{P_{\mathrm{proximal}}} = \frac{P_{\mathrm{distal}}}{P_{\mathrm{aorta}}}$$

The FFR is derived from coronary artery pressure measurements using a 0.014-inch pressure wire. Two types of pressure wires are available: 5-Star WaveWire (Radi Medical, Uppsala, Sweden) and SmartWire (Volcano Therapeutics, Rancho Cordova, CA). In both, the super-miniaturized pressure transducer is positioned at the proximal end of the distal radio-opaque tip.

Before proceeding with wire insertion, the patient should be fully heparinized. The pressure wire is zeroed and the pressure transducer of the fluid-filled catheter is carefully fixed to the table at the correct height, usually 5 cm below the sternum at the estimated height of the aortic root. The pressure transducer is then advanced to the tip of the catheter or within the very proximal coronary artery, where pressures from the wire and the catheter should be equal. If not equal, and if the height of the pressure transducer appears correct, electronic equalization of the pressures can be applied.

The wire transducer is then advanced distal to the lesion, ideally on continuous monitoring to note any pressure drop across the stenosis. At times, this is impossible due to the tortuosity of the vessel or due to lesion complexity. In this case, the wire can be disconnected to facilitate torquing and reconnected after the lesion is crossed. By reconnecting the wire immediately after crossing the lesion with the tip of the wire, the pressure transducer (which is positioned 3 cm proximal to the tip) is still proximal to the lesion and, thus, shifts in the recorded pressure can be excluded. If the pressure wire, which is never as steerable as a normal guidewire, even after disconnection cannot manage to cross the lesion, an over-the-wire balloon can be used with

Table 7 Fractional flow reserve criteria for clinical decision making

Inducible ischemia (including left main disease)	< 0.75
Universally accepted threshold for deferred intervention	> 0.80
Post-AMI reversible ischemia	< 0.75
End-point for balloon angioplasty	≥ 0.90
End-point for stenting	≥ 0.94

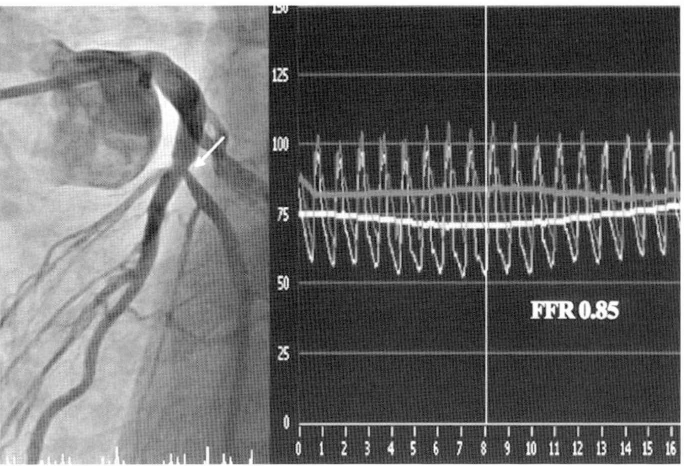

Figure 1 Intermediate ostial lesion of the first diagonal branch. A pressure wire was inserted and maximal hyperemia was achieved using intracoronary injection of 96 μg of adenosine. At peak hyperemia, average pressures were 85 mmHg in the proximal coronary artery and 72 mmHg distal to the lesion (FFR 0.85). Treatment was limited to an occluded circumflex (LCx).

wire exchange before measurements. Proximal pressure is recorded via the guiding catheter, avoiding pressure damping by gently withdrawing it into the ascending aorta (17).

Pharmacological hyperemia is induced using the same agents described for CFR. FFR is calculated at maximal hyperemia as the ratio of mean distal to mean aortic pressure through simultaneous recordings. Its normal value is one and, obviously, any decrease of FFR reflects the effect of epicardial stenoses. A cutoff value of 0.75 has been established based on comparative studies with noninvasive investigations, and indicates that an epicardial lesion with a coexisting FFR ≤0.75 can cause myocardial ischemia, and requires treatment (Table 7) (18–27). An FFR ≥ 0.80 indicates that intervention should be deferred as it would not improve myocardial perfusion or prognosis (Fig. 1); the results of a small randomized trial, now prolonged to five years follow-up suggest that deferral of angioplasty in patients with FFR > 0.75 is safe and results in an excellent clinical outcome (28–31).

FFR is also useful when assessing borderline in-stent restenosis. In these cases, angiographic quantification is notoriously unreliable and physiologic assessment is invaluable (Fig. 2). The same cutoff values seem to apply to restenosis.

Pitfalls in FFR calculation are described in Table 8.

Table 8 Pitfalls in fractional flow reserve calculation

- Pressure damping by the guiding catheter, which can lead to underestimation of lesion severity by limiting the maximal flow and, consequently, the maximal pressure gradient.
- Inaccurate proximal (aortic pressure) readings through the fluid filled catheter due to an open Y connector: avoid this by using catch or copilot types of connectors and withdrawing introducer needle.
- Use of catheters with side-holes precludes the detection of the modified waveform characteristic of pressure damping, provides a proximal pressure which is a mixture of the aortic and the proximal coronary pressure and causes spilling of medication into the aorta if an intracoronary route of injection is used.
- Submaximal coronary vasodilatation (Table 4).
- Signal drift, an artificial electronic drop in pressure measured by the wire.
- Missed maximal hyperemic response to adenosine due to late return to pressure readings after intracoronary injection or inappropriate averaging of multiple beats if conventional recorders with physiological signals are used.

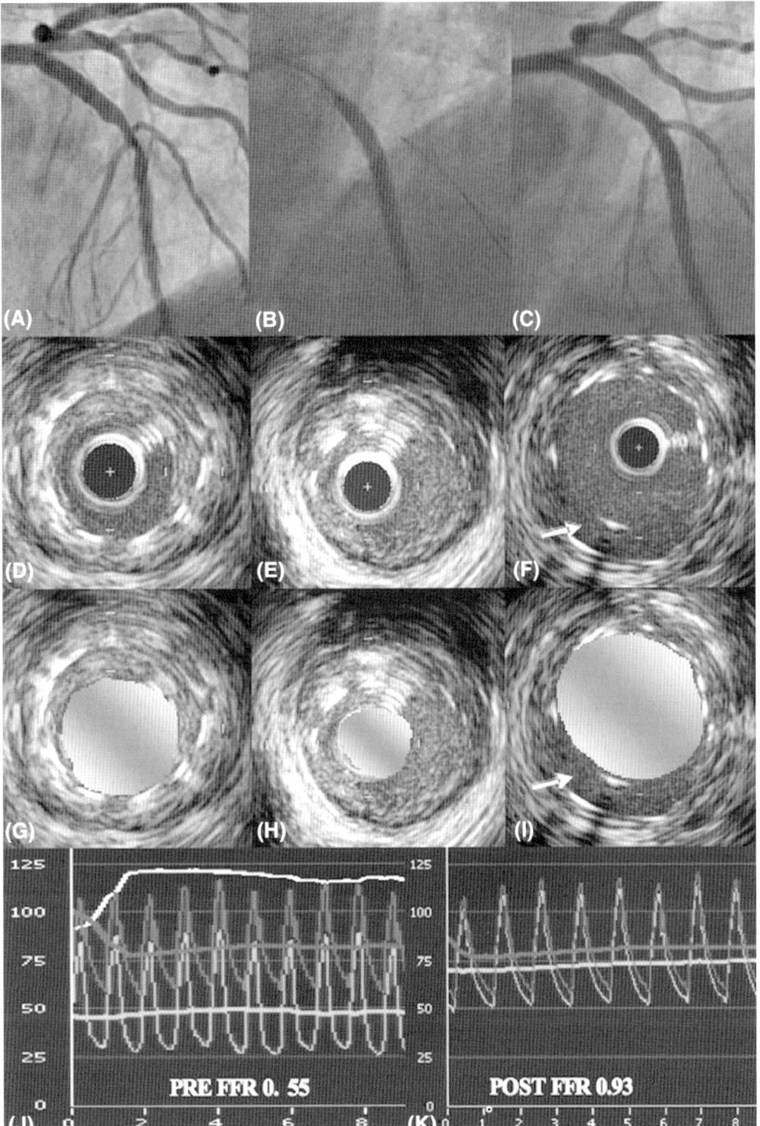

Figure 2 Intermediate in-stent restenosis within the LAD (**A**). Intravascular ultrasound demonstrated significant intimal hyperplasia within the proximal portion of the stent (**D,G**) and at the proximal edge (**E,H**). At maximal hyperemia, pressure distal to the stent was 45 mmHg and within the proximal LAD 82 mmHg, with a fractional flow reserve of 0.55 (**J**). The lesion was treated with deployment of a drug eluting stent to cover the entire length of the previous stent (**B,C**). Intravascular ultrasound showed optimal deployment of the new stent (**F,I**), with an adequate luminal area. An area of intimal hyperplasia trapped between the old and the new stent can been seen (*arrow*). Postprocedural Fractional flow reserve was 0.93.

It is essential to examine the morphology of the pressure tracings at all times to recognize pressure damping by the guiding catheter. Moreover, signal drift can be distinguished from a pressure drop distal to a significant lesion because in the latter case, a significant diastolic gradient will be present, especially during hyperemia, with a systolic gradient that will be much smaller. If signal drift is suspected, FFR can be estimated during pullback using the proximal pressure measured with the guidewire.

Limitations of FFR:

- FFR measures the current potential to induce ischemia on maximal effort but cannot predict the potential of a lesion to cause acute ischemic events in the future (sudden death, acute myocardial infarction).
- FFR only assesses fixed stenoses and cannot rule out ischemia due to variant angina.
- Severe anemia or myocardial hypertrophy can increase the threshold of FFR for ischemia.

As discussed earlier, FFR and CFR provide complementary information on the status of the coronary circulation (Fig. 3). Recently, a thermodilution technique was developed and validated to measure CFR as well as FFR using a single pressure wire with a thermistor (32–34). This is based on the principle that flow can be calculated with thermodilution based on the vascular volume and mean transit time (TT). By using nitrates prior to this technique, the vascular volume (V) can be considered constant at rest and during hyperemia and thus can be eliminated from the equation, leaving only mean transit time.

$$CFR = \frac{F_{rest}}{F_{hyperaemia}} = \frac{\frac{V_{hyperaemia}}{TT_{hyperaemia}}}{\frac{V_{rest}}{TT_{rest}}}$$

When vessels are pretreated with nitrates

$$V_{rest} = V_{hyperemia}$$

and thus

$$CFR = \frac{TT_{rest}}{TT_{hyperemia}}$$

Therefore, CFR can be calculated as the ratio of mean transit times at rest and at maximal hyperemia. Thermodilution is performed by injecting 3 to 4 mL of normal saline at room temperature in the coronary artery with the pressure transducer and thermistor, distal to the lesion. Injections are repeated three times at rest and three times during hyperemia, and mean transit times are calculated automatically. This method permits simultaneous CFR and FFR calculations using a information on the status of the coronary vasculature.

In conclusion, FFR is an accurate index for functional evaluation of intermediate stenoses, it can avoid abusive revascularization, and it shortens the length of hospitalization and makes the interventional cardiologists more autonomous in their decisions.

PRESSURE PULLBACK AND THE PHYSIOLOGIC ASSESSMENT OF MULTIPLE LESIONS

Pressure pullback during hyperemia can be used to assess the FFR of a single lesion or of multiple stenoses in a single vessel. Pullback can be performed at baseline, but it is more sensitive when performed during the steady state of maximal hyperemia. Intracoronary papaverine (20 mg with a peak action of 23 ± 5 seconds and a plateau phase of 22 ± 7 seconds), intravenous ATP (140 μg/kg/min in the peripheral vein with a peak action of 104 ± 36 seconds), and intravenous adenosine (140 μg/kg/min, peak action of 112 ± 48 seconds) can induce a steady hyperemic state, long enough for pullback to be performed. The effect of intracoronary ATP and adenosine is too short and should not be used for pullback. Femoral vein infusion is preferable in patients with borderline CFR, as response time is less variable compared to peripheral venous infusion.

Pressure pullback is underutilized in clinical practice, because operators dislike having to cross the lesion with the wire more than once. Nevertheless, it has to be emphasized that the pressure transducer is situated 3 cm proximal to the tip of the wire and, thus, pullback could be performed without pulling back the entire length of the wire and without having to re-cross the lesion.

When assessing multiple lesions in a single vessel, the pullback technique permits identification of the most significant stenosis to be treated first. Complex formulae (35) are also available to calculate the hemodynamic significance of tandem lesions with FFR, without the need for pressure pullback. The simplest and most frequently used approach is to assess FFR distal to all stenoses and treat the lesion that angiographically appears most severe first. Thereafter, based on the result of the repeat FFR, it can be decided whether the remaining lesion(s) should be treated or not.

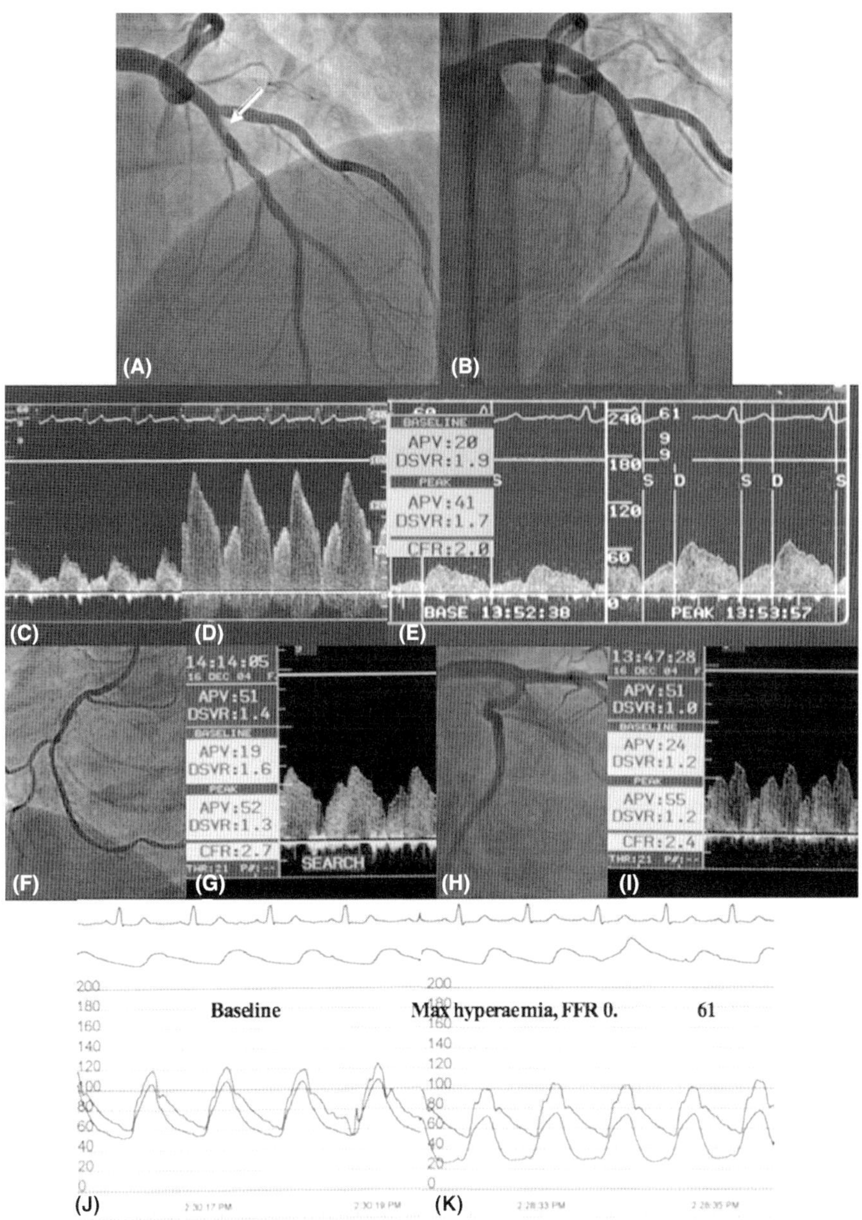

Figure 3 Eccentric, hazy lesion of the mid-LAD of uncertain significance on angiography (**A,B**). A Dopplerwire was inserted and a significant increase in velocity was seen when the wire was advanced from the proximal vessel (**C**) into the plaque (**D**). Intracoronary adenosine was given and CFR was calculated at 2.0, suggesting that the lesion could be hemodynamically significant (**E**). Coronary flow reserve was also calculated in the RCA (**F**,**G**) and LCx (**H**,**I**), that were lesion-free on angiography. rCFR in the LAD using the RCA as a reference was 0.74 and when LCx was used as a reference, was 0.83. The Dopplerwire was then exchanged for a pressure wire. A mild trans-stenotic gradient was already seen at baseline (**J**). At maximal hyperemia, the trans-stenotic gradient increased and fractional flow reserve was 0.61. The lesion was thus treated. This example highlights the limitations of coronary flow reserve and relative coronary flow reserve.

SPECIAL SITUATIONS

Assessment of fractional flow reserve in the left main coronary artery

It is widely accepted that a >50% stenosis of the left main stem (LMS) is an indication for surgical treatment. Nevertheless, angiographic evaluation of lesions within the LMS can be very challenging. In fact, one study showed that the LMS was the coronary segment with the greatest inter-observer variability (36). Objective, physiologic evaluation of borderline LMS lesions is therefore essential to assist clinical decision making. Studies using FFR have shown the safety of deferring surgery in patients with a LMS lesion and an FFR > 0.75.

Assessment of fractional flow reserve in vessels supporting myocardial territories of previous infarction

There have been concerns that FFR could be inaccurate in areas of previous myocardial infarctions. In fact, in these areas there has been a decrease in viable myocardium, and resistance vessels could be impaired and respond abnormally to vasodilatatory stimuli. Nevertheless, studies have shown that FFR is still reliable in identifying reversible ischemia in the partially infarcted areas (37). An FFR of > 0.80 at least six days after myocardial infarction suggests that intervention can be deferred, even when the lesion appears angiographically severe. Myocardial necrosis and distal microvascular disease cause a reduction in blood flow. No significant pressure drop can, therefore, develop even across an anatomically significant lesion.

In the acute setting of myocardial infarction, severe microvascular impairment makes FFR unreliable, and decision-making should be based on symptoms and electrocardiographic changes.

Assessment of fractional flow reserve in left ventricular hypertrophy

A disproportion between myocardial mass and the vascular bed is often present in left ventricular hypertrophy and can affect myocardial reserve. In this case, FFR could underestimate the potential of a lesion to cause ischemia. Even though a specific cutoff value for patients with left ventricular hypertrophy has not been established, this should be higher than the standard 0.75. Operators should, thus, be careful when interpreting FFR values in patients with significant left ventricular hypertrophy.

COMBINED PRESSURE AND FLOW ASSESSMENT

Gould and Young, with their pioneering work, demonstrated that the relationship between pressure gradient (ΔP) through a stenosis and flow velocity (V) is curvilinear and is described by the formula (38–42):

$$\Delta P = aV + bV^2$$

where a and b are constants related to the stenosis. Therefore, assessment of lesion severity is best performed based on both pressure gradient and flow velocity, unlike CFR and FFR that use either one or the other. Instantaneous diastolic measurement of intracoronary flow velocity and pressure gradient across a lesion provides a $V/\Delta P$ relation that can accurately assess the severity of coronary stenoses. Diastolic measurements are preferable in order to avoid the sudden changes in coronary flow velocity that occur in systole. Instantaneous measures do not require maximal hyperemia or maximal microvascular dilation and are independent of hemodynamic status.

A major limitation of this technique is that it requires acquisition of instantaneous pressure and flow readings with two separate wires, increasing procedural time, costs, and risks. A combined pressure and flow wire is now available (ComboWire XT, Volcano Therapeutics) and can be used for this purpose.

Curves and parameters obtained using average values of ΔP and V were also shown to be powerful descriptors of coronary hemodynamics. The stenosis resistance index calculated during hyperemia (hSRv) is a parameter that can be calculated using the mean stenosis pressure gradient and the average peak flow velocity (43,44):

$$\text{hSRv} = \frac{\Delta P}{\text{APV}}$$

In the hands of its proposers, hSRv was proven to be a stronger predictor of reversible ischemia compared to FFR and CFR. It is independent of baseline hemodynamic conditions and possesses an unequivocal normal value of zero in the absence of stenosis. Moreover, it is less affected by fluctuations in hyperemic flow velocity, secondary to insufficient drug delivery or microvascular dysfunction compared to FFR, since changes in peak flow affect pressure gradient and flow velocity in a similar way. The slope between baseline and maximal hyperemic $V/\Delta P$ ratio also has a high diagnostic accuracy for ischemia compared to FFR and CFR (45).

With indices based on average values of pressure gradient and velocity, lesion severity can still be underestimated if maximal hyperemia is not achieved. Instantaneous $V/\Delta P$ parameters are, therefore, preferable.

The superiority of $V/\Delta P$ parameters may cause a shift away from FFR and CFR in the near future, with the advent of dual sensor wires with Doppler and pressure transducers.

INTRAVASCULAR ULTRASOUND

Intravascular ultrasound (IVUS) was introduced over a decade ago as a complementary investigation to angiography. It is performed using miniaturized flexible ultrasound probes with a diameter of 2.8Fr (Atlantis–Boston Scientific) or 2.9Fr (Eagle-Eye, Volcano Endosonics). The probes are compatible with conventional 6Fr guiding catheters and use a monorail approach. A single spinning high-frequency piezoelectric crystal or multiple (64) sequentially-activated microcrystals produce a 360 degree cross-sectional image of the vessel. The transducer is advanced manually into the distal coronary artery over a standard intracoronary wire through the guiding catheter. The transducer is then withdrawn automatically through the target stenoses at a constant speed of 0.5 mm/sec while images are recorded. Intracoronary nitroglycerine (100–200 μg) has to be injected prior to IVUS assessment. At the end of an IVUS procedure, an angiographic run of the coronary artery is recorded to check for vessel disruption due to the instrumentation.

A 30 to 40 MHz, transducer has an axial resolution of 0.08 to 0.1 mm and a lateral resolution of 0.20 to 0.25 mm. The mechanical system with the large 40 MHz crystal has greater resolution and dynamic range. Both systems can create online longitudinal reconstruction of the vessel when imaging is obtained during pullback. The multi-element probe has a longer monorail segment reducing the risk of wire looping and provides blood colour encoding. A recent addition of this system has been elastography and tissue characterization(46–57).

IVUS provides 360-degree tomographic images of the vessel circumference and is thus superior to angiography, which shows a projected silhouette of the lumen. No calibration is required during IVUS examination and bidimensional measurements can be performed easily and accurately. IVUS is particularly helpful in evaluating vessel segments that are inadequately visualized on angiography such as bifurcations and ostia, as well as lesions that are eccentric or "hazy" and of uncertain severity. IVUS studies have shown that the majority of atherosclerotic lesions are eccentric but significant discrepancy exists between apparent angiographic eccentricity and IVUS findings (58). It is especially important that eccentric lesions are identified and appropriately assessed, as this not only affects the decision to treat, but also the technique used for revascularization and the periprocedural risk.

Percent area stenosis and lesion length with IVUS have shown inverse correlation with FFR in intermediate lesions, while MLD and minimal lumen area (MLA) are positively correlated to FFR (Table 9). Nowadays, MLA is the parameter most commonly used in assessing lesion severity, as it is not affected by lesion eccentricity and requires no normal reference. The cutoff value that best fits a FFR < 0.75 is MLA $\leq 3.0\,mm^2$ (59), whereas a MLA $> 4\,mm^2$ has been suggested as a safe cutoff for deferring treatment (60).

IVUS is also extremely helpful when assessing left main stem lesions (LMS). It provides information on lesion severity and plaque characteristics, especially in the presence of unusual angiographic morphology. The most commonly used cutoff value for significant LMS stenosis is a minimum lumen area of less than $9\,mm^2$, even though a recent long-term followup study

Table 9 Comparison between intravascular ultrasound and fractional flow reserve

IVUS	*FFR*
Enables characterization of lesion morphology and guidance for the intervention (device selection, balloon sizing, stent)	Provides a functional assessment by measuring functional severity (and thus may not be sensitive to subtle changes in stent expansion)
MLA measured by IVUS can be a good anatomic predictor of the physiological impact of a coronary lesion	Good correlation with noninvasive means of assessment of ischemia, such as exercise testing, perfusion scanning or positron emission tomography
IVUS thresholds for significant lesions are: For epicardial proximal coronary arteries: MLA <3–$4\,\text{mm}^2$ For left main stem: MLA $<7.5\,\text{mm}^2$	FFR thresholds are: FFR $<$ 0.75 the lesion can induce ischemia FFR $>$ 0.80, the lesion is not able to cause ischemia FFR 0.75–0.80 is the narrow grey zone
Not routinely feasible in most catheter labs, time consuming	Rapidly obtainable index (FFR), not time consuming
More expensive, requires high level of expertize in image interpretation	Easy technique when the few potential pitfalls are understood
Minimal risks, low complication rates, does not require medication other than GTN	Low risk procedure, requires use of expensive drugs for inducing hyperemia
Requires guidewire and catheter insertion and may induce ischemia during interrogation treatment	Requires low profile guidewire insertion that can be subsequently used for lesion

suggests that deferral of revascularization when MLA $\geq 7.5\,\text{mm}^2$ is safe (61), while Jasti et al. recently reported even a smaller cutoff of MLA $\geq 5.9\,\text{mm}^2$ (62).

64-SLICE COMPUTED TOMOGRAPHY

Multislice computed tomography (CT), also known as helical or spiral CT, is performed using a rotating scanner that spins at high velocity around the patient emitting radiation and acquiring images. This is a highly sensitive imaging modality, which became even more accurate with the advent of thinner slice detectors, 64-slice detectors. Already with less sophisticated scanners, a good correlation had been found between CT and angiography or IVUS in the assessment of both native vessels and bypass grafts, but still not good enough for CT to replace traditional angiography (63). Recent data using 64-slice scanners to assess coronary atherosclerosis suggest that sensitivity and specificity of noninvasive angiography have improved significantly (99% and 95%, respectively) when compared to traditional angiography (64). A recent study, comparing 64-slice CT to IVUS in the assessment of intermediate coronary stenoses, demonstrated good correlation between the two modalities ($r = 0.83$, $P < 0.001$). The sensitivity of CT was 94% but specificity 81%, with an accuracy of 90% (65).

Even though noninvasive angiography using 64-slice detectors appears promising, more data are warranted before it is used routinely in the assessment of patients with suspected coronary artery disease. Moreover, arrhythmias such as atrial fibrillation, ectopic beats or even sinus tachycardia can produce artifacts. Overestimation of lesion severity can occur if vessels are heavily calcified, whereas accuracy declines with increases in body mass index (66). Finally, no automated quantitative coronary angiography software is still available and lesion severity is assessed by visual estimation.

ASSESSMENT OF INTERMEDIATE LESIONS IN CURRENT PCI GUIDELINES

Current PCI guidelines state that patients with intermediate lesions and no documented ischemia or prior stress imaging should undergo physiologic assessment. Lesions with a FFR below 0.75 (or a CFR of < 2 according to ACC guidelines) should undergo treatment. Those with an FFR above 0.80 should not be treated, as "plaque sealing" or stenting of hemodynamically nonsignificant lesions is to be avoided. The ESC guidelines underline the concept of the "grey area" in the FFR values (between 0.75 and 0.80), in which false positive or negative investigations are to be expected. Nevertheless, unlike other diagnostic tests, the FFR "grey zone" is quite narrow, making this index highly suitable for clinical decision making.

CONCLUSIONS

The physiologic and intravascular ultrasound assessment of angiographically intermediate coronary stenoses without documented myocardial ischemia is still important in the decision-making process in interventional cardiology.

Even though deferral of intervention based on IVUS parameters has been shown to be safe, in current practice guidelines IVUS does not seem to have a primary role in the assessment of the severity of intermediate lesions. Physiologic assessment with FFR or CFR is the recommended approach. Parameters based on both pressure gradient and flow velocity can improve clinical decision making and may substitute FFR and CFR in the near future.

Drug-eluting stents have the potential to completely change our approach to intermediate stenoses. The concept of treating a lesion only if flow limiting is based on the procedural risks, and especially on the risk of restenosis. If restenosis is abolished by drug-eluting stents or, in the future, biodegradable drug-eluting stents are developed to avoid the possible risk of late thrombosis and complications related to the need for long-term double antiplatelet therapy, we may resurrect the concept of "plaque sealing," not recommended and potentially detrimental with bare-metal stents. If the treatment of intermediate stenoses is based not on their present potential to cause ischemia but on the risk of future events, the pendulum may swing from FFR and other functional methods of assessment of lesion severity to IVUS or other morphologic techniques, such as optical coherence tomography, which are more likely to identify vulnerable plaques (Table 10).

Table 10 Techniques proposed for identifying vulnerable lesions
Intravascular ultrasound
Elastography
Virtual histology
Angioscopy
Thermography
Optical coherence tomography
Magnetic resonance
64-slice CT

REFERENCES

1. Smith SC Jr, Dove JT, Jacobs AK, et al. ACC/AHA guidelines for percutaneous coronary intervention (revision of the 1993 PTCA guidelines)-executive summary: a report of the American College of Cardiology/American Heart Association task force on practice guidelines (Committee to revise the 1993 guidelines for percutaneous transluminal coronary angioplasty) endorsed by the Society for Cardiac Angiography and Interventions. Circulation 2001; 103:3019–3041.
2. Silber S, Albertsson P, Aviles FF, et al. Guidelines for percutaneous coronary interventions. The Task Force for Percutaneous Coronary Interventions of the European Society of Cardiology. Eur Heart J 2005; 26:804–847.
3. Fischer JJ, Samady H, McPherson JA, et al. Comparison between visual assessment and quantitative angiography versus fractional flow reserve for native coronary narrowings of moderate severity. Am J Cardiol 2002; 90:210–215.
4. Pijls NHJ, De Bruyne BD. Coronary Pressure. 2nd ed. London: Kluwer Academic Publishers, 2000.

5. Gould KL, Lipscomb K, Hamilton GW. Physiologic basis for assessing critical coronary stenosis. Instantaneous flow response and regional distribution during coronary hyperemia as measures of coronary flow reserve. Am J Cardiol 1974; 33:87–94.
6. Gould KL, Lipscomb K. Effects of coronary stenosis on coronary flow reserve and resistance. Am J Cardiol 1974; 34:48–55.
7. De Bruyne B, Pijls NH, Barbato E, et al. Intracoronary and intravenous adenosine 5′-triphosphate, adenosine, papaverine, and contrast medium to assess fractional flow reserve in humans. Circulation 2003; 107:1877–1883.
8. Parham WA, Bouhasin A, Ciaramita JP, et al. Coronary hyperemic dose responses of intracoronary sodium nitroprusside. Circulation 2004; 109:1236–1243.
9. Donohue TJ, Kern MJ, Aguirre FV, et al. Assessing the hemodynamic significance of coronary artery stenoses: analysis of translesional pressure-flow velocity relations in patients. J Am Coll Cardiol 1993; 22:449–458.
10. Miller DD, Donohue TJ, Younis LT, et al. Correlation of pharmacological 99mTc-sestamibi myocardial perfusion imaging with poststenotic coronary flow reserve in patients with angiographically intermediate coronary artery stenoses. Circulation 1994; 89:2150–2160.
11. Heller LI, Cates C, Popma J, et al. Intracoronary Doppler assessment of moderate coronary artery disease: comparison with 201Tl imaging and coronary angiography. FACTS Study Group. Circulation 1997; 96:484–490.
12. Kern MJ. Coronary physiology revisited: practical insights from the cardiac catheterization laboratory. Circulation 2000; 101:1344–1351.
13. Gould KL, Kirkeeide RL, Buchi M. Coronary flow reserve as a physiologic measure of stenosis severity. J Am Coll Cardiol 1990; 15:459–474.
14. Baumgart D, Haude M, Goerge G, et al. Improved assessment of coronary stenosis severity using the relative flow velocity reserve. Circulation 1998; 98:40–46.
15. de Bruyne B, Bartunek J, Sys SU, et al. Simultaneous coronary pressure and flow velocity measurements in humans: feasibility, reproducibility, and hemodynamic dependence of coronary flow velocity reserve, hyperemic flow versus pressure slope index, and fractional flow reserve. Circulation 1996; 94:1842–1849.
16. Pijls NH, van Son JA, Kirkeeide RL, et al. Experimental basis of determining maximum coronary, myocardial, and collateral blood flow by pressure measurements for assessing functional stenosis severity before and after percutaneous transluminal coronary angioplasty. Circulation 1993; 87:1354–67.
17. Pijls NH, Kern MJ, Yock PG, et al. Practice and potential pitfalls of coronary pressure measurement. Catheter Cardiovasc Interv 2000; 49:1–16.
18. De Bruyne B, Bartunek J, Sys SU, et al. Relation between myocardial fractional flow reserve calculated from coronary pressure measurements and exercise-induced myocardial ischemia. Circulation 1995; 92:39–46.
19. Pijls NH, Van Gelder B, Van der Voort P, et al. Fractional flow reserve. A useful index to evaluate the influence of an epicardial coronary stenosis on myocardial blood flow. Circulation 1995; 92:3183–3193.
20. Pijls NH, De Bruyne B, Peels K, et al. Measurement of fractional flow reserve to assess the functional severity of coronary-artery stenoses. N Engl J Med 1996; 334:1703–1708.
21. Bartunek J, Marwick TH, Rodrigues AC, et al. Dobutamine-induced wall motion abnormalities: correlations with myocardial fractional flow reserve and quantitative coronary angiography. J Am Coll Cardiol 1996; 27:1429–1436.
22. Abe M, Tomiyama H, Yoshida H, et al. Diastolic fractional flow reserve to assess the functional severity of moderate coronary artery stenoses: comparison with fractional flow reserve and coronary flow velocity reserve. Circulation 2000; 102:2365–2370.
23. Chamuleau SA, Meuwissen M, van Eck-Smit BL, et al. Fractional flow reserve, absolute and relative coronary blood flow velocity reserve in relation to the results of technetium-99 m sestamibi single-photon emission computed tomography in patients with two-vessel coronary artery disease. J Am Coll Cardiol 2001; 37:1316–1322.
24. Pijls NH. Is it time to measure fractional flow reserve in all patients? J Am Coll Cardiol 2003; 41:1122–1124.
25. Bech GJ, Pijls NH, De Bruyne B, et al. Usefulness of Fractional Flow Reserve to Predict Clinical Outcome After Balloon Angioplasty. Circulation 1999; 99:883–888.
26. Bech GJ, De Bruyne B, Pijls NH, et al. Fractional flow reserve to determine the appropriateness of

angioplasty in moderate coronary stenosis: a randomized trial. Circulation 2001; 103:2928–2934.
27. Lopez-Palop R, Pinar E, Lozano I, et al. Utility of the fractional flow reserve in the evaluation of angiographically moderate in-stent restenosis. Eur Heart J 2004; 25:2040–2047.
28. Kern MJ, Donohue TJ, Aguirre FV, et al. Clinical outcome of deferring angioplasty in patients with normal translesional pressure-flow velocity measurements. J Am Coll Cardiol 1995; 25: 178–187.
29. Bech GJ, De Bruyne B, Bonnier HJ, et al. Long-term follow-up after deferral of percutaneous transluminal coronary angioplasty of intermediate stenosis on the basis of coronary pressure measurement. J Am Coll Cardiol 1998; 31:841–847.
30. Schiele F, Legalery P, Seronde MF, et al. One-year outcome of patients submitted to routine fractional flow reserve assessment to determine the need for angioplasty. http://www.escardio.org/ knowledge/congresses/abol/presentation? id = 25208.
31. Berger A, Botman KJ, MacCarthy PA, et al. Long-term clinical outcome after fractional flow reserve-guided percutaneous coronary intervention in patients with multivessel disease. J Am Coll Cardiol 2005; 46:438–442.
32. De Bruyne B, Pijls NH, Smith L, et al. Coronary thermodilution to assess flow reserve: experimental validation. Circulation 2001; 104: 2003–2006.
33. Pijls NH, De Bruyne B, Smith L, et al. Coronary thermodilution to assess flow reserve: validation in humans. Circulation 2002; 105:2482–2486.
34. Barbato E, Aarnoudse W, Aengevaeren WR, et al. Validation of coronary flow reserve measurements by thermodilution in clinical practice. Eur Heart J 2004; 25:219–223.
35. Pijls NH, De Bruyne B, Bech GJ, et al. Coronary pressure measurement to assess the hemodynamic significance of serial stenoses within one coronary artery: validation in humans. Circulation 2000; 102:2371–2317.
36. Cameron A, Kemp HG Jr, Fisher LD, et al. Left main coronary artery stenosis: angiographic determination. Circulation 1983; 68:484.
37. De Bruyne B, Pijls NH, Bartunek J, et al. Fractional flow reserve in patients with prior myocardial infarction. Circulation 2001; 104:157–162.
38. Gould KL. Pressure-flow characteristics of coronary stenoses in unsedated dogs at rest and during coronary vasodilation. Circ Res 1978; 43: 242–253.
39. Gould KL. Quantification of coronary artery stenosis in vivo. Circ Res 1985; 57:341–353.
40. Serruys PW, Di Mario C, Meneveau N, et al. Intracoronary pressure and flow velocity with sensor-tip guidewires: a new methodologic approach for assessment of coronary hemodynamics before and after coronary interventions. Am J Cardiol 1993; 71:41D–53D.
41. Di Mario C, de Feyter PJ, Slager CJ, de Jaegere P, Roelandt JR, Serruys PW. Intracoronary blood flow velocity and transstenotic pressure gradient using sensor-tip pressure and Doppler guidewires: a new technology for the assessment of stenosis severity in the catheterization laboratory. Catheter Cardiovasc Diagn 1993; 28:311–319.
42. Marques KM, Spruijt HJ, Boer C, Westerhof N, Visser CA, Visser FC. The diastolic flow-pressure gradient relation in coronary stenoses in humans. J Am Coll Cardiol 2002; 39:1630–1636.
43. Meuwissen M, Siebes M, Chamuleau SAJ, et al. Hyperemic stenosis resistance index for evaluation of functional coronary lesion severity. Circulation 2002; 106:441–446.
44. Siebes M, Verhoeff BJ, Meuwissen M, de Winter RJ, Spaan JA, Piek JJ. Single-wire pressure and flow velocity measurement to quantify coronary stenosis hemodynamics and effects of percutaneous interventions. Circulation 2004; 109:756–762.
45. Meuwissen M, Verhoeff BJ, Chaumleau SAJ, et al. The diagnostic value of the flow velocity-pressure gradient slope for assessment of functional coronary lesion severity. Abstract, ESC Congress 2005. Available at: http://www.escardio.org/knowledge/congresses/abol/presentation?id = 22865
46. Topol EJ, Nissen SE. Our preoccupation with coronary luminology: the dissociation between clinical and angiographic findings in ischemic heart disease. Circulation 1995; 92:2333–2342.
47. Tobis JM, Mallery JA, Gessert J, et al. Intravascular ultrasound cross-sectional arterial imaging before and after balloon angioplasty in vitro. Circulation 1989; 80:873–882.
48. Tobis JM, Mallery JA, Mahon D, et al. Intravascular ultrasound imaging of human coronary arteries in vivo: analysis of tissue characterizations with comparison to in vitro histological specimens. Circulation 1991; 83:913–926.

49. Yock PG, Fitzgerald PJ, Linker DT, et al. Intravascular ultrasound guidance for catheter-based coronary interventions. J Am Coll Cardiol 1991; 17:39B–45B.
50. Colombo A, Hall P, Nakamura S, et al. Intracoronary stenting without anticoagulation accomplished with intravascular ultrasound guidance. Circulation 1995; 91:1676–1688.
51. Tobis J, Colombo A. IVUS and coronary stenting. Catheter Cardiovasc Diagn 1996; 39:346.
52. Fitzgerald PJ, Oshima A, Hayase M, et al. Final results of the Can Routine Ultrasound Influence Stent Expansion (CRUISE) study. Circulation 2000; 102:523–530.
53. Mudra H, Klauss V, Blasini R, et al. Ultrasound guidance of Palmaz-Schatz intracoronary stenting with a combined intravascular ultrasound balloon catheter. Circulation 1994; 90:1252– 1261.
54. Nakamura S, Colombo A, Gaglione A, et al. Intracoronary ultrasound observations during stent implantation. Circulation 1994; 89:2026–2034.
55. Karrillon GJ, Morice MC, Benveniste E, et al. Intracoronary stent implantation without ultrasound guidance and with replacement of conventional anticoagulation by antiplatelet therapy: 30–day clinical outcome of the French Multicenter Registry. Circulation 1996; 94:1519–1527.
56. Moussa I, Moses J, Di Mario C, et al. Does the specific intravascular ultrasound criterion used to optimize stent expansion have an impact on the probability of stent restenosis? Am J Cardiol 1999; 83:1012–1017.
57. Kern MJ, Dupouy P, Drury JH, et al. Role of coronary artery lumen enlargement in improving coronary blood flow after balloon angioplasty and stenting: a combined intravascular ultrasound Doppler flow and imaging study. J Am Coll Cardiol 1997; 29:1520–1527.
58. Mintz GS, Popma JJ, Pichard AD, et al. Limitations of angiography in the assessment of plaque distribution in coronary artery disease: a systematic study of target lesion eccentricity in 1446 lesions. Circulation 1996; 93:924–931.
59. Takagi A, Tsurumi Y, Ishii Y, Suzuki K, Kawana M, Kasanuki H. Clinical potential of intravascular ultrasound for physiological assessment of coronary stenosis: relationship between quantitative ultrasound tomography and pressure-derived fractional flow reserve. Circulation 1999; 100: 250–255.
60. Abizaid AS, Mintz GS, Mehran R, et al. Long-term follow-up after percutaneous transluminal coronary angioplasty was not performed based on intravascular ultrasound findings: importance of lumen dimensions. Circulation 1999; 100: 256–261.
61. Fassa AA, Wagatsuma K, Higano ST, et al. Intravascular ultrasound-guided treatment for angiographically indeterminate left main coronary artery disease: a long-term follow-up study. J Am Coll Cardiol 2005; 45:204–211.
62. Jasti V, Ivan E, Yalamenchili V, et al. Correlations between fractional flow reserve and intravascular ultrasound in patients with an ambiguous left main coronary artery stenosis. Circulation 2004; 110:2831–2836.
63. Caussin C, Daoud B, Ghostine S, et al. Comparison of lumens of intermediate coronary stenosis using 16-slice computed tomography versus intravascular ultrasound. Am J Cardiol 2005; 96: 524–528.
64. Mollet NR, Cademartiri F, van Mieghem CA, et al. High-resolution spiral computed tomography coronary angiography in patients referred for diagnostic conventional coronary angiography. Circulation 2005; 112:2318–2323.
65. Caussin C, Ghostine S, Pesenti-Rossi D, et al. Quantification of coronary intermediate stenosis using 64-slice computed tomography compared to intravascular ultrasound. Abstract, ESC Congress 2005. Available at: http://www.escardio.org/knowledge/congresses/abol/presentation?id = 24425.
66. Raff GL, Gallagher MJ, O'Neill WW, Goldstein JA. Diagnostic accuracy of noninvasive coronary angiography using 64-slice spiral computed tomography. J Am Coll Cardiol 2005; 46: 552–557.

12

Approach to patients with impaired renal function

Eugenia Nikolsky and Roxana Mehran

INTRODUCTION

Coronary artery disease (CAD) is a frequent comorbidity and a common cause of mortality in patients with chronic renal insufficiency (CRI). The reasons are multifactorial and include high-risk demographic characteristics of patients with CRI; metabolic changes contributing to accelerated atherosclerosis (lipid and carbohydrate abnormalities, glucose intolerance, insulin resistance, secondary hyperparathyroidism, increased levels of homocystein, and carnitine deficiency); propensity to a hypercoagulable state (enhanced fibrinogen activity and platelet aggregation); specifics of hemodynamic changes (volume and pressure overload); anemia; and electrolyte disturbances as well as impaired pharmacokinetics and pharmacodynamics of medications.

A significant proportion of patients with CRI require coronary revascularization. In a pooled analysis of contemporary primary percutaneous coronary intervention (PCI) trials, CRI at baseline was present in approximately 25% of the patients (1). Among patients undergoing PCI for acute myocardial infarction (MI), about 20% of the study population had baseline CRI (2).

DEFINITION OF RENAL FUNCTION IMPAIRMENT

It is important to recognize that the use of serum creatinine solely is not a reliable indicator of renal damage and should not be used to assess the level of kidney function. By consensus, glomerular filtration rate (GFR) is the best measure of overall kidney function (3). The GFR is equal to the sum of the filtration rates in all of the functioning nephrons, and estimation of the GFR gives a rough measure of the number of functioning nephrons. The normal level of GFR varies according to age, gender, and body size. Normal GFR in young adults is approximately 120 to 130 m/L min per 1.73 m2 and declines with age.

Estimation of GFR is used to assess the degree of renal impairment. *Chronic renal insufficiency is defined as estimated glomerular filtration rate (eGFR) $\leq$60 mL/min per 1.73 m^2 representing loss of half or more of the normal kidney function, or the presence of persistent proteinuria with an albumin/creatinine ratio $>$30 mg/g in the urine samples.* Several formulas based on easily obtained variables have been developed to estimate the GFR; these include the

Cockcroft–Gault and Modification of Diet in Renal Disease (MDRD) equations:

- The *Cockcroft–Gault Equation* takes into account the increase in creatinine production with increasing weight and the decline in creatinine production with age. The value obtained must be multiplied by 0.85 in women.

  Creatinine clearance (mL/min) = (140 − Age) × Body weight (kg)/Serum creatinine (μg/dL) × 72

- The *Modification of Diet in Renal Disease (MDRD) equation* is based on data obtained from the MDRD study. In addition to the serum creatinine, the equation uses age, serum albumin concentration, and blood urea nitrogen value to estimate the GFR:

  $$\text{eGFR, mL/min per } 1.73\,\text{m}^2 = 170 \times \text{Serum creatinine } (\mu\text{g/dl})^{-0.999} \times \text{Age}^{-0.176} \times \text{Serum urea } (\mu\text{g/dl})^{-0.170} \times \text{Albumin } (\text{g/dl})^{0.318} (\times 0.762 \text{ if female}) \times (1.180 \text{ if African American})$$

- The *simplified or abbreviated Modification of Diet in Renal Disease (MDRD) equation*:

  $$\text{eGFR, mL/min/}1.73\,\text{m}^2 = 186 \times (\text{Serum creatinine [mg/dL]})^{-1.154} \times [\text{Age}^{-0.203} \times (0.742 \text{ if female}) \times (1.210 \text{ if African American}]$$

The website (http://www.kidney.org/professionals/kdoqi/gfr_calculator.cfm) is available for quick calculation of either creatinine clearance or eGFR applying one of the proposed equations.

EARLY POST-PCI OUTCOMES IN PATIENTS WITH CRI

The presence of impaired renal function is associated with less favorable demographic characteristics including a larger proportion of elderly population and females, and a higher prevalence of hypertension, diabetes mellitus, cerebrovascular and/or peripheral vascular disease, and congestive heart failure, as well as prior MI and coronary artery bypass grafting (CABG) (4–8). Angiographic features of patients with CRI frequently include multivessel CAD, vein graft disease, more complex lesions, and lower ejection fractions (4–8). However, the rate of angiographic success in large PCI series was not related to the renal function and exceeded 95% (5,6).

Nevertheless, short-term prognosis post-PCI is remarkably worse in patients with CRI. In the PCI arm of the randomized Bypass Angioplasty Revascularization Investigation (BARI) trial, patients with versus without CRI had almost 10 times higher in-hospital mortality (6.7% vs. 0.7%, respectively; $P < 0.05$) (7). Similar data were obtained in the later series on 362 patients with CRI (serum creatinine >1.5 mg/dl) compared with 2,972 patients with preserved renal function (serum creatinine ≤1.5 mg/dl) (10.1% vs. 1.1%) (4). Notably, in-hospital mortality was similarly high in patients with both mild and severe CRI (serum creatinine 1.6 to 2.0 mg/dl and >2.0 mg/dl, respectively) (11.5% vs. 9.9%) (4).

In the contemporary PCI era, CRI remains a significant predictor of worse short-term prognosis. In the second Randomized Evaluation in PCI Linking Bivalirudin to Reduced Clinical Events (REPLACE-2) trial that included patients with stable and unstable angina and/or provokable ischemia, 30-day mortality was significantly higher among 886 patients with CRI compared to 4,824 patients without CRI (1.6% vs. 0.1%; $P < 0.001$) (9). The same was true regarding 30-day MI (8.5 vs. 6.4%; $P = 0.02$) and the triple endpoint of death/MI/target vessel revascularization (TVR) (9.5% vs. 7.0%; $P = 0.01$). Likewise, in the do Tirofiban and ReoPro Give Similar Efficacy Outcome (TARGET) trial, patients in the lowest quartile of creatinine clearance (<70 mL/min) compared to those in the highest quartile (>114 mL/min) had significantly higher rates of composite endpoint of death/MI/urgent TVR (7.3% vs. 5.8%; $P = 0.005$) (10). Finally, in the randomized Controlled Abciximab and Device Investigation to Lower Late Angioplasty Complications (CADILLAC) trial, 30-day mortality among patients undergoing primary PCI for acute MI was strikingly higher in patients with versus without baseline CRI (7.5% vs. 0.8%; $P < 0.0001$) with incremental increase in mortality for each 10 mL/min decline in baseline creatinine clearance (2). In all of these trials, after adjusting for demographic, clinical, and procedural factors, CRI consistently represented a significant predictor of in-hospital mortality (4–7,9).

Patients with CRI compared to individuals with preserved renal function more frequently develop PCI-related complications including pulmonary edema (11.9% vs. 2.3%), stroke (1.4% vs. 0.5%), and access site vascular repair (9.4 vs. 4.4%), contributing to the prolonged in-hospital stay (4,6).

HEMORRHAGIC COMPLICATIONS IN RELATION TO CRI

Due to alteration in the coagulation system and impaired response to medications, patients with CRI are prone to periprocedural bleeding complications. In the REPLACE-2 trial, patients with CRI had more than double the incidence of major bleeding (6.1% vs. 2.5%; $P < 0.0001$) and CRI was a significant predictor of major bleeding (odds ratio 1.72; $P = 0.03$) irrespective of antithrombotic regimen (bivalirudin or unfractionated heparin plus planned platelet glycoprotein IIb/IIIa receptor inhibitors) (9). In the above-mentioned TARGET trial as well, patients in the lowest quartile of creatinine clearance compared to those in the highest quartile had significantly increased risk of major bleeding (1.6% vs. 0.3%, respectively) and red blood cell transfusions (5.3% vs. 2%) (10). Finally, in the CADILLAC trial, hemorrhagic complications and transfusion requirements were increased more than twofold in patients with CRI (11).

ADJUNCTIVE PHARMACOTHERAPY IN PATIENTS WITH CRI

Knowledge of drug metabolism is especially important when considering the choice of anticoagulation regimen in patients with CRI. ***One should bear in mind that many antithrombotic medications are cleared renally.***

Heparin

Therapeutic doses of unfractionated heparin are cleared by a combination of rapid, saturable mechanisms and slower, nonsaturable, dose-independent mechanisms of renal clearance (12). Though the presence of CRI generally does not require dose adjustment of unfractionated heparin during PCI, enhanced propensity to bleeding complications in ***patients with CRI necessitates close intraprocedural monitoring of anticoagulation.***

There are no data on the use of low molecular weight heparins in the catheter laboratory because large randomized studies excluded patients with advanced CRI. These agents are cleared primarily by the renal route, and their half-life is extended in patients with renal failure. Due to the inability to closely monitor anticoagulation during the procedure, low molecular weight heparins probably should not be used in the catheter laboratory in patients with CRI.

Direct thrombin inhibitors

Bivalirudin (Angiomax®) is cleared from plasma by a combination of renal mechanisms and proteolytic cleavage, with a half-life in patients with normal renal function of 25 min. Drug elimination is clearly related to renal function. Study of pharmacokinetics and pharmacodynamics of bivalirudin showed that its clearance was very close in patients with normal renal function (creatinine clearance ≥90 mL/min) and in patients with mild CRI (creatinine clearance 60 to 89 mL/min), but was reduced by 45% in patients with moderate CRI (creatinine clearance 30 to 59 mL/min), by 68% in patients with severe CRI (creatinine clearance <30 mL/min), and by 77% in dialysis-dependent patients (13).

Given the specifics of bivalirudin's pharmacodynamics and pharmacokinetics, the following regimen of administration of bivalirudin in patients with CRI is recommended:

> An intravenous bolus of 0.75 mg/kg regardless of renal function followed by an infusion of 1.75 mg/kg/h for the duration of the PCI procedure in patients with moderate renal impairment (creatinine clearance 30–59 mL/min); 1.0 mg/kg/h in patients with severe renal impairment (creatinine clearance <30 mL/min); and 0.25 mg/kg/h in patients on hemodialysis.

In the randomized REPLACE II trial, among patients with impaired renal function (creatinine clearance <60 mL/min), bivalirudin demonstrated suppression of ischemic events at 30-day follow-up to the degree provided by heparin and glycoprotein IIb/IIIa inhibition (9.7% vs. 9.4%, respectively) (9). In addition, treatment with bivalirudin was associated with a trend toward lower incidence of protocol-defined major bleeding (5.1% vs. 7.1%; $P = 0.20$) and a significant reduction in composite of major plus minor bleeding by TIMI criteria (3.2% vs. 7.1%; $P = 0.009$)(9). In a meta-analysis of three randomized trials of bivalirudin versus heparin among patients treated with PCI, there was greater absolute benefit of bivalirudin in terms of reduction of ischemic and bleeding complications in patients with worse degrees of renal impairment (2.2%, 5.8%, 7.7%, and 14.4% for patients with normal renal function, mild, moderate and severe renal impairment, respectively) (1).

Platelet glycoprotein IIb/IIIa receptor inhibitors

Abciximab is rapidly cleared from the circulation by the reticuloendothelial system and increases the risk of bleeding in patients with CRI to the magnitude not exceeding that in patients without renal impairment. In the PCI series from the Mayo Clinic, there was no significant interaction between creatinine clearance and either major or minor bleeding with abciximab (14).

In contrast to abciximab, eptifibatide and tirofiban undergo renal clearance, requiring appropriate dosing adjustments in patients with renal insufficiency. In the Enhanced Suppression of Platelet IIb/IIIa Receptor with Intregrilin Therapy (ESPRIT) trial, eptifibatide was documented to be at least as effective in patients with *mild* CRI as in patients with normal renal function without increasing bleeding risk (15). In the subanalysis from the TARGET trial, there was a trend toward greater benefit of abciximab over tirofiban regarding 30-day ischemic complications in patients with creatinine clearance <70 ml/min (6.0% vs. 8.7%; $P = 0.07$) (10). Abciximab, compared with tirofiban, was also associated with an increased risk of minor bleeding in patients with creatinine clearance <70 mL/min (7.2% vs. 3.4%; $P = 0.004$) (10).

Given that the use of dialysis is an exclusion criterion from the randomized PCI trials, no data are available on the use of platelet glycoprotein IIb/IIIa receptor inhibitors in patients with end-stage renal disease.

LONG-TERM OUTCOMES POST-PCI IN RELATION TO CRI

Impaired renal function is associated with unfavorable prognosis post-PCI (7,8,16,17). In the BARI trial, patients with even mild CRI experienced doubling of mortality during a seven-year period compared to patients with preserved renal function (7). In the Mayo Clinic's PCI prospective registry on 5,327 patients, one-year mortality after successful intervention was 1.5%, 3.6%, 7.8%, and 18.3% in patients with creatinine clearance ≥70, 50 to 69, 30 to 49, and <30 ml/ min, respectively. As expected, the mortality rate was the highest in patients on dialysis (19.9%) (5). In the same study, by multivariate analysis, moderate or severe renal insufficiency was associated with a greater risk of death than even diabetes (5). Furthermore, in the contemporary Prevention of Restenosis with Tranilast and its Outcomes (PRESTO) PCI trial, the risk of death at 9 months was 2.7 times higher in the lowest versus the highest creatinine clearance group (<60 mL/min vs. >89 mL/min) (8). Finally, in patients undergoing primary PCI for acute MI, presence of CRI was associated with a striking increase in short-term and late mortality, similar to the excess risk of anterior versus nonanterior MI location (11).

RESTENOSIS AND REPEAT REVASCULARIZATION IN PATIENTS WITH CRI

Two large-scale trials provided similar results, showing that patients with CRI are not at increased risk of restenosis after bare-metal stent implantation. In the PRESTO trial, patients with mild or moderate CRI (baseline serum creatinine <1.8 mg/dl) had paradoxically lower rates of restenosis post-PCI (83% of the patients received stent) and TVR compared to patients with preserved renal function (8). At 9-month angiographic follow-up performed in 2,556 of 11,484 patients (22%), those in the lowest quartile of creatinine clearance (<60 mL/min) had 32% restenosis rate compared with 37% in patients in the highest quartile of creatinine clearance (>89 mL/min) ($P = 0.02$) (8). Likewise, in the bare-metal stent arm of the randomized TAXUS IV trial, by multivariate analysis, an *increase* for each 10 mL/min in creatinine clearance was independently associated with the risk of 9-month binary restenosis (odds ratio = 1.14; $P = 0.009$) (18).

Drug-eluting stents in patients with CRI

In the subanalysis from the TAXUS-IV pivotal randomized trial comparing outcomes after implantation of the polymer-based slow-release paclitaxel-eluting stent versus bare-metal stent in patients with stable and unstable angina and provokable ischemia, implantation of paclitaxel-eluting stent resulted in strikingly lower rates of 9-month angiographic restenosis in patients with (2.1% vs. 20.5%; $P = 0.009$) and without (9.2% vs. 27.8%; $P < 0.0001$) baseline CRI, translating into lower rates of 1-year TLR in the TAXUS arm compared with the bare-metal stent arm, both in patients with CRI (3.3% vs. 12.2%, respectively; $P = 0.01$) and without CRI (4.7% vs. 15.8%, respectively; $P < 0.0001$) (18). In the Cypher Registry Experience at Washington Hospital Center with Drug-eluting Stents (C-REWARDS), patients with CRI had significantly lower rates of 6-month TLR when treated with sirolimus-eluting stent compared with bare-metal stents (7.1% vs. 22.1%; $P = 0.02$) (19).

In two studies, CRI was identified as an independent predictor of stent thrombosis after drug-eluting stent implantation (20,21) while there were no such concerns in the TAXUS-IV trial (18).

CONTRAST-INDUCED NEPHROPATHY AND DIALYSIS POST-PCI

Patients with CRI are at increased risk of contrast-induced nephropathy (CIN) (22). It is defined as an absolute (≥0.5 mg/dl) or relative (≥25%) increase in serum creatinine level after the exposure to contrast agent compared to baseline value, when alternative explanations for renal impairment have been excluded (23,24). Further deterioration of renal function after exposure to contrast medium has been shown to worsen prognosis of patients with CRI (25).

Rates of CIN are extremely high in patients with CRI, ranging from 14.8% to 55% (23,24). The higher the baseline creatinine value, the greater the risk of CIN. In one study, CIN occurred in only 2% of patients with baseline plasma creatinine ≤1.2 mg/dl, 10.4% in patients with serum creatinine of 1.4 to 1.9 mg/dl, and 68% in patients with serum creatinine level of ≥2.0 mg/dl (26).

A curvilinear relationship was found between estimated creatinine clearance and risk of renal failure requiring dialysis in patients undergoing diagnostic coronary angiography with or without angioplasty (Fig. 1) (22,23). Below a threshold estimated creatinine clearance of 25 mL/min, risk of dialysis increases rapidly (22,23).

Impaired renal function is frequent in patients with other risk factors for the development of CIN (Table 1). Assessment of cumulative risk is important to identify an individual patient's risk to develop CIN. ***A simple CIN risk score (Fig. 2) was proposed based on the readily available information, and is recommended for both clinical and investigational purposes (27).*** The occurrence of CIN was found to be 7.5% to 57.3% for a low (≤5) and high (≥16) risk score, respectively, with corresponding rates of dialysis 0.04% to 12.6% (27).

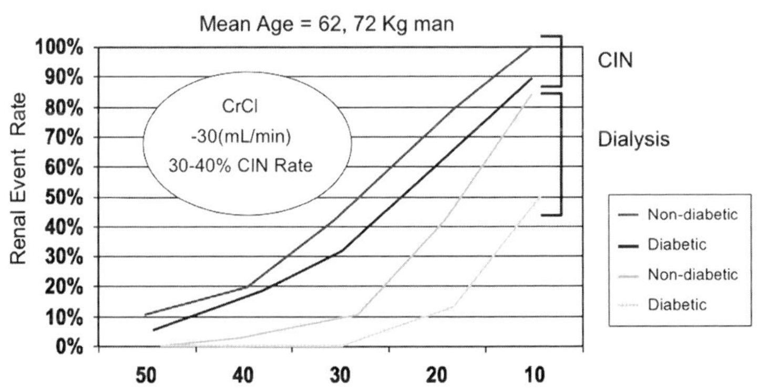

Figure 1 Validated risk of acute renal failure requiring dialysis after diagnostic angiography and/or angioplasty. A mean contrast dose of 250 mL and a mean age of 65 years is assumed. *Abbreviations*: CrCl, creatinine clearance; CIN, contrast induced nephropathy. *Source*: From Ref. 23. (*See color insert.*)

Table 1 Risk factors for the development of contrast-induced nephropathy

Fixed (nonmodifiable) risk factors	*Modifiable risk factors*
Pre-existing renal failure	Volume and type of contrast medium
Diabetes mellitus	Multiple contrast injections within 72 hours
Advanced congestive heart failure	Hemodynamic instability
Reduced left ventricular ejection fraction	Dehydration
Acute myocardial infarction	Anemia
Cardiogenic shock	Intra-aortic balloon pump
Renal transplant	Low serum albumin level (<35 g/L)
	Angiotensin converting enzyme inhibitors
	Diuretics
	Nephrotoxic drugs [nonsteroidal anti-inflammatory agents (NSAIDS), antibiotics, cyclosporine, etc.]

Choice of contrast media in patients with CRI

Within the variety of currently available contrast agents with low osmolarity, there are certain differences in nephrotoxic effect that seem to be more evident with ionic than nonionic agents. In one randomized study of 307 patients with baseline renal insufficiency (serum creatinine ≥1.5 mg/dl), the degree of renal function deterioration was less with the nonionic agent iopamidol than with the ionic agent diatrizoate, as measured by the mean of the maximal increase in serum creatinine (0.20 ± 0.44 vs. 0.38 ± 0.73 mg/dl; $P < 0.0001$) and the incidence of CIN (8% vs. 19%; $P < 0.01$) (28). However, another randomized study failed to show a significant difference in the rates of CIN in the group exposed to iopamidol versus diatrizoate, either in low- or high-risk patients (29). To address this issue in a larger trial, the Nephrotoxicity in High-Risk Patients Study of Iso-Osmolar and Low-Osmolar Non-Ionic Contrast Media (NEPHRIC) study was performed (30).

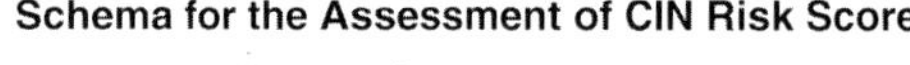

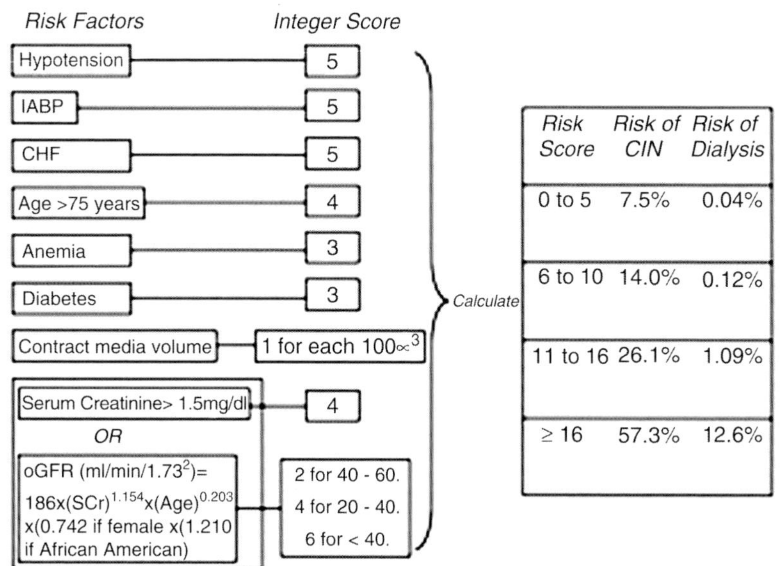

Figure 2 Scheme to define CIN risk score. CHF denotes congestive heart failure class III–IV by the New York Heart Association classification and/or history of pulmonary edema. eGFR denotes estimated glomerular filtration rate. *Anemia*: baseline hematocrit value <39% for men and <36% for women. *Hypotension*: systolic blood pressure <80 mmHg for at least 1 hour requiring inotropic support with medications or IABP within 24 hours periprocedurally. *Source*: From Ref 27.

Table 2 Randomized trials assessing various treatment modalities in prevention of contrast-induced nephropathy

Treatment	*Supporting studies*	*No effect/Deleterious effect*
Hydration	Solomon et al. *N Engl J Med* 1994; 331:1416–1420	Briguori et al. J Am Coll Cardiol 2002; 40:298–303
N-acetyl-L-cysteine	Conesa et al. *Am J Physiol Regul Integr Comp Physiol* 2001; 281: R730–737 Tepel et al. *N Engl J Med* 2000; 343: 180–184 Diaz-Sandoval et al. *Am J Cardiol* 2002; 89:356–358 Shyu et al. *Am J Cardiol* 2002; 40:1383–1388	Vallero et al. G Ital Nefrol 2002; 19:529–533 Allaqaband et al. *Catheter Cardiovasc Interv* 2002; 57:279–283 Durham et al. Kidney Int 2002; 62:2202–2207
Dopamine	Kapoor et al. *Int J Cardiol* 1996; 53:233–236	Gare et al. J Am Coll Cardiol 1999; 34:1682–1688 Hans et al. Am Surg 1998; 64:432–436 Abizaid et al. Am J Cardiol 1999; 83:260–263, A5
Fenoldopam	Tumlin et al. *Am Heart J* 2002; 143:894–903	Allaqaband et al. Catheter Cardiovasc Interv 2002; 57:279–283 Stone et al. JAMA. 2003; 290:2284–2291
Theophylline	Huber et al. *Radiology* 2002; 223:772–779 Kolonko et al. *J Nephrol* 1998; 11:151–156 Kapoor et al. *Nephrol Dial Transplant* 2002; 17:1936–1941	Erley et al. Kidney Int Suppl 1998; 67:S192–194 Shammas et al. J Invasive Cardiol 2001; 13:738–740 Abizaid et al. Am J Cardiol 1999; 83:260–263, A5
Atrial natriuretic peptide		Kurnik et al. Am J Kidney Dis 1998; 31:674–680
Calcium channel blockers	Neumayer et al. *Nephrol Dial Transplant* 1989; 4:1030–1036	Carraro et al. Nephrol Dial *Transplant* 1996; 11:444–448 Khoury et al. Pharmacotherapy 1995; 15:59–65 Spangberg-Viklund et al. Scand J Urol Nephrol 1996; 30:63–68
Prostaglandin E1	Sketch et al. *Am J Ther* 2001; 8:155–162	
Captopril	Gupta et al. *Indian Heart J* 1999; 51:521–526	
Hemodialysis		Vogt et al. Am J Med 2001; 111:692–698 Lehnert et al. *Nephrol Dial Transplant* 1998; 13:38–362 Berger et al. Dtsch Med *Wochenschr* 2001; 126:162–166 Huber et al. Invest Radiol 2002; 37:471–481 Sterner G et al. *Scand J Urol Nephrol* 2000; 34:323–326
Hemofiltration	Marenzi et al. *N Engl J Med* 2003; 349:1333–1340	

This was a randomized, double-blind, prospective, multicenter study comparing the nephrotoxicity of iohexol, a nonionic monomer, to iodixanol, a nonionic dimer. A total of 129 subjects with diabetes mellitus and serum creatinine concentrations of 1.5 to 3.5 mg/dl undergoing coronary or aortofemoral angiography were enrolled. Significantly more patients assigned to iohexol (17/65; 26%) experienced a serum creatinine increase of 0.5 mg/dl or more, compared with patients in the iodixanol group (2/64 patients; 3%). No patient in the iodixanol group had an increase in serum creatinine of ≥1.0 mg/dl, compared to 10 patients (15%) in the iohexol group (30).

In a meta-analysis of 45 trials, the greater increase in serum creatinine after administration of high- compared with low-osmolar contrast media was seen in patients with pre-existing CRI (31).

It is controversial whether the strategy of gadolinium-based contrast administration may reduce rates of renal function deterioration as compared to the iodinated contrast agents in patients with CRI (32,33).

Volume of contrast agent

Volume of contrast medium is a main modifiable risk factor for CIN, and it is especially crucial in patients having other risk factors. In our study on a diabetic population, CIN developed in approximately every fifth, fourth, and second patient who received 200 to 400 mL, 400 to 600 mL, and >600 mL of contrast, respectively, and each 100 mL increment in contrast volume resulted in a 30% increase in the odds of CIN (odds ratio = 1.30; 95% confidence internal, 1.16–1.46) (34).

Prevention of CIN

In an attempt to minimize the harmful effects of contrast medium, multiple preventive modalities have been investigated and are summarized in Table 2. ***Adequate hydration is so far the only established way to reduce CIN (35).*** In patients with CRI undergoing angiography, hydration with 0.45% saline provided better protection against renal function deterioration than did hydration with 0.45% saline plus mannitol or furosemide (35). In patients with mild to moderate CRI, different modes of fluid administration (intravenous versus oral) were shown to produce similar effects (36). Isotonic saline was found to be superior over half-isotonic saline in reducing rates of CRI (0.7% versus 2%, respectively) (37). ***Bear in mind that patients with CRI and impaired left ventricle performance should be hydrated cautiously.*** In our institution, the recommended regimen of hydration in the presence of CRI is 1 cc/kg/h for 12 hours pre- and post-PCI for patients with normal ejection fraction and volume replacement matching urine output to maintain euvolemic state for 12 hours pre- and post-PCI for patients with moderately or severely reduced ejection fraction.

In a prospective, single-center, randomized trial of 119 patients, preventive hydration with sodium bicarbonate before and after iopamidol administration was more effective than hydration with sodium chloride for prophylaxis of CIN (38).

In a small, single-center, randomized study of 114 patients with CRI (serum creatinine >2 mg/dl), hemofiltration was shown to prevent deterioration of renal function and to reduce rates of initiation of dialysis post-PCI and one-year mortality in patients with CRI undergoing PCI (39). Prophylactic hemodialysis does not diminish the risk of CIN and may actually increase it (40).

Studies from our institution highlighted the negative impact of periprocedural hypotension and the use of an intra-aortic balloon pump in the development of CIN (27,41). The detrimental influence of prolonged hypotension on kidney function is well known; however, even relatively short periods of hypotension may be hazardous.

When a contrast agent is administered to patients treated with a nephrotoxic drug [nonsteroidal anti-inflammatory drugs (NSAIDs), several antibiotics, cyclosporine, cisplatin, etc.], the cumulative toxic effect on renal function may emerge. NSAIDs are well known to induce renal arteriolar vasoconstriction by inhibition of prostaglandin synthesis and have been shown to predispose to the nephrotoxic effect of radiocontrast media.

Finally, repeated use of contrast media within a short period of time (2 to 4 weeks) should be avoided if possible.

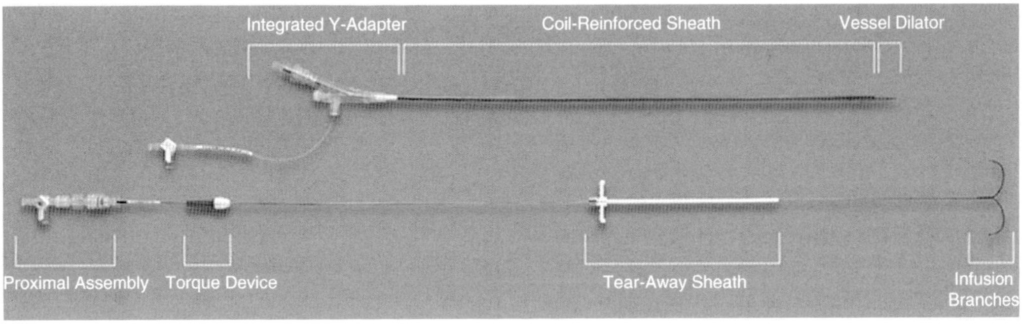

Figure 3 Benephit™ Infusion System (FlowMedica, Inc., Fremont, CA).

Targeted renal therapy

Targeted renal therapy is a novel catheter-based approach aimed at delivery of renal vasodilator agents such as fenoldopam, a selective dopamine-1 receptor agonist, and nesiritide, a B-type natriuretic peptide, directly to the kidneys via the renal arteries using Benephit™ Infusion System (FlowMedica, Inc., Fremont, CA) to maximize the beneficial kidney effects of drugs while minimizing systemic side effects (Fig. 3). Ongoing trials are addressing the issue of whether local drug delivery will allow the reduction of CIN rates in patients undergoing contrast medium exposure (42).

CONCLUSION

Chronic renal insufficiency is a frequent comorbidity in patients undergoing PCI. There is a remarkable body of evidence indicating that renal impairment, even mild, in patients undergoing PCI confers a clinically significant risk for excess mortality and morbidity. Estimation of creatinine clearance or GFR should be an essential part of the pre-PCI patient evaluation. Patients with impaired renal function are at increased risk of CIN, known to further worsen the prognosis of patients with CRI. To minimize dye- induced renal damage, patients should undergo adequate periprocedural hydration accounting for the left ventricle performance. Temporary periprocedural discontinuation of nephrotoxic agents is essential. Nonionic contrast agents provide lower rates of CIN and are therefore preferred in patients with impaired renal function. Undoubtedly, the amount of contrast should be minimized. Patients with baseline CRI warrant close surveillance and intensive medical management for early recognition of disease progression.

REFERENCES

1. Chew DP, Bhatt DL, Kimball W, et al. Bivalirudin provides increasing benefit with decreasing renal function: a meta-analysis of randomized trials. Am J Cardiol 2003; 92:919–923.
2. Stone GW, Grines CL, Cox DA, et al. The Controlled Abciximab and Device Investigation to Lower Late Angioplasty Complications (CADILLAC) Investigators. Comparison of angioplasty with stenting, with or without abciximab, in acute myocardial infarction. N Engl J Med 2002; 346:957–966.
3. Levey AS, Coresh J, Balk E, et al. National Kidney Foundation. National Kidney Foundation practice guidelines for chronic kidney disease: evaluation, classification, and stratification. Ann Intern Med 2003; 139:137–147.
4. Rubenstein MH, Harrell LC, Sheynberg BV, Schunkert H, Bazari H, Palacios IF. Are patients with renal failure good candidates for percutaneous coronary revascularization in the new device era? Circulation 2000; 102:2966–2972.
5. Best PJ, Lennon R, Ting HH, et al. The impact of renal insufficiency on clinical outcomes in patients undergoing percutaneous coronary interventions. J Am Coll Cardiol 2002; 39:1113–1119.
6. Gruberg L, Dangas G, Mehran R, et al. Clinical outcome following percutaneous coronary interventions in patients with chronic renal failure. Catheter Cardiovasc Interv 2002; 55:66–72.

7. Szczech LA, Best PJ, Crowley E, et al. Bypass Angioplasty Revascularization Investigation (BARI) Investigators. Outcomes of patients with chronic renal insufficiency in the bypass angioplasty revascularization investigation. Circulation. 2002; 105:2253–2258.
8. Best PJ, Berger PB, Davis BR, et al. PRESTO Investigators. Impact of mild or moderate chronic kidney disease on the frequency of restenosis: results from the PRESTO trial. J Am Coll Cardiol 2004; 44:1786–1791.
9. Chew DP, Lincoff AM, Gurm H, et al. REPLACE-2 Investigators. Bivalirudin versus heparin and glycoprotein IIb/IIIa inhibition among patients with renal impairment undergoing percutaneous coronary intervention (a subanalysis of the REPLACE-2 trial). Am J Cardiol 2005; 95:581–585.
10. Berger PB, Best PJ, Topol EJ, et al. The relation of renal function to ischemic and bleeding outcomes with 2 different glycoprotein IIb/IIIa inhibitors: the do Tirofiban and ReoPro Give Similar Efficacy Outcome (TARGET) trial. Am Heart J 2005; 149:869–875.
11. Sadeghi HM, Stone GW, Grines CL, et al. Impact of renal insufficiency in patients undergoing primary angioplasty for acute myocardial infarction. Circulation 2003; 108:2769–2775.
12. Hirsh J, Anand SS, Halperin JL, Fuster V. American Heart Association. Guide to anticoagulant therapy. Heparin: a statement for healthcare professionals from the American Heart Association. Circulation 2001; 103:2994–3018.
13. Robson R. The use of bivalirudin in patients with renal impairment. J Invasive Cardiol 2000; 12(suppl F):33F–36F.
14. Best PJ, Lennon R, Gersh BJ, et al. Safety of abciximab in patients with chronic renal insufficiency who are undergoing percutaneous coronary interventions. Am Heart J 2003; 146:345–350.
15. Reddan DN, O'Shea JC, Sarembock IJ, et al. Treatment effects of eptifibatide in planned coronary stent implantation in patients with chronic kidney disease (ESPRIT Trial). Am J Cardiol 2003; 91:17–21.
16. Nikolsky E, Mehran R, Turcot D, et al. Impact of chronic kidney disease on prognosis of patients with diabetes mellitus treated with percutaneous coronary intervention. Am J Cardiol 2004; 94: 300–305.
17. Rinehart AL, Herzog CA, Collins AJ, Flack JM, Ma JZ, Opsahl JA. A comparison of coronary angioplasty and coronary artery bypass grafting outcomes in chronic dialysis patients. Am J Kidney Dis 1995; 25:281–290.
18. Halkin A, Mehran R, Casey CW, et al. Impact of moderate renal insufficiency on restenosis and adverse clinical events after paclitaxel-eluting and bare metal stent implantation: results from the TAXUS-IV Trial. Am Heart J 2005; 150:1163–1170.
19. Kuchulakanti PK, Torguson R, Chu WW, et al. Impact of chronic renal insufficiency on clinical outcomes in patients undergoing percutaneous coronary intervention with sirolimus-eluting stents versus bare metal stents. Am J Cardiol 2006; 97:792–797.
20. Iakovou I, Schmidt T, Bonizzoni E, et al. Incidence, predictors, and outcome of thrombosis after successful implantation of drug-eluting stents. JAMA 2005; 293:2126–2130.
21. Kuchulakanti PK, Chu WW, Torguson R, et al. Correlates and long-term outcomes of angiographically proven stent thrombosis with sirolimus- and paclitaxel-eluting stents. Circulation 2006; 113:1108–1113.
22. McCullough PA, Wolyn R, Rocher LL, Levin RN, O'Neill WW. Acute renal failure after coronary intervention: incidence, risk factors, and relationship to mortality. Am J Med 1997; 103:368–375.
23. McCullough PA, Sandberg KR. Epidemiology of contrast-induced nephropathy. Rev Cardiovasc Med 2003; 4(suppl 5):S3–S9.
24. Mehran R, Nikolsky E. Contrast-induced nephropathy: definition, epidemiology, and patients at risk. Kidney Int Suppl 2006; (100): S11–S15.
25. Gruberg L, Mintz GS, Mehran R, et al. The prognostic implications of further renal function deterioration within 48 h of interventional coronary procedures in patients with pre-existent chronic renal insufficiency. J Am Coll Cardiol 2000; 36:1542–1548.
26. Hall KA, Wong RW, Hunter GC, et al. Contrast-induced nephrotoxicity: the effects of vasodilator therapy. J Surg Res 1992; 53:317–320.
27. Mehran R, Aymong ED, Nikolsky E, et al. A simple risk score for prediction of contrast-induced nephropathy after percutaneous coronary intervention: development and initial validation. J Am Coll Cardiol 2004; 44:1393–1399.
28. Taliercio CP, Vlietstra RE, Ilstrup DM, et al. A randomized comparison of the nephrotoxicity of

iopamidol and diatrizoate in high risk patients undergoing cardiac angiography. J Am Coll Cardiol 1991; 17:384–390.

29. Schwab SJ, Hlatky MA, Pieper KS, et al. Contrast nephrotoxicity: a randomized controlled trial of a nonionic and an ionic radiographic contrast agent. N Engl J Med 1989; 320:149–153.
30. Aspelin P, Aubry P, Fransson SG, Strasser R, Willenbrock R, Berg KJ. Nephrotoxicity in High-Risk Patients Study of Iso-Osmolar and Low-Osmolar Non-Ionic Contrast Media Study Investigators. Nephrotoxic effects in high-risk patients undergoing angiography. N Engl J Med 2003; 348: 491–499.
31. Barrett BJ, Carlisle EJ. Meta-analysis of the relative nephrotoxicity of high- and low-osmolarity iodinated contrast media. Radiology 1993; 188:171–178.
32. Sam AD 2nd, Morasch MD, Collins J, Song G, Chen R, Pereles FS. Safety of gadolinium contrast angiography in patients with chronic renal insufficiency. J Vasc Surg 2003; 38:313–318.
33. Rieger J, Sitter T, Toepfer M, Linsenmaier U, Pfeifer KJ, Schiffl H. Gadolinium as an alternative contrast agent for diagnostic and interventional angiographic procedures in patients with impaired renal function. Nephrol Dial Transplant 2002; 17:824–828.
34. Nikolsky E, Mehran R, Turcot D, et al. Impact of chronic kidney disease on prognosis of patients with diabetes mellitus treated with percutaneous coronary intervention. Am J Cardiol 2004; 94: 300–305.
35. Solomon R, Werner C, Mann D, D'Elia J, Silva P. Effects of saline, mannitol, and furosemide to prevent acute decreases in renal function induced by radiocontrast agents. N Engl J Med 1994; 331:1416–1420.
36. Taylor AJ, Hotchkiss D, Morse RW, McCabe J. PREPARED: Preparation for Angiography in Renal Dysfunction: a randomized trial of inpatient vs. outpatient hydration protocols for cardiac catheterization in mild-to-moderate renal dysfunction. Chest 1998; 114:1570–1574.
37. Mueller C, Buerkle G, Buettner HJ, et al. Prevention of contrast media-associated nephropathy: randomized comparison of 2 hydration regimens in 1620 patients undergoing coronary angioplasty. Arch Intern Med 2002; 162:329–336.
38. Merten GJ, Burgess WP, Gray LV, et al. Prevention of contrast-induced nephropathy with sodium bicarbonate: a randomized controlled trial. JAMA 2004; 291:2328–2334.
39. Marenzi G, Marana I, Lauri G, et al. The prevention of radiocontrast-agent-induced nephropathy by hemofiltration. N Engl J Med 2003; 349: 1333–1340.
40. Vogt B, Ferrari P, Schonholzer C, et al. Prophylactic hemodialysis after radiocontrast media in patients with renal insufficiency is potentially harmful. Am J Med 2001; 111:692–698.
41. Dangas G, Iakovou I, Nikolsky E, et al. Contrast-induced nephropathy after percutaneous coronary interventions in relation to chronic kidney disease and hemodynamic variables. Am J Cardiol 2005; 95:13–19.
42. Ng MK, Tremmel J, Fitzgerald PJ, Fearon WF. Selective renal arterial infusion of fenoldopam for the prevention of contrast-induced nephropathy. J Interv Cardiol 2006; 19:75–79.

13

Drug-eluting stent restenosis

John Cosgrave and George Dangas

INTRODUCTION

Drug-eluting stents (DESs) have been enthusiastically adopted by the interventional community following encouraging data from randomized trials (1,2). As with many new technologies initial enthusiasm is being dampened by more realistic results from complex patient and lesion subsets. There is no doubt that DESs represent a vast improvement; however, we must realize that they are not a magic bullet and restenosis remains a real problem. We will present data on the incidence, etiology, treatment, and prognosis of this challenging lesion cohort. While many new stents and drugs are under investigation or have recently come to the market, we will focus on the two initially commercially available platforms—the sirolimus-eluting (SES) Cypher™ stent (Cordis/Johnson & Johnson, Warren, NJ) and the paclitaxel-eluting (PES) Taxus™ stent (Boston Scientific, Natick, MA).

RATE OF RESTENOSIS

Data from the randomized trials (Table 1) of DESs have revealed in-stent angiographic restenosis rates in single figures. Despite these encouraging results it must be realized that these represent selected cohorts and may not reflect the true incidence in the real world. Indeed, when we consider bifurcation lesions, chronic total occlusions, and patients with diabetes mellitus, the incidence of restenosis can be as high as 20% (3,4). While there is no doubt that drug-eluting stents have dramatically reduced the incidence of restenosis, this very fact has also encouraged the percutaneous treatment of increasingly complex patients and lesions. Coupled with the widespread utilization of DESs and the numbers of percutaneous interventions (PCIs) performed per year, this means that even if restenosis rates are less than 10% (somewhat optimistic), the problem of DES restenosis has the potential to be a significant one. **If we estimate that over 2.5 million PCIs were performed worldwide in 2006 and that DESs reduced overall restenosis to 8%, there would still be a large number (150,000 cases based on a DES usage of 75%).**

MECHANISMS OF RESTENOSIS

When considering DES restenosis the pathophysiology of bare metal stent restenosis remains pertinent as the actual stent platforms have changed little (5). **The success of DESs in abrogating the proliferative response depends on a combination of stent scaffolding, homogeneous drug elution controlled by the**

Table 1 Restenosis rates from randomized trials

	DES-treated patients	*Angiographic follow-up*	*In stent restenosis*	*In segment restenosis*	*TLR*
SIRIUS	533	65.6%[a]	3.2%	8.9%	4.1%
E SIRIUS	175	92%	3.9%	5.9%	4%
SES Smart	128	96%	4.9%	9.8%	7%
TAXUS IV	662	44%[b]	5.5%	7.9%	3%
TAXUS V	577	86%	13.7%	18.9%	8.6%
TAXUS VI	219	96%	9.1%	12.4%	6.8%

[a]350 SES patients underwent angiographic follow-up, which was 86% of a pre-specified cohort but only 65.6% of the total cohort.
[b]292 PES patients underwent angiographic follow-up, which was 76.4% of a pre-specified cohort but only 44% of the total cohort.

polymer, and drug efficacy. Therefore, a number of issues may relate particularly to DES restenosis and our understanding of this phenomenon has been greatly enhanced by intravascular ultrasound, albeit in small sub-studies (Table 2). Another important concept is that stent-based drug delivery can lead to large concentration gradients with the amount of drug in the tissue varying from nil to several times the mean over extremely short distances (6). This means that relatively subtle alterations may have profound implications for effective drug delivery.

Table 2 Etiology and risk factor for DES restenosis

Etiology	*Risk factors*
Stent under-expansion	Advancing age
Stent over-expansion	Female sex
Strut fracture	Diabetes mellitus
Non-uniform strut distribution	Prior CABG
Mural thrombus	Bifurcations
Non-uniform drug deposition	Chronic total occlusions
Localized hypersensitivity	Reference vessel diameter
Drug efficacy	Stent length

Stent under-expansion

An under-expanded stent may not achieve complete apposition to the endothelium and more drug may be lost in the blood stream and less eluted into the vessel wall (Fig. 1). Under-expansion has been implicated in SES restenosis and an analysis from the TAXUS IV study has shown a decrease in target lesion revascularization in stents deployed at higher pressures (7,8). **In a study of IVUS guided stent implantation, Cheneau et al. demonstrated that only 15% of the stents were adequately expanded at 14 atm whereas 60% were adequately expanded at 20 atm (9).** Despite the poor stent expansion the apposition to the vessel wall was in fact good at 14 atm. Another study of 2.5 mm stent implantation in 200 lesions without post-dilation showed that the stents only achieved 75 ± 10% of the predicted minimal stent diameter and 66 ± 17% of the predicted minimal stent area (predicted by manufacturers' compliance charts). A significant number of stents (24% of SESs and 28% of PESs) did not achieve a final minimal stent area of 5 mm^2, a cut off often associated with the development of restenosis (10). In an IVUS analysis of 13 restenotic lesions (11 in stent), stent under-expansion was demonstrated in 7 (64%) stents (11).

It is realized that much of these data are derived from small studies; however, we feel that many stents benefit from high pressure

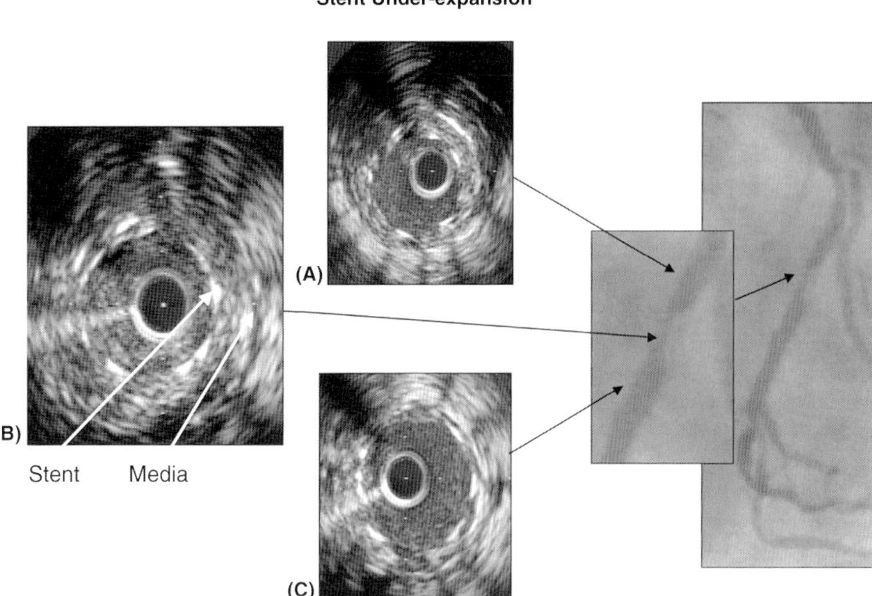

Figure 1 IVUS images from a restenotic circumflex lesion showing under-expansion. (**A**) Proximal to lesion demonstrating adequate expansion. (**B**) Restenotic segment demonstrating under-expansion. (**C**) Distal to lesion demonstrating adequate expansion.

implantation usually with a non-compliant balloon.

Stent over-expansion

Paradoxically not only is under-expansion a potential risk for restenosis but likewise over-expansion may cause problems. In the early period of DES implantation, the largest stent available was the 3 mm SES; in a study from Milan these 3 mm stents were post-dilated with a 3.5 mm balloon and the TLR rate was 13% (12). **Stent over-expansion may lead to strut fracture or polymer disruption, which impairs homogeneous drug delivery (13).** It is also possible that in the absence of a mechanical stent problem, the drug dose on the smaller stent may be inadequate for the surface area of a larger vessel. Despite this interesting and reasonable hypothesis no data, are currently available to support it. With the advent of a greater range of stent sizes, the problem of over-dilation will become a historical one.

STRUT FRACTURE

Due to the concept of complete lesion coverage advocated with DESs, longer stents are being increasingly implanted. **Longer stents are exposed to greater radial forces and are also more affected by vessel flexion and subsequent deformity (Fig. 2).** These factors can compromise stent integrity and it is no surprise that strut fracture has been reported in a 33-mm SES with focal restenosis (13). Fourteen cases of strut fracture were recently reported, all occurring in the mid-portion of the stent. The majority of the stents were implanted in angulated sections of coronary arteries. Focal restenosis at the site of the strut fracture was found in 6 (43%) of the cases (14). Despite this association it is unlikely that mechanical stent problems account for the majority of cases of restenosis.

Non-uniform distribution of stent struts

Local vessel factors such as the degree of calcification or plaque consistency and burden imply that not all stents are symmetrically implanted. This may lead to inhomogeneous drug distribution due to the variability in distance between the stent struts (Fig. 3). **An in vitro study showed that non-uniform circumferential stent strut distribution affected local drug concentrations (6).**

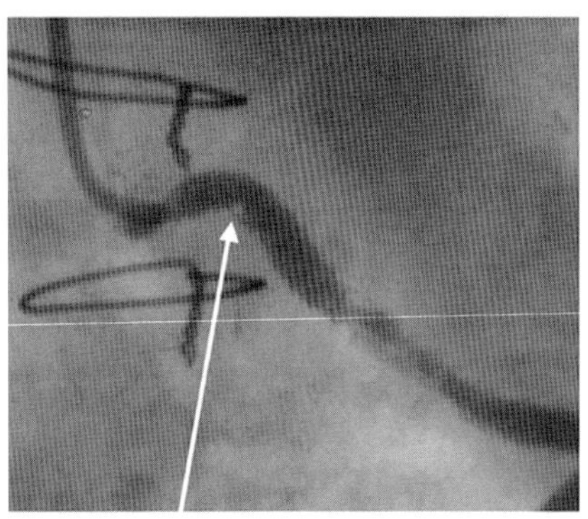

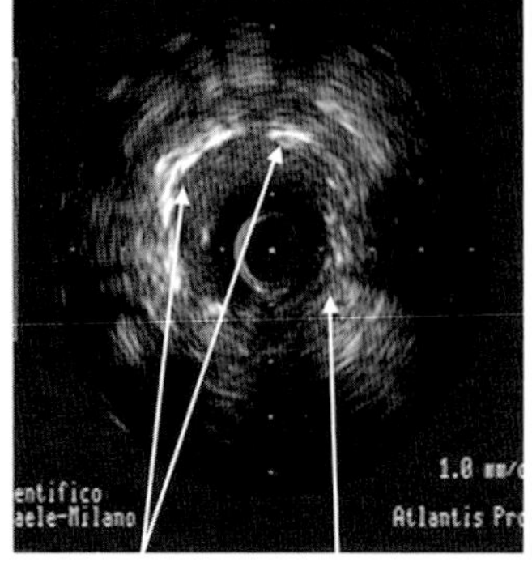

Figure 2 IVUS image showing strut fracture at a "hinge" point (indicated by the arrow on the angiogram) in a saphenous vein graft. No stent struts are visible between 1 and 6 o'clock. The absence or paucity of stent struts is the classic IVUS finding of strut fracture.

An IVUS study compared 24 SES restenotic lesions with 25 SES controls without restenosis (15). The number of visible stent struts and the maximum inter-strut angle were measured. The restenotic segments had fewer visible stent struts and a greater inter-strut angle than normal cross sections in the same stents and compared to the non-restenotic SES. This study also found that the maximum neo-intimal hyperplasia occurred at the site of the maximum inter-strut angle.

MURAL THROMBUS

It is not surprising that the milieu into which the drug is released also affects the drug distribution. In particular mural thrombus, which is

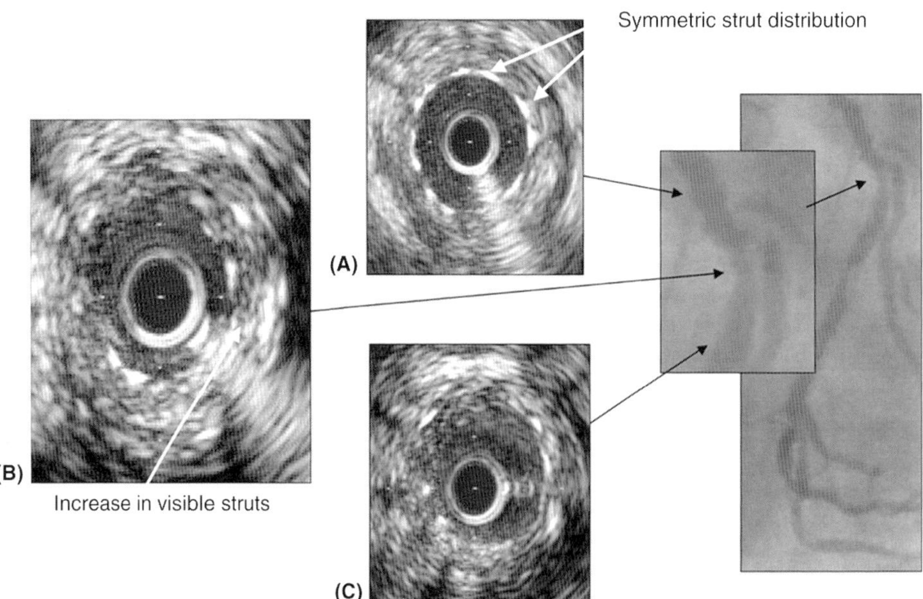

Figure 3 IVUS images from a restenotic circumflex lesion. (**A**) Proximal to lesion demonstrating normal strut symmetry. (**B**): Restenotic segment demonstrating asymmetric strut distribution with an increase in visible struts between 2 and 7 o'clock and a corresponding decrease between 9 and 12. (**C**) Distal to lesion demonstrating acceptable strut symmetry.

often formed at the time of stent implantation, can have a number of different effects (16). An in vitro study examined the effect of clot consistency on paclitaxel diffusion. Blood clots retained 3 times the amount of paclitaxel as surrounding solutions. Paclitaxel diffusion was fastest in fibrin-rich thrombus and the higher the proportion of red cells, the slower the diffusion. A computational model was used to predict the potential of thrombus to absorb, retain, and release drug. **The authors postulated the thrombus between the stent struts and the vessel wall could reduce uptake by 10 times, whereas thrombus overlying the stent struts could protect them from drug washout by the bloodstream.** While this hypothesis is fascinating, it is currently unclear precisely how much clinical relevance it has.

NON-UNIFORM DRUG DEPOSITION

It is often assumed that the most important method of drug delivery to the vessel wall is by simple diffusion from areas of strut to arterial wall contact, suggesting that it is only the drug on the abluminal surface of the stent that is effective. This somewhat simplistic approach fails to take into account the effect of drug loss into the blood stream from the adluminal surface. Alterations in the pattern of blood flow often caused by the stent itself may have an important role in determining arterial wall drug deposition by creating areas of stagnation and drug pooling. These concepts are impossible to study even in an animal model, however Balakrishnan et al. have developed a "coupled computational fluid dynamics and mass transfer model."

Using this model, they suggest that only 11% of total drug deposition is accounted for by direct strut artery contact, while 43% is derived from the adluminal surface (17). Another interesting finding was that non-apposed struts can still deliver a significant amount of drug. This is reassuring when we consider how common malapposition is. In this model greater separation of the struts led to greater variability in drug concentrations with peaks and troughs, which could of course decrease efficacy. This concurs with one of the IVUS studies of restenotic lesions (15). Mathematical models such as this one can give us a better understanding of drug elution and cause us to question some of our core precepts, however the clinical relevance of these theories has yet to be defined.

LOCALIZED HYPERSENSITIVITY

As DESs are composed of a polymer and a drug in conjunction with the stent platform, the possibility of a localized hypersensitivity reaction to any of these components exists.

Autopsy findings from a patient who died following a thrombosis in a SES revealed an aneurysmal vessel with an extensive inflammatory infiltrate involving the intima, media, and adventitia consisting of lymphocytes, plasma cells, macrophages, and eosinophils (18). Recently data from the Research on Adverse Drug Events And Reports (RADAR) project have been published (19). From 5,783 reports in the Food and Drug Administration (FDA) database, 262 cases demonstrated hypersensitivity symptoms of which only two could definitely be attributed to clopidogrel. From a variety of sources the authors identified 17 cases that were felt to be probably or definitely related to stent implantation rather than concomitant medications. In four of these cases a stent thrombosis was the cause of death and autopsy data were available. **Eosinophilic infiltrates consistent with localized hypersensitivity were demonstrated.** As with all cases of hypersensitivity, it is often difficult to know what is the precise cause, however we know that metal allergies have caused problems with bare metal stents. The increasing complexity of stents with drug and polymer means that a role for hypersensitivity in the etiology of DES restenosis must be considered.

DRUG EFFICACY

Despite all the complex theories about variations in drug deposition we must acknowledge that even if the drug is deposited in an optimal fashion some patients may be resistant to its effects. **Rapamycin resistance has been described in different cell lines due to receptor mutations or down regulation of transcription proteins (20). In vitro, some tumor cells have**

demonstrated paclitaxel resistance mediated by increased production of P-glycoprotein or via mutations in β-tubulin (21). Interestingly polymorphisms in the gene that encodes for proteins involved in paclitaxel metabolism (ATP binding cassette sub-family B member 1, also known as MDR1 and P-glycoprotein 170) have recently been shown to be associated with increased late loss in PES. The CT and TT genotypes had a higher incidence of binary restenosis and a higher late loss than the CC genotype (22). It is currently unclear how relevant drug resistance is in the etiology of DES restenosis, however this certainly warrants further investigation.

LATE RESTENOSIS

Despite reassuring long-term results from both the FIM and RAVEL studies, concerns exist about the possibility of a late catch-up phenomenon similar to that seen following brachytherapy (23–25). A porcine model has demonstrated significant advantage in terms of neo-intimal area at 30 days for SES compared to bare metal stents. However this advantage was not sustained at 90 or 180 days with similar degrees of neo-intimal proliferation in both stents (26). A recent case report has confirmed the occurrence of this phenomenon in humans; two patients with normal angiography at 7 months presented with recurrent symptoms 18 and 20 months after the index procedure (27). In both cases the previously patent stents demonstrated significant restenosis.

We have recently analyzed follow-up data on our first year of SES implantation: restenosis occurred in 160 lesions (23.5%); of these, 29 (4.3%) occurred after 1 year. In 20 patients a 6–9 month angiography was normal, and 9 patients who were asymptomatic subsequently developed late onset symptoms and angiography demonstrated restenosis. The mean time of documentation was 629 ± 221 days. Insulin-requiring diabetes mellitus was associated with late restenosis and interestingly the reference vessel diameter (RVD) at baseline was larger in the late restenosis group. This association with RVD may simply imply that it takes longer for a sufficient neo-intimal tissue volume to develop in larger vessels.

PREDICTORS OF RESTENOSIS

Data from Patrick Serruys' group reported on a selected high risk cohort of 238 patients from their overall experience (28). The restenosis rate was 7.9% and ostial location, diabetes mellitus, total stent length, reference vessel diameter, and lesion location in the left anterior descending coronary artery were all significantly associated with the occurrence of restenosis. In another study of high risk groups, a total of 263 lesions were analyzed (29). They found that the only predictors of restenosis were female sex and lesion length > 30 mm. In an analysis of 1,795 unselected patients following SES or PES implantation from Korea, the incidence of restenosis was 8.8%. Multivariate analysis revealed that post-intervention minimal lumen diameter, lesion length, and the use of PES rather than SES were associated with restenosis (30). The largest published cohort to date comprised 1845 patients with 2093 lesions (31). In this paper which included a number of patients from randomized comparative trials of both SESs and PESs as well as non-randomized SES data, the angiographic follow-up was 81% with a restenosis rate of 13%. Univariate analysis revealed that advancing age, female sex, prior coronary artery bypass surgery, complex lesions, chronic total occlusions, smaller vessels, longer lesions, stent length, final diameter stenosis, and PES implantation were all associated with restenosis. Using a multivariate model, female sex, prior coronary artery bypass surgery, chronic total occlusions, smaller vessels, maximum balloon inflation pressure, stent type, and final diameter stenosis all remained associated with restenosis. Of particular interest is the lack of association of diabetes mellitus with restenosis in this study, however we still feel that diabetes remains an important risk factor. Important problems with this study are the non-sequential time period during which SESs and PESs were used and the lack of baseline data regarding PES and SES patients to allow the reader to evaluate the different characteristics of the lesions and patients.

While the treatment of bifurcation lesions and chronic total occlusions were not shown to be predictors of restenosis in most of these studies, there is no doubt that both are associated with increased risk. In bifurcations the problem at the ostium of the side branch is the major offender while the increased risk with long stents frequently utilized in CTO is the corresponding risk factor (albeit less powerful than reference vessel size but still important) (32). **In essence the predictive factors of DES restenosis are similar to those for bare metal stents: diabetic patients, smaller vessels, longer stents, and complex lesions are more likely to undergo restenosis (Table 2).**

PATTERNS OF RESTENOSIS

The pattern of restenosis in the bare metal stent era is well described; the seminal paper by Mehran et al. described a useful categorization of restenosis (33). Pattern I included focal and multi-focal lesions less than 10 mm in length; pattern II was defined as >10 mm but within the stent margins (diffuse); pattern III, >10 mm and extending outside the stent (proliferative); and pattern IV was occlusive restenosis (Fig. 4). Not only was this classification easy to use but it also had significant clinical impact as it closely correlated with outcomes following treatment of restenosis with recurrence rates as low as 9% with a focal presentation and as high as 50% with an occlusive pattern. In the Mehran et al. series of 288 lesions, 42% were focal, 21% diffuse, 30% proliferative, and 7% occlusive. When classifying DES restenosis it is often difficult to differentiate between occlusive restenosis and clinically silent late stent thrombosis. While both will appear angiographically similar, the pathology is markedly different.

Two early reports of non-randomized data described the pattern of restenosis following SES implantation. **The majority of restenoses demonstrated a focal pattern** with 8 of 14 lesions being focal and the remaining 6 multifocal in the Milan experience and 12 of 14 lesions focal from the Rotterdam experience (34,35). With regard to PES implantation Iakovou et al. showed a 50% incidence of focal restenosis (36). These initial encouraging data were confirmed by both the SIRIUS (87% focal) and TAXUS IV (62% focal) studies (2,37). It must be realized that all these observations are either based on small numbers of lesions or on highly selected cohorts.

Recent data from our center (38) analyzed the largest cohort of restenotic lesions to date and included an unselected "real world" population. In the SES cohort of 150 lesions, 71% were focal, 16.7% diffuse, 0.7% proliferative, and 11.3% occlusive. **While the predominant pattern in the PES cohort of 149 lesions was also focal (51.7%), there was a significantly higher incidence of diffuse (26.2%) and occlusive restenosis (21.5%).** Similar to SES, proliferative restenosis is extremely rare (0.6%).

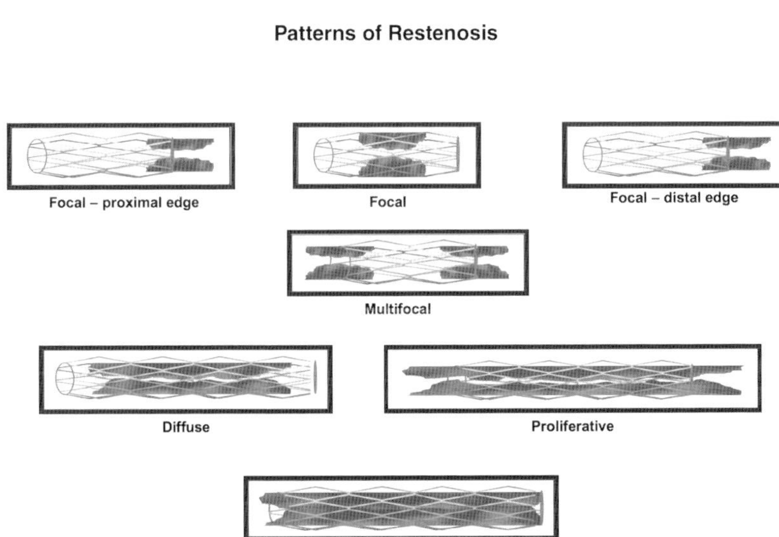

Figure 4 A classification for the pattern of restenosis. Focal <10mm in length, diffuse >10mm but within the stent, proliferative >10mm and extending beyond the stent margins, occlusive total occlusion of the stent. *Source*: From Ref. 33.

An interesting observation from this study is the location of restenosis when it occurs. For both stents focal restenosis occurred much more frequently at the margins of the stent and was significantly more likely to occur proximally than distally (61.0% vs. 16.9%, $p < 0.001$ for PES and 45.8% vs. 16.8%, $p < 0.001$ for SES). For lesions within the stent margins focal is more likely than diffuse restenosis for SES, whereas the opposite is the case for PES.

The increased occurrence of proximal edge restenosis with both stents seems counter-intuitive, one would expect that the proximal vessel would be larger and hence less prone to restenosis and less susceptible to baro-trauma. Perhaps this phenomenon is related to drug leaching from the stent proximally with consequently greater deposition distally (17). Balakrishnan et al. using a complex computational model have suggested that tissue segments beneath distal struts have a higher drug concentration than proximal struts.

TREATMENT OF RESTENOSIS

The treatment options for DES restenosis are similar to those for bare metal restenosis: balloon angioplasty (POBA), cutting balloon, athero-ablation, repeat stent implantation (or brachytherapy). Unfortunately there is a paucity of data to guide the interventional community and our decisions are currently being made on a best-guess basis. A number of basic statements seem logical based on data from our experience of bare metal restenosis. Cutting balloons are unlikely to be superior to POBA apart from the advantages seen in procedure times due to less balloon slippage (39). It seems reasonable to assume that if a DES has failed, implantation of a bare metal stent is unlikely to be successful particularly as it has not been shown to be better than POBA for bare metal stent restenosis (40,41). While brachytherapy seems attractive, it is not widely available particularly in Europe and the concerns about the long-term results will probably apply to the subset of DES restenosis as well (25). Another important issue to consider is the possibility of late stent thrombosis. Delayed endothelial healing is increasingly apparent following DES implantation and is a predisposing factor for thrombosis. Perhaps the "double-whammy" of an anti-proliferative drug followed by brachytherapy may be too great a burden for the endothelium to bear. Radiation dosing may need to be altered as the drug treated vessel may behave differently and we do not know what effect VBT will have on the non-resorbable polymer.

Initial published data on the treatment of 27 SES restenotic lesions, the majority treated with repeat DES implantation (44% SES and 41% PES), were somewhat disappointing. Most of the lesions were focal or multi-focal with only seven diffuse and one total occlusion. Angiographic follow-up was available for 21 lesions, which revealed a recurrence rate of 42.9% (42). **The following factors were associated with recurrence of the treated SES restenosis: prior brachytherapy, prior POBA restenosis, hyperlipidemia, treatment of the SES restenosis with POBA, and rapid onset SES restenosis.** For de novo lesions treated with SES that restenosed, the recurrence rate was 18.2%. Neither diabetes mellitus nor the pattern of restenosis influenced outcomes in this small study.

In the SIRIUS trial percutaneous target lesion revascularization (TLR) was required in 22 patients (43). The majority of the lesions were focal (91%); 18 received a bare metal stent (the only stents allowed), three were treated with POBA, and one with brachytherapy. A second restenosis that required revascularization occurred in 5 patients (23%).

Our own experience with DES restenosis encompasses 321 lesions (210 SES and 111 PES) treated prior to June 2005. When we compare the outcomes of repeat DES implantation and POBA for focal lesions, the restenosis rates are 16.7% and 27.7%, respectively ($p = 0.17$) and the TLR rates are 8.8% and 12.4% respectively ($p = 0.49$). Following the treatment of non-focal lesions the results are more disappointing with restenosis rates of 40.5% and 62.5%, respectively ($p = 0.15$) and TLR rates 21.1% and 22.6%, respectively ($p = 1.0$). If we consider the possibility of drug resistance in the etiology of restenosis, it is reasonable to speculate that implantation of a different DES would be superior to the same DES. Considering this hypothesis we found a restenosis rate of 12.9% compared to 19.1%, respectively, in focal lesions and a corresponding small improvement in TLR rates (6.4% compared with 10.3%). For non-focal lesions there was no difference in restenosis (40% and 41.2%) and again a small non-significant advantage for implanting a different DES in TLR rates (19.1% compared to 24.2%). **Not surprisingly the outcomes for focal lesions were better and repeat stent implantation, with a different DES seemed the best option.** These data must be interpreted cautiously as this was a non-randomized retrospective analysis; nevertheless it represents the largest cohort of DES restenotic lesions to date. One important observation from our data is that the percutaneous treatment of DES restenosis appears safe and in particular repeat DES implantation is not associated with any episodes of stent thrombosis in our series.

Two other studies have addressed the concept of implanting the same or different DES. One study reported the results of 150 SES restenotic lesions treated with PES implantation. The majority of the lesions were focal and the TLR rates were significantly higher in the non-focal group (30% vs. 11%, $p = 0.014$). Non-fatal subacute thromboses occurred in 2 cases, one each in focal and diffuse subtypes (both patients were receiving dual anti-platelet therapy) (44). The other study reported results of 108 SES and PES restenotic lesions, of which 64 received the same stent, 22 a different DES, 19 POBA, 2 bare metal stents, and 1 VBT. The overall TLR rate was 26% and there were no differences between the treatment groups in the clinical endpoints analyzed (45).

Case-based suggestions for the treatment of DES restenosis

While we have given an overview of restenosis following DES implantation, we would like to give some pertinent examples of how we approach this problem in our daily practice. While this approach is not strictly evidence based, we feel it is appropriate until further data become available. Where possible IVUS assessment is extremely helpful as the underlying pathology may guide the therapeutic decisions. Other critical issues are the importance of the vessel that has restenosed and, of course, the clinical situation of the patient. It seems unwise to embark on aggressive therapeutic strategies in asymptomatic patients with, for example, restenosis in a diagonal branch. In many cases further therapy is not necessary and we need to resist the oculo-stenotic reflex.

In our practice, our interventional approach to DES restenosis is the following:

- Focal in-stent or edge restenosis: IVUS optional, implantation of the same or different DES.
- Diffuse restenosis or stent occlusion: IVUS evaluation (to detect stent under-sizing) and implantation of a different DES (Fig. 5).

CHALLENGING SUB-GROUPS

We have already mentioned the importance of stent under-expansion and have suggested routine high-pressure dilation with a non-compliant balloon. Unfortunately this does not always work and we must consider other options. Sometimes the best option is to accept a sub-optimal result particularly in small vessels or asymptomatic patients. If, on the other hand, something needs to be done we can suggest two options. **The first is rotablation followed by repeat high pressure dilation and repeat DES implantation. The other option is to use laser atherectomy followed by high-pressure dilation and repeat DES implantation.** Fortunately this situation is rare but we have had two or three cases where rotablation was the only effective therapeutic modality.

A relatively rare problem is restenosis in an aorto-ostial location where a single stent may not provide adequate scaffolding to prevent elastic recoil. Similarly a single stent may not be sufficient in lesions with a large tissue burden as plaque prolapse can be problematic. **We have recently published our experience with the "sandwich" technique, which involves the placement of two stents one within the other with almost complete overlap (46).** While we do not routinely recommend this approach, it certainly has a niche application when implantation of the first stent gives a sub-optimal result.

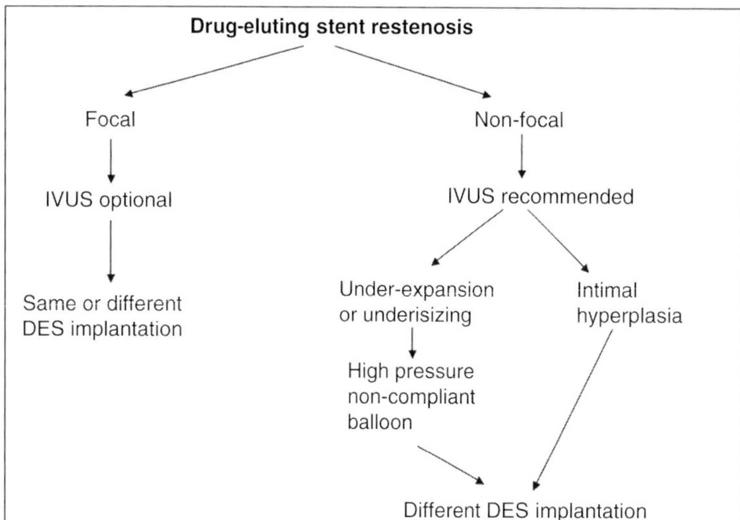

Figure 5 Suggested treatment paradigm for DES restenosis.

PROGNOSIS OF DES RESTENOSIS

There is no doubt that a focal pattern of restenosis in a bare metal stent conveyed a reasonably good prognosis with low recurrence rates regardless of the therapy used. With the increase in the proportion of focal restenosis, particularly following SES implantation, this observation could have significant clinical implications. We have recently studied the prognostic implications of the pattern of restenosis following both SES and PES implantation (47). We identified 250 lesions (66.4% SES and 33.6% PES); 163 were focal (65.2%) and 87 were non-focal (34.8%) lesions. **The rate of recurrent restenosis was 17.8% in the focal group and 51.1% in the non focal group (p = 0.0001).** The incidence of TLR also increased with the type of restenosis treated (9.8% and 23%, respectively; $p = 0.007$). An adjusted multivariate analysis revealed that a non-focal pattern remained associated with both the occurrence of restenosis and TLR (odds ratio, 5.1; 95% CI, 1.1–23; $p = 0.03$, and odds ratio, 3.61; 95% CI, 1.2–10.9); $p = 0.02$, respectively).

CONCLUSIONS

Despite the excellent results of DES, restenosis remains a significant issue particularly in complex patient and lesion subsets. The pathology of DES restenosis is probably very similar to that seen following bare metal stents, although we must consider the possibility of hypersensitivity to either the drug or the polymer. The etiology of restenosis is multi-factorial but is likely to be due to either inhomogeneous drug deposition for a variety of reasons or smooth muscle cell drug resistance, a poorly explored concept. Risk factors for the development of restenosis are diabetes mellitus, lesion length, reference vessel diameter, bifurcation lesions and chronic total occlusions. **Unlike bare metal stents the predominant pattern is focal, which is associated with a better prognosis.** Little data are available on the optimal therapeutic strategy but it seems reasonable to use POBA or repeat DES implantation for focal lesions and repeat DES implantation for non-focal lesions. Whatever therapeutic modality is utilized we should realize that most of the treatment options we have discussed seem superior to historical data from the bare metal stent era.

REFERENCES

1. Moses JW, Leon MB, Popma JJ, et al. Sirolimus-eluting stents versus standard stents in patients with stenosis in a native coronary artery. N Engl J Med 2003; 349:1315–1323.

2. Stone GW, Ellis SG, Cox DA, et al. A polymer-based, paclitaxel-eluting stent in patients with coronary artery disease. N Engl J Med 2004; 350:221–231.
3. Stone GW, Ellis SG, Cannon L, et al. Comparison of a polymer-based paclitaxel-eluting stent with a bare metal stent in patients with complex coronary artery disease: a randomized trial. JAMA 2005; 294:1268–1270.
4. Cosgrave J, Agostoni P, Ge L, et al. Clinical outcome following aleatory implantation of paclitaxel-eluting or sirolimus-eluting stents in complex coronary lesions. Am J Cardiology 2005; 96(12): 1663–1668.
5. Costa MA, Simon DI. Molecular basis of restenosis and drug-eluting stents. Circulation 2005; 111: 2257–2273.
6. Hwang CW, Wu D, Edelman ER. Physiological transport forces govern drug distribution for stent-based delivery. Circulation 2001; 104:600–605.
7. Fujii K, Mintz GS, Kobayashi Y, et al. Contribution of stent underexpansion to recurrence after sirolimus-eluting stent implantation for in-stent restenosis. Circulation 2004; 109(9):1085–1088.
8. Kutcher MA, Applegate RJ, Hermiller J, et al. Optimal stent implantation pressure in the drug-eluting-stent era: observations from the taxus iv study. Am J Cardiol 2004; 94(suppl 6A):213E.
9. Cheneau E, Satler LF, Escolar E, et al. Underexpansion of sirolimus-eluting stents: incidence and relationship to delivery pressure. Catheter Cardiovasc Interv 2005; 65(2):222–226.
10. de Ribamar Costa J, Mintz GS, Carlier SG, et al. Assessing drug-eluting stent expansion: lessons learned from intravacular ultrasound. (abstr). J Am Coll Cardiol. 2006; 47(suppl B):11B.
11. Kim BK, Oh S, Jeon DW, et al. Is stent underexpansion the main cause of in-stent restenosis after sirolimus-eluting stent implantation? an intravascular ultrasound study [abstr]. J Am Coll Cardiol 2006; 47(4 Suppl B):12B.
12. Iakovou I, Stankovic G, Montorfano M, et al. Is overdilatation of 3.0 mm sirolimus-eluting stent associated with a higher restenosis rate? Catheter Cardiovasc Interv 2005; 64(2):129–133.
13. Sianos G, Hofma S, Ligthart JMR, et al. Stent fracture and restenosis in the drug-eluting stent era. Catheter Cardiovasc Inter 2004; 61:111–116.
14. Yoon YW, Hong BK, Kwon HM, et al. Delayed strut fracture of sirolimus-eluting stent (CYPHER®) and related restenosis: A significant problem or an occasional observation? [abstr]. J Am Coll Cardiol 2006; 47(suppl B):3B.
15. Takebayashi H, Mintz GS, Carlier SG, et al. Nonuniform strut distribution correlates with more neointimal hyperplasia after sirolimus-eluting stent implantation. Circulation 2004; 110:3430–3434.
16. Hwang CW, Levin AD, Jonas M, Li PH, Edelman ER. Thrombosis modulates arterial drug distribution for drug-eluting stents. Circulation 2005; 111:1619–1626.
17. Balakrishnan B, Tzafriri AR, Seifert P, Groothuis A, Rogers C, Edelman ER. Strut position, blood flow, and drug deposition implications for single and overlapping drug-eluting stents. Circulation 2005; 111:2958–2965.
18. Virmani R, Guagliumi G, Farb A, et al. Localized hypersensitivity and late coronary thrombosis secondary to a sirolimus-eluting stent: should we be cautious? Circulation 2004; 109(6):701–705.
19. Nebeker JR, Virmani R, Bennett CL, et al. Hypersensitivity cases associated with drug-eluting coronary stents: a review of available cases from the Research on Adverse Drug Events and Reports (RADAR) project. J Am Coll Cardiol 2006; 47(1):175–181.
20. Huang S, Bjornsti MA, Houghton PJ. Rapamycins: mechanism of action and cellular resistance. Cancer Biol Ther 2003; 2(3):222-232.
21. Orr GA, Verdier-Pinard P, McDaid H, Horwitz SB. Mechanisms of Taxol resistance related to microtubules. Oncogene 2003; 22(47):7280–7295.
22. Ahn CM, Park S, Hong JA, Lee JH, Ko YG, Choi D, et al. Association of the polymorphism in the drug transporter gene ABCB1 with in-stent restenosis of Paclitaxel eluting stents in the Korean subjects [abstr]. J Am Coll Cardiol 2006; 47(4 suppl B):22B.
23. Sousa JE, Costa MA, Abizaid A, et al. Four-year angiographic and intravascular ultrasound follow-up of patients treated with sirolimus-eluting stents. Circulation 2005; 111(18):2326–2329.
24. Fajadet J, Morice MC, Bode C, et al. Maintenance of long-term clinical benefit with sirolimus-eluting coronary stents: three-year results of the RAVEL trial. Circulation 2005; 111(8):1040–1044.
25. Waksman R, Ajani AE, White RL, et al. Five-year follow-up after intracoronary gamma radiation therapy for in-stent restenosis. Circulation 2004; 109(3):340–344.
26. Carter AJ, Aggarwal M, Kopia GA, et al. Long-term effects of polymer-based, slow-release,

sirolimus-eluting stents in a porcine coronary model. Cardiovasc Res 2004; 63:617–624.

27. Wessely R, Kastrati A, Schömig A. Late restenosis in patients receiving a polymer-coated sirolimus-eluting stent. Ann Intern Med 2005; 143(5): 392–394.
28. Lemos PA, Hoye A, Goedhart D, et al. Clinical, angiographic, and procedural predictors of angiographic restenosis after sirolimus-eluting stent implantation in complex patients: an evaluation from the Rapamycin-Eluting Stent Evaluated At Rotterdam Cardiology Hospital (RESEARCH) study. Circulation 2004; 109(11):1366–1370.
29. Berenguer A, Mainar V, Bordes P, Valencia J, Gomez S, Lozano T. Incidence and predictors of restenosis after sirolimus-eluting stent implantation in high-risk patients. Am Heart J 2005; 150:536–542.
30. Lee CW, Park DW, Lee BK, et al. Predictors of restenosis after placement of drug-eluting stents in one or more coronary arteries. Am J Cardiol 2006; 97(4):506–511.
31. Kastrati A, Dibra A, Mehilli J, et al. Predictive factors of restenosis after coronary implantation of sirolimus- or paclitaxel-eluting stents. Circulation 2006; 113(19):2293–2300.
32. Colombo A, Moses JW, Morice MC, et al. Randomized study to evaluate sirolimus-eluting stents implanted at coronary bifurcation lesions. Circulation 2004; 109(10):1244–1249.
33. Mehran R, Dangas G, Abizaid AS, et al. Angiographic patterns of in-stent restenosis: classification and implications for long-term outcome. Circulation 1999; 100:1872–1878.
34. Lemos PA, Saia F, Ligthart JM, et al. Coronary restenosis after sirolimus-eluting stent implantation: morphological description and mechanistic analysis from a consecutive series of cases. Circulation 2003; 108(3):257–260.
35. Colombo A, Orlic D, Stankovic G, et al. Preliminary observations regarding angiographic pattern of restenosis after rapamycin-eluting stent implantation. Circulation 2003; 107:2178–2180.
36. Iakovou I, Schmidt T, Ge L, et al. Angiographic patterns of restenosis after paclitaxel-eluting stent implantation. J Am Coll Cardiol 2005; 45(5): 805–806.
37. Popma JJ, Leon MB, Moses JW, et al. Quantitative assessment of angiographic restenosis after sirolimus-eluting stent implantation in native coronary arteries. Circulation 2004; 110: 3773–3780.
38. Corbett SJ, Cosgrave J, Melzi G, et al. Patterns of restenosis after drug-eluting stent implantation: Insights from a contemporary and comparative analysis of sirolimus- and paclitaxel-eluting stents. Eur H J 2006; 27(19):2330–2337.
39. Albiero R, Silber S, Di Mario C, et al. RESCUT Investigators. Cutting balloon versus conventional balloon angioplasty for the treatment of in-stent restenosis: results of the restenosis cutting balloon evaluation trial (RESCUT). J Am Coll Cardiol 2004; 43(6):943–949.
40. Alfonso F, Zueco J, Cequier A, et al. Restenosis Intra-stent: Balloon Angioplasty Versus Elective Stenting (RIBS) Investigators. A randomized comparison of repeat stenting with balloon angioplasty in patients with in-stent restenosis. J Am Coll Cardiol 2003; 42(5):796–805.
41. Mehran R, Dangas G, Abizaid A, et al. Treatment of focal in-stent restenosis with balloon angioplasty alone versus stenting: Short- and long-term results. Am Heart J 2001; 141(4):610–614.
42. Lemos PA, van Mieghem CA, Arampatzis CA, et al. Post-sirolimus-eluting stent restenosis treated with repeat percutaneous intervention. Late angiographic and clinical outcomes. Circulation 2004; 109:2500–2502.
43. Moussa I, Moses JW, Kuntz RE, et al. The fate of patients with clinical recurrence after sirolimus-eluting stent implantation (a two-year follow-up analysis from the SIRIUS Trial). Am J Cardiol 2006; 97(11):1582–1584.
44. Damani SB, Lee SS, Sawhney N, et al. Paclitaxel-eluting stents are more effective in treating focal patterns of sirolimus-eluting stent restenosis compared to non-focal patterns of sirolimus-eluting stent restenosis [abstr]. J Am Coll Cardiol 2006; 47(suppl B):44B.
45. Shelton M, Moore A, Shelton MC, Ligon R, Mishkel G. Treatment of in-stent restenosis in drug eluting stents: Have stent sandwiches solved the problem? [abstr]. J Am Coll Cardiol 2006; 47(suppl B):44B.
46. Morici N, Cosgrave J, Iakovou I, et al. Sandwich drug-eluting stenting: A novel method to treat high-risk coronary lesions. J Invasive Cardiol 2006; 18(1):2–5.
47. Cosgrave J, Melzi G, Biondi-Zoccai GL, et al. Drug-eluting stent restenosis: The pattern predicts the outcome. J Am Coll Cardiol 2006; 47(12):2399–2404.

14

Intravascular ultrasound in the drug-eluting stent era

Gary S. Mintz

INTRODUCTION

In the bare-metal stent (BMS) era, serial (post-intervention and follow-up) intravascular ultrasound (IVUS) was crucial to understanding how stents worked, why they failed, and how to improve their effectiveness. Acute and chronic stent under-expansion was common, chronic stent recoil was rare, and late lumen loss was almost entirely the result of intimal hyperplasia (IH).

The importance of IVUS now can be extended to the drug-eluting stent (DES). This review will focus on the two DESs with the most clinical experience: Cypher® (Johnson & Johnson, New Brunswick, NJ) and Taxus® (Boston Scientific, Natick, MA). Most of the IVUS data, especially the clinical IVUS data, have been based on analyses of Cypher stents. It is not clear whether these data and clinical experience can be simply extrapolated to Taxus stents and, especially, to the next generation of DES.

IVUS FINDINGS IN DES THROMBOSIS

Fujii et al. (1) reported 15 patients who developed Cypher stent thrombosis and compared them with 45 matched controls. The minimum stent area (MSA) measured $4.3 \pm 1.6\,mm^2$ in Cypher thrombosis (vs. $6.2 \pm 1.9\,mm^2$ in controls, $p < 0.001$); stent expansion (MSA divided by the mean reference lumen area) was smaller ($65 \pm 18\%$ vs. $85 \pm 14\%$, $p < 0.001$); and a residual edge stenosis [reference minimum lumen area $<4\,mm^2$ with a plaque burden (plaque/ external elastic membrane) $>70\%$] was more common in the thrombosis group (67% vs. 9%, $p < 0.001$). However, there was no difference in the rate of acute or late stent malapposition between the two groups. In an unpublished study of 12 drug-eluting stent thromboses (eight Cypher and four Taxus) from the Washington Hospital Center, the MSA measured $<5.0\,mm^2$ in eight (Ashesh Bush, MD, personal communication). While these numbers are small, they are consistent with reports of BMS thromboses in which MSA and stent expansion were smaller, calcification was rare, and dissections were common when BMS thromboses were compared to non-thrombosed stents. An example is shown in Figure 1.

There is concern regarding the frequency of late stent thrombosis in DES-treated patients. In a study of 13 patients (eight of which had Cypher stents and five had Taxus stents) with late (>12 months) stent thrombosis, Cook et al. (2) reported that stent expansion ($60 \pm 26\%$) was less than in control patients without late DES thrombosis ($81 \pm 18\%$); incomplete stent apposition, associated with a larger peri-stent

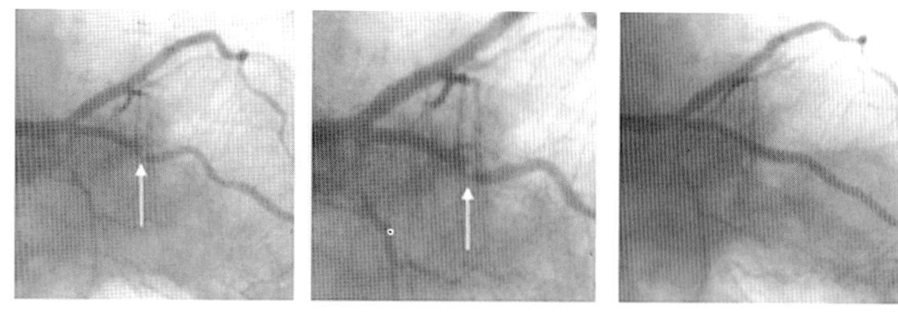

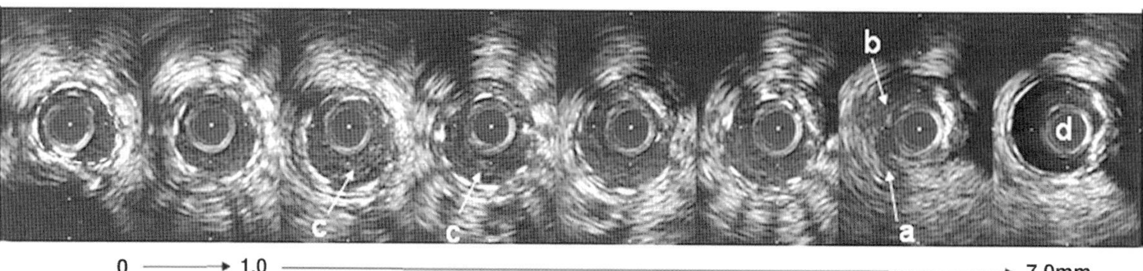

Figure 1 This patient presented with thrombosis of a 2.5 mm Cypher® stent four days after implantation. Note the filling defect (*white arrows*) in the ramus branch in (**A**) and in the magnified view (**B**). IVUS imaging (**D**) showed a perforation in the arterial wall (*a*) and a dissection plane abutting the IVUS catheter (*b*) just distal to the distal edge of the stent as well as the mottled, heterogeneous, hypoechoic in-stent tissue (*c*) representing stent thrombosis. (The dissection flap *b* is difficult to see because it abuts the IVUS catheter.) The minimum stent CSA (*dotted white line*) measured 3.5 mm^2 with a minimum diameter of 2.0 mm. [The distal reference lumen CSA (*d*) measured 5.0 mm^2.] Another stent was implanted overlapping the first and extending distally; the result is shown in (**C**). *Source*: From Mintz GS. Intracoronary ultrasound. London: Taylor and Francis Group; 2005 with permission.

external elastic membrane (EEM) cross-sectional area (CSA), was more common (77% vs. 12%). However, the authors did not state whether malapposition was acute and persistent or new and acquired, and this report contrasted with the report by Hong et al. (3) who found that late stent malapposition (LSM) occurred in 13.2% of 538 Cypher stents and 8.4% of 167 Taxus stents, but that there were no adverse events from implantation to when LSM was detected at 6 months or during the subsequent 12 months.

IVUS FINDINGS IN LATE DES MALAPPOSITION

The definition of late stent malappostion (LSM) is separation of at least one stent strut from the arterial wall intima, not overlapping a side-branch, with evidence of blood flow (speckling) behind the strut, and where the post-implantation IVUS revealed complete apposition of the stent to the vessel wall. It is most commonly caused by positive remodeling (a peri-stent increase in EEM CSA), either in the absence of or greater than any increase in peri-stent intimal hyperplasia. An example is shown in Figure 2.

Cypher

In SIRIUS, LSM was seen in 8.7% of Cypher stents versus no controls ($p < 0.05$). There were no deleterious clinical events in any of these 19 patients at 12 months post-stent implantation (4). A longer-term follow-up IVUS study from RAVEL indicated that malapposition discovered at 6-months post-implantation, in general, neither progressed nor regressed over the subsequent 12 months (5). However, exaggeration of the mechanisms responsible for LSM can cause aneurysm formation.

Taxus

In TAXUS-II, LSM at 6 months was seen in 8.0% of slow-release and 9.5% of moderate-release Taxus stents ($p = 0.3$ vs. 5.4% in controls). LSM detected at 6 months was not associated with adverse events at 12 months (including no stent thromboses) (6). In a subset of patients studied at

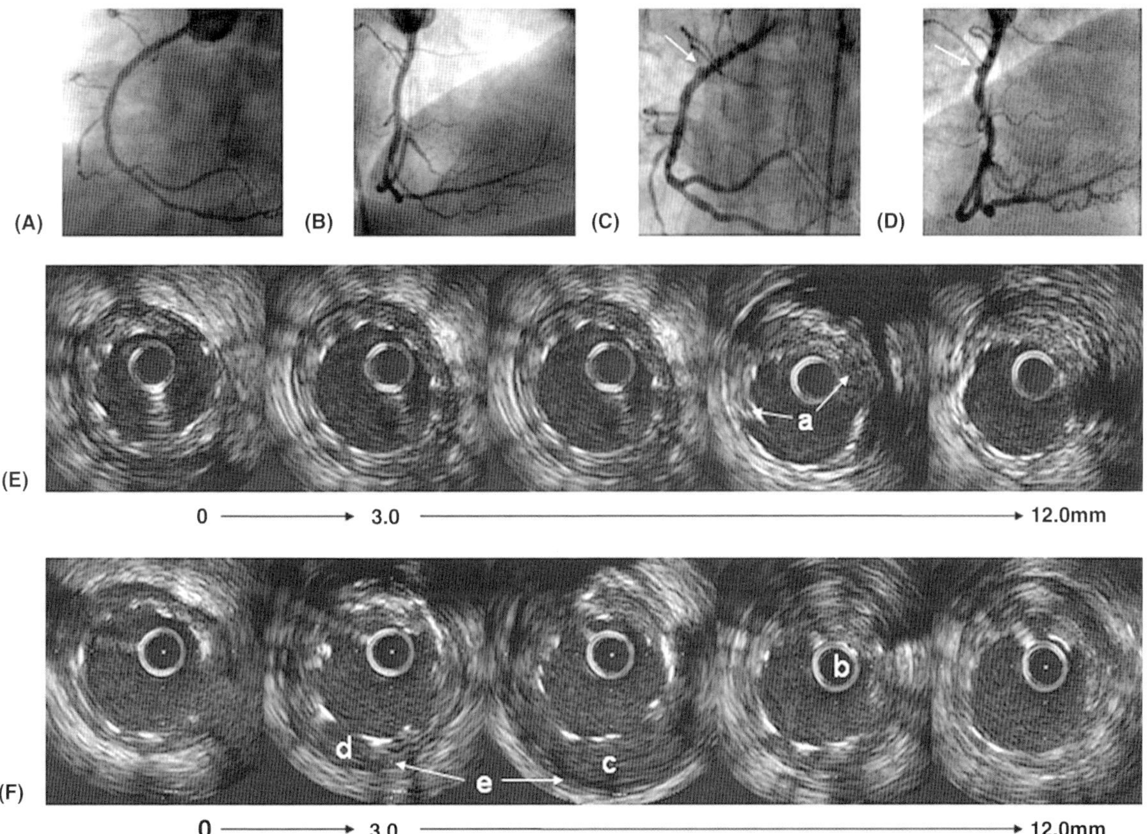

Figure 2 This patient underwent Cypher® stent implantation into a right coronary stenosis; the final angiogram is shown in (**A**) and (**B**). At follow-up (**C** and **D**) there was a focal angiographic aneurysm in the proximal right coronary (*white arrows*). The final (post stent implantation) IVUS is shown in (**E**), and the follow-up IVUS is shown in (**F**). Note the plaque prolapse (*a*) that is not present on the same image slice at follow-up (*b*). Also note the late stent malapposition (*c* and *d*) that involves the arc of normal vessel wall (*e*). At the site of maximum late stent malapposition (*c*), there has been an increase in EEM CSA from 17.8 mm^2 to 28.9 mm^2, along with an increase in effective lumen CSA (intra-stent lumen CSA plus area of malapposition) from 8.8 mm^2 to 16.8 nn^2. The stent CSA (8.8 mm^2) and the peri-stent P&M CSA (8.9 mm^2) have not changed. *Source*: From Mintz GS. Intracoronary ultrasound. London: Taylor and Francis Group; 2005, with permission.

2 years, the incidence of LSM was 0% in the slow-release group (down from 9.3%) and 2.4% in the moderate-release group (down from 9.8%) (7).

In TAXUS-IV, LSM was seen in 1.1% of slow-release Taxus stents versus 2.2% of controls (8). In TAXUS-V, LSM was seen in 8.7% of slow-release Taxus stents versus 4.1% of controls ($p = 0.3$) (9), and in TAXUS-VI, LSM was seen in 16.7% of moderate-release Taxus stents versus 4.3% of controls ($p = 0.018$). Finally, in a meta-analysis of TAXUS-IV, V, and VI, 9-month LSM was more common in Taxus than in control stents (8.4% vs. 3.5%, $p < 0.02$); this was predominantly driven by non-FDA approved moderate-release Taxus stent use. In TAXUS-VI, LSM was associated with less IH than fully apposed stents. One year later, there were no major adverse cardiac events (including stent thromboses) in any patient with LSM (10).

Asian Medical Center experience

In the report by Hong et al. the frequency of LSM increased after directional coronary atherectomy before stenting (25%); after primary stenting in acute myocardial infarction (MI) (32%), suggesting that thrombus dissolution may be important in infarct lesions that develop LSM); and in chronic total occlusions (27.5%). Independent predictors of LSM were total stent length, primary stenting in acute MI, and occlusions. In the subgroup of elective stenting after conventional balloon predilation, the only independent predictor of LSM was total stent length.

IVUS FINDINGS IN DES RESTENOSIS

Stent underexpansion as a cause of Cypher restenosis

In a substudy of SIRIUS where adequate patency was defined as a follow-up IVUS minimum lumen CSA >4 mm^2, Sonoda et al. (11) reported that the post-intervention MSA that best separated "adequate" from "inadequate" patency at follow-up was 5.0 mm^2. The positive predictive value for this cutoff point was 90%, suggesting that Cypher failure in SIRIUS was mostly due to stent underexpansion at the time of implantation.

In a study of 550 patients with 670 native coronary artery lesions treated with Cypher stents, Hong et al. (12) reported that the IVUS cut-offs that best predicted angiographic restenosis were an MSA of 5.5 mm^2 and a stent length of 40 mm. When patients were divided into subgroups, angiographic restenosis rates were 0.4% (MSA > 5.5 mm^2 and stent length < 40 mm); 2.4% (MSA < 5.5 mm^2 and stent length < 40 mm); 8.6% (MSA > 5.5 mm^2 and stent length > 40 mm); and 17.7% (MSA < 5.5 mm^2 and stent length > 40 mm (12).

These two studies were supported by two smaller, single-center "registries." In one IVUS study of 33 Cypher failures reported by Takebayashi et al. (13) an MSA <5.0 mm^2 was observed in 67%. In another study of 26 DES failures (21 Cypher stents and 5 Taxus stents) reported by Kim et al. (14), MSA measured 4.6 ± 1.5 mm^2; 61% had an MSA <5.0 mm^2 and 38% had an MSA <4.0 mm^2. However, in an analysis of 48 Cypher restenoses by Sano et al. (15), while 71% of stents had an MSA <5.0 mm^2 somewhere within the stent, this occurred at the minimum lumen site in only 46.9%.

It is important not to focus on a single MSA. While the studies by Sonoda et al. and Hong et al. reported the single MSA that *best separated restenosis from no restenosis*, it is important to note that the sensitivity of this single cut-off was only 75%, and an increasingly larger MSA was still associated with fewer restenotic events in both of these studies (Fig. 3). In support of this, in one study of patients with ostial LAD stenoses treated with Cypher stents, a final stent CSA of 7.4 ± 1.4 mm^2 was associated with only a 5.1%

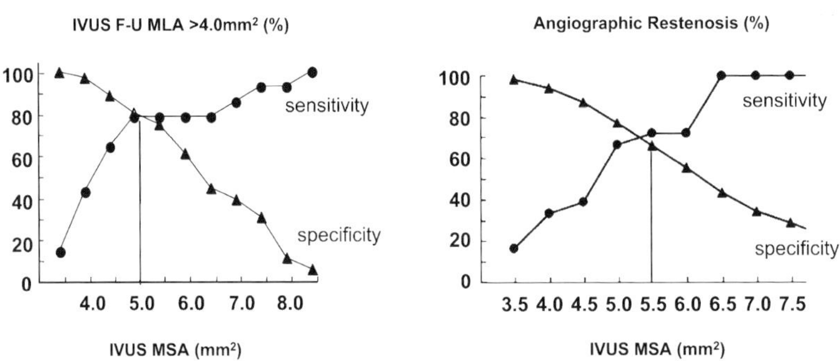

Figure 3 In (**A**) in 72 patients from the SIRIUS trial, the sensitivity and specificity curves identified different optimal thresholds of minimum stent area (MSA) to predict adequate follow-up IVUS minimum lumen area (MLA, defined as a lumen CSA 5 4.0 mm^2). However, the sensitivity of this threshold was 76%, the specificity 83%, the positive predictive value 90%, and the accuracy 78%. (**B**) was from a study by Hong et al. in which a 6-month follow-up angiography was performed in 449 patients (81.6%) with 543 lesions (81.1%) from the initial cohort of 550 patients with 670 native coronary lesions. Similar sensitivity and specificity curve analysis showed that the final minimum stent area by IVUS and IVUS-measured stent length that best separated angiographic restenosis from non-restenosis were 5.5 mm^2 and 40 mm, respectively. *Source*: From Refs. 11 and 12.

frequency of angiographic restenosis with no target lesion revascularizations (16).

Other causes of Cypher restenosis

Cypher stent failure has been attributed to strut fractures (17). The IVUS diagnosis of strut fracture requires documentation of stent struts present immediately post-procedure that are no longer seen at follow-up and not merely a paucity of struts at follow-up, or the nearly complete circumferential lack of stent struts within a single restenotic stent at follow-up. However, it is not clear whether Cypher strut fracture is a common or uncommon cause of restenosis. To date, serial IVUS documented stent strut fracture as a cause of Cypher restenosis has been documented and reported in the literature in less than ten cases. An example is shown in Figure 4.

Cypher stent failure has also been attributed to gaps between adjacent stent struts (17). Nonuniform stent strut distribution has been noted since the earliest days of BMS implantation; the uniformity and homogeneity of strut

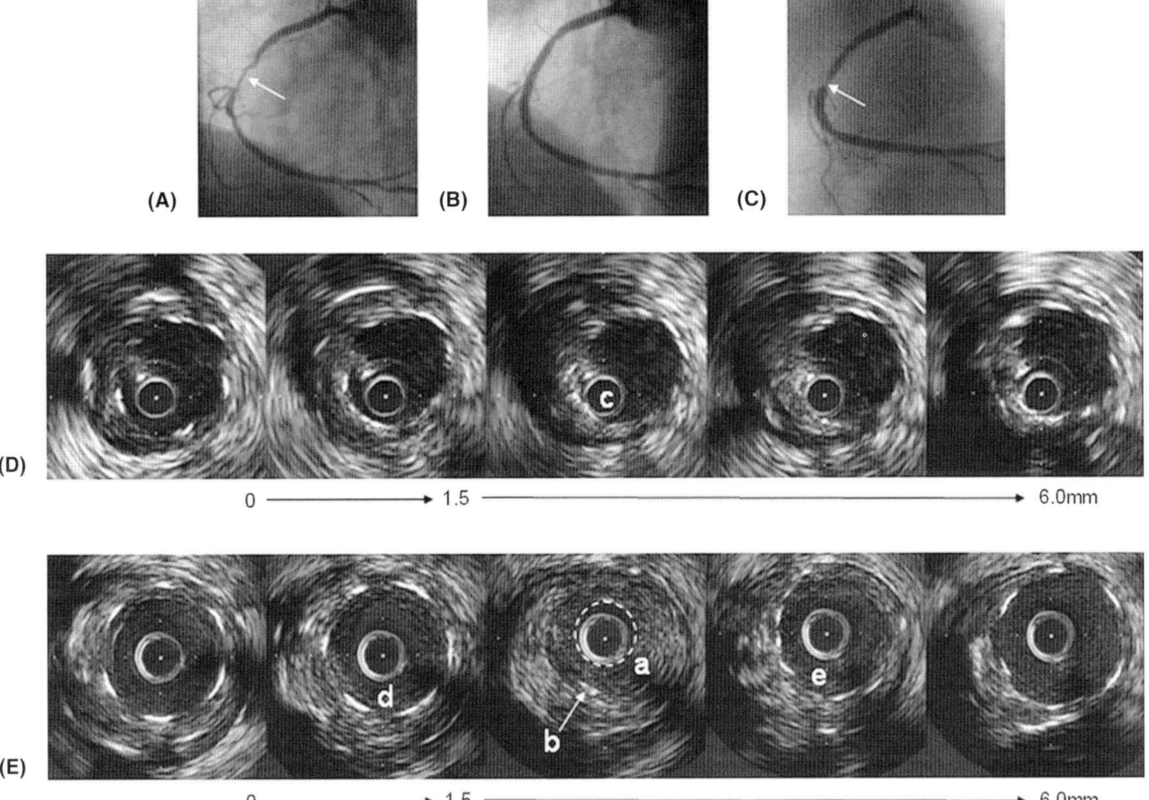

Figure 4 This long right coronary artery stenosis (*arrow* in **A**) was treated with two overlapping Cypher® stents (33 mm and 15 mm in length) with the final result shown in (**B**). At 7 month follow-up, there was focal in-stent restenosis (*arrow* in **C**). (**D**) shows the final (post-stent implantation) IVUS, and (**E**) shows the follow-up IVUS. The two imaging sequences show identical image slices. Note the superior resolution (sharpness) of (**E**) that was recorded using a 40 MHz transducer compared to (**D**) that was recorded using a 30 MHz transducer. At the site of focal intimal hyperplasia (*a*), the minimum lumen CSA (*dotted line*) measured 2.0 mm^2, and there was a paucity of stent struts (actually, only one stent strut, *b*) compared to the same image slice (*c*) on the post-intervention study. The intimal hyperplasia was very focal and extended for less than 2 mm proximally (*d*) and distally (*e*). This is an example of focal intra-sirolimus-eluting stent restenosis, possibly from strut fracture (struts were apparent at implantation that were not seen at follow-up). *Source*: From Mintz GS. Intracoronary ultrasound. London: Taylor and Francis Group; 2005, with permission.

distribution is unpredictable. It is, however, important to note that the IVUS appearance of stent strut distribution can be affected by transducer angle. In 24 Cypher restenoses, Takebayashi et al. (18) reported that the minimum lumen site had a larger maximum interstrut angle and fewer stent struts even when normalized for the number of stent cells compared to non-restenotic sites within the same stent and to non-restenotic Cypher stents. By implication, circumferential stent strut distribution affected the dose of sirolimus delivered to the arterial wall and, therefore, the amount of IH. In a subsequent report, Sano et al. (15) reported that there were fewer stent struts in restenotic lesions with adequate stent expansion than in lesions with stent underexpansion (MSA $<5.0\,\text{mm}^2$ at the minimum lumen site).

It is also important to distinguish between strut fracture and gaps between adjacent stent struts. It is easy to confuse the two if only follow-up IVUS studies are available and if there is a paucity rather than an absence of struts at follow-up.

Cypher edge restenosis

Of 31 Cypher failures in SIRIUS, 27 restenoses were focal and 19 were at the stent edges. Sakurai et al. (19) reported that larger reference plaque burdens and larger edge stent CSA/reference minimum lumen CSAs were associated with Cypher edge restenosis suggesting that incomplete lesion coverage—landing the stent edge within a plaque (even a secondary plaque)—contributed to edge restenosis. An example of Cypher edge restenosis is shown in Figure 5.

Restenosis after Cypher treatment of BMS restenosis

Recurrence is more common after Cypher treatment of BMS restenosis than after de novo Cypher implantation (20). In one study reported by Fujii et al. (21), nine of 11 patients who failed Cypher stent treatment of BMS restenosis had an MSA $<5.0\,\text{mm}^2$ versus five of 19 non-recurrences ($p = 0.003$); seven recurrent lesions had an MSA $<4.0\,\text{mm}^2$ versus four non-recurrences ($p = 0.02$); and a gap between Cypher stents was identified in three recurrences versus one non-recurrence (21).

Taxus

There are no data regarding predictors of Taxus stent failure (i.e., the importance of stent underexpansion), Taxus strut fracture, effect of non-uniform Taxus strut distribution, Taxus edge restenosis, or failure after Taxus treatment of BMS restenosis. However, considering that Taxus stents are associated with more intimal hyperplasia than Cypher stents, it is logical to conclude that Taxus stents should be expected to achieve better long-term results than Cypher stents.

CLINICAL USES OF IVUS IN THE DES ERA

When should IVUS be used?

There are no studies specifically addressing the clinical utility of IVUS in the DES era. In particular, there are no randomized angiographic versus IVUS trials. However, patients at higher risk for Cypher stent thrombosis (22,23) or restenosis have been described (20). Ostial lesions, diabetic patients, small vessels, long lesions, bifurcations, and treatment of in-stent restenosis are associated with higher rates of Cypher stent restenosis (20). Patients at high risk for stent thrombosis have renal failure, limitations to use of dual antiplatelet therapy, bifurcation lesions, diabetes, or poor ventricular function (16). Whenever these risk factors are present or when consequences of failure would be significant [i.e., unprotected left main coronary artery (LMCA) lesions], IVUS should be used to select the optimal stent size and length, and stent dimensions should be optimized for vessel size rather than settling for an MSA of $5.0–5.5\,\text{mm}^2$.

Assessment and treatment of intermediate stenoses

In the BMS era, intermediate lesions were routinely assessed with IVUS or invasive physiology. A pre-intervention IVUS minimum lumen CSA $\geq 4.0\,\text{mm}^2$ had a diagnostic accuracy of 92% in predicting a coronary flow reserve ≥ 2.0 (24). Nishioka et al. (25) found that the IVUS minimum lumen area had a diagnostic accuracy of 93% versus stress myocardial perfusion imaging. Takagi et al. (26) found similar results when the IVUS minimum lumen area was compared to fractional flow reserve measured by the pressure wire.

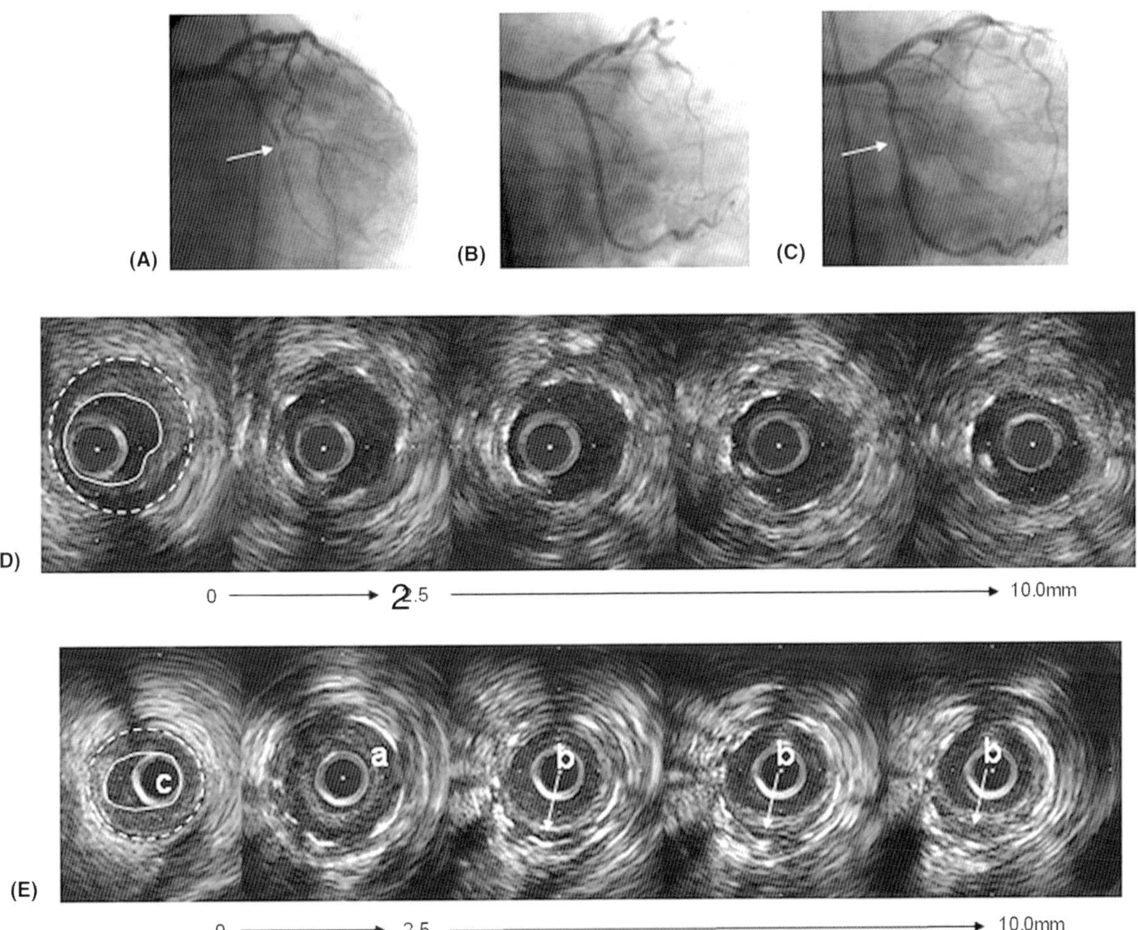

Figure 5 This left circumflex stenosis (*arrow* in **A**) was treated with implantation of an 18 mm long Cypher® stent. The final angiographic result is shown in (**B**). At 9 month follow-up, there was focal restenosis (*arrow* in **C**). (**D**) shows the final (post-stent implantation) IVUS, and (**E**) shows the follow-up IVUS. Note the focal proximal edge intimal hyperplasia (*a*) that extends distally (*b*). In addition, there is a decrease in proximal edge EEM CSA from 10.5 mm^2 (*dotted line* in **D**) to 6.9 mm^2 (*dotted line* in *c* in **E**), as well as a decrease in lumen CSA from 4.6 mm^2 (*solid line* in **D**) to 2.4 mm^2 (*solid line* in *c* in **E**). This is an example of focal proximal edge sirolimus-eluting stent restenosis from a combination of intimal hyperplasia precisely at the edge of the stent (*a*) and a decrease in EEM CSA more proximally (*c*). *Source*: From Mintz GS. Intracoronary ultrasound. London: Taylor and Francis Group; 2005, with permission.

In support of these studies, percutaneous intervention was deferred based on IVUS findings in 300 patients. Events occurred in 24 patients. There was an important difference between lesions with minimum lumen CSA above and below 4.0 mm^2. In 248 lesions with a minimum lumen CSA $\geq$4.0 mm^2, the event rate was only 4.4% and the revascularization rate was only 2.8% (27).

Moses et al. (28) reported 167 patients with intermediate lesions (angiographic diameter stenosis <50%) from SIRIUS, TAXUS-IV, and FUTURE I/II. At one year patients treated with DES had similar rates of cardiac death or myocardial infarction (3.4% vs. 5.4% in BMS, $p = 0.49$), fewer target vessel revascularizations (3.4% vs. 20.3%, $p = 0.0004$), major adverse cardiac events (5.6% vs. 25.4%, $p = 0.0003$), and binary angiographic restenoses (1.8% vs. 34.0%, $p < 0.0001$). No patient in either group developed stent thrombosis (28). Stenting of borderline lesions was safe with a rate of one-year events similar to deferred intervention, putting in question the need for IVUS or physiologic assessment of intermediate non-left main coronary lesions. Conversely, routine drug-eluting stent implantation was not better than judicious decision making, and it was presumably more expensive. IVUS can also unmask occult stenoses that may warrant treating with a second or a longer first drug-eluting stent (29). Whether invasive assessment of intermediate lesions makes sense may ultimately depend on the frequency and consequences of later (beyond 1 year) events—that is, late stent thrombosis.

Assessment and treatment of left main coronary artery (LMCA) disease

The most common criterion used in decisions for revascularization for LMCA disease is a minimum lumen CSA below 6.0 mm^2. This is based both on Murray's law [assuming that each daughter vessel (the LAD and the LCX) requires a minimum lumen CSA of 4.0 mm^2] (30) and the study by Jasti et al. (31) correlating IVUS with fractional flow reserve. We also reported 122 patients who underwent angiographic and IVUS assessment of left main coronary artery disease severity, who did not have subsequent catheter or surgical intervention and who were followed for at least 1 year. There were three distinct predictors of cardiac events: diabetes, a major epicardial vessel or bypass graft with an angiographic diameter stenosis ≥50% left untreated, and left main coronary artery lesion site minimum lumen diameter measured by IVUS (32).

There has been one published study of IVUS use during DES treatment of LMCA disease. In this study of 102 patients treated with Cypher stents, IVUS guidance was used in 86%; MSA measured 9.6 ± 2.6 mm^2, and target lesion revascularization at 1 year was performed in two Cypher stent patients (2.0%) (33). The low rate of Cypher failure in this study may be related to optimizing Cypher stent dimensions and expansion.

Adequate DES expansion

As noted, the single criterion that best predicted an adequate IVUS minimum lumen CSA at follow-up or freedom from angiographic restenosis was a minimum stent CSA of 5.0–5.5 mm^2. Is this adequate in all situations? First, there was still a stepwise relationship between a larger minimum stent CSA and a lower restenosis rate (Fig. 3). Second, the SIRIUS trial enrolled relatively low-risk patients. Third, even this modest cut-off was often not achieved. Interventionalists routinely rely on the manufacturer-supplied compliance chart to target final stent dimensions based on stent size and inflation pressure. However, a critical IVUS analysis showed DES achieved only 75 ± 10% of predicted minimal stent diameter and 66 ± 17% of predicted minimal stent CSA, and approximately 25% of DES implanted into >3.0 mm vessels did not achieve a final minimal stent CSA of >5.0 mm^2 (34). Thus, stent implantation guided by manufacturer-supplied charts can be associated with an unpredictably smaller final stent size.

Whenever there are risk factors for DES failure (restenosis or thrombosis), the minimum stent CSA should be optimized for the size of the vessel rather than settling for just a minimal stent CSA of 5.0–5.5 mm^2. Conversely, an MSA of 5.0 mm^2 may not be achievable in small vessels since it corresponds to a 0% residual stenosis in a 2.5 mm vessel and a negative residual stenosis in a <2.5 mm vessel, but it still can be vessel-size optimized; stent expansion (MSA/reference lumen area) in smaller vessels may be the best predictor of an adequate lumen at follow-up (35).

Stent CSA can be optimized by appropriate stent sizing based on pre-intervention IVUS followed by adjunct high-pressure balloon inflations guided by iterative IVUS. The safest paradigm is to size the stent to the largest reference lumen diameter whether proximal or distal to the lesion. More aggressive approaches (i.e., reference midwall sizing, discounted "media-to-media" sizing, etc.) must be balanced against a higher rate of acute complications including dissection or perforation.

Acute DES apposition

Apposition is different from expansion; the two terms and concepts are not interchangeable. Expansion refers to either the absolute MSA or the MSA relative to a pre-defined standard (i.e., the reference lumen CSA). Apposition refers to contact between the stent and vessel wall. Lack of expansion and apposition can occur together or separately, but they have different implications and technical solutions. Optimal expansion requires repeated adjunct inflations at higher pressures with or without larger balloon sizes to overcome resistance of the vessel/lesion to dilation. Conversely, because there is only blood between the malapposed stent strut and vessel wall, achieving full apposition just requires a larger balloon, sized to the intimal diameter and inflated at low pressures.

Full stent-vessel wall apposition appeared to be *less* important than adequate stent expansion. In the study by Hong et al. (3), post-procedure (acute) incomplete stent apposition was observed in 51 DES-treated lesions (7.2%). There were no major adverse cardiac events (including target lesion revascularization), and maximum intrastent IH CSA at follow-up measured $1.2 \pm 0.5\,mm^2$, similar to what was reported for stents with complete apposition[3]. In another IVUS study by Kimura et al. (36) of Cypher stents that were incompletely apposed at implantation, there was more IH at follow-up at the site of *complete* malapposition, resolution than at the site of *persistent* stent malapposition, and no patient developed angiographic restenosis. In TAXUS-II, eight of 13 acute stent malappositions in the slow-release group resolved; all acute stent malappositions in the moderate-release group resolved; and at 12 months of follow-up, acute stent malapposition was not associated with an increase in adverse clinical events (7). Thus, initial concerns that acute incomplete stent apposition would affect drug delivery to the vessel wall and lead to DES failure appeared to be unfounded, and aggressive adjunct inflations to eliminate acute stent malapposition seemed unwarranted. There are two possible explanations for the lack of a relationship between acute stent vessel wall malapposition and subsequent restenosis: Stent vessel wall apposition may be necessary to develop intimal hyperplasia, and, as demonstrated by Balakrishnan et al. (37), the overall tissue uptake of the drug was not just determined by the stent struts that are in direct contact with the arterial wall. Local blood flow and location of drug on the strut were far more important in determining arterial wall drug deposition and distribution than were drug load or arterial wall contact with coated strut surfaces.

Full DES lesion coverage

In the DES era the restenosis penalty of increasing stent length is much lower than in the BMS era leading to the concept of full lesion coverage. DES stent length should be based on the distance between the proximal and distal reference sites; this is best measured using IVUS and motorized transducer pullback. However, this does not mean that these references will be normal; atherosclerotic arteries are diffusely diseased. Rather, the goal is to identify proximal and distal cross-sections with the largest lumen and least plaque and to measure the distance between these two sections to avoid placing the stent edge into a plaque, a predictor of increased edge effects (38). Selecting the correct DES length the first time should be cost effective compared to having to implant a second, expensive, overlapping stent. It may be associated with fewer acute complications (39). However, it is even more important to achieve adequate stent expansion in long or multiple DES (12).

Treatment of bare-metal ISR with DES

DES treatment of bare-metal ISR is associated with a higher recurrence than de novo DES implantation; analysis of failures shows stent under-expansion or gaps between multiple DES (20,21,40). Thus, when treating bare-metal ISR, it is necessary to optimize stent expansion and to cover the entire length of the ISR lesion leaving neither gaps nor uncovered edges.

DES treatment of bifurcation lesions

In the DES era it may be necessary to pay more attention to the side branch than in the BMS era. Pre-intervention IVUS of the side branch can determine whether or not the side branch is involved, whether it is diseased but not stenotic, or whether it is stenotic. Post-intervention imaging of the side branch can determine whether the side branch has been compromised (after provisional stenting) or whether there is

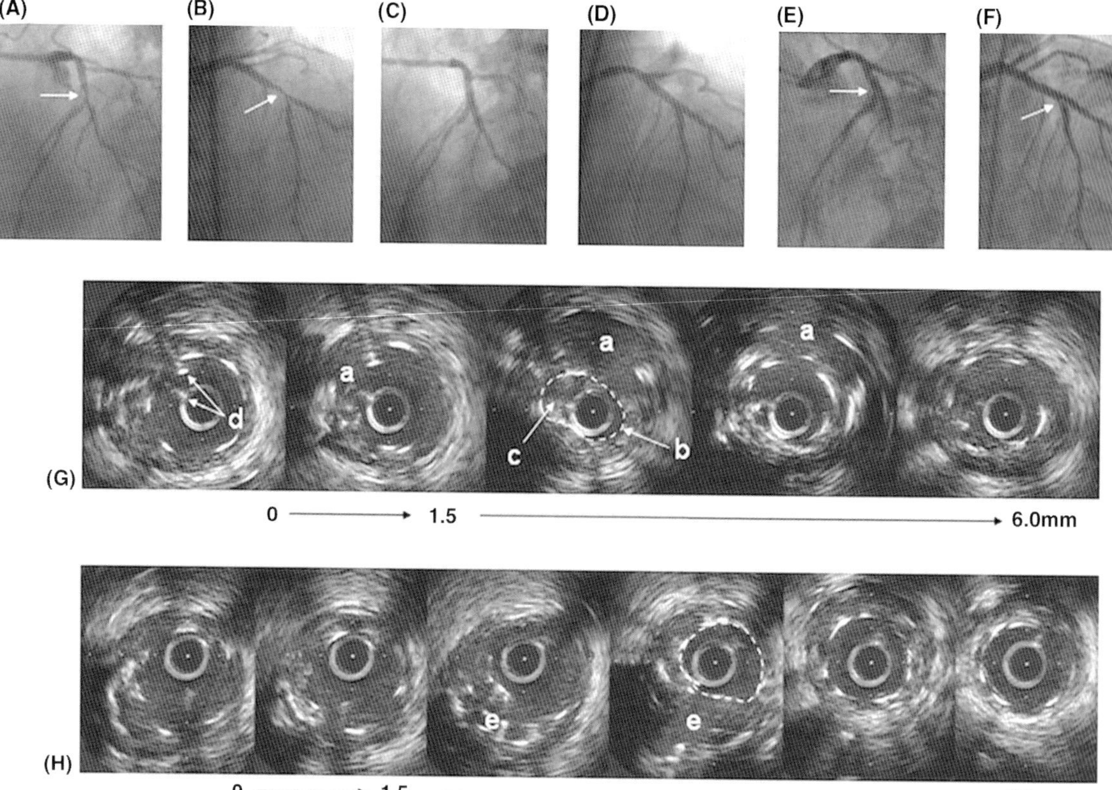

Figure 6 (**A**) and (**B**) (*arrows*) show a left anterior descending artery diagonal branch stenosis prior to bifurcation stenting. (**C**) and (**D**) show the lesion after implantation of a Cypher® stent into each branch. (**E**) and (**F**) (*arrows*) show restenosis in the left anterior descending just distal to the diagonal branch. (**G**) is the IVUS imaging of the left anterior descending; note the relationship to the diagonal branch stent (*a*). The minimum stent CSA (*dotted line* in *b*) within the left anterior descending measured 3.0 mm^2, the minimum lumen CSA measured 2.0 mm^2, and the intimal hyperplasia CSA (*c*) measured 1.0 mm^2. Also note the two guidewires in the left anterior descending proximal to the diagonal branch. (**H**) is the imaging of the diagonal branch; note the relationship to the left anterior descending stent (*e*). The minimum stent CSA (*dotted line* in *f*) within the diagonal branch measured 5.0 mm^2 with a lack of intimal hyperplasia. *Source*: From Mintz GS. Intracoronary ultrasound. London: Taylor and Francis Group; 2005, with permission.

adequate side branch in addition to adequate main vessel expansion (after deliberately stenting both branches). However, the side branch *cannot* be adequately assessed from the main vessel; it is necessary to image the side branch directly using IVUS. A recent analysis of LAD/diagonal bifurcation lesions treated with the crush technique found the MSA at the side branch ostium in 68% where it measured $<4\,mm^2$ in 44% and $<5\,mm^2$ in 82% (41). An example of restenosis in a bifurcation lesion treated with two Cypher stents is shown in Figure 6.

DES failure

Currently, IVUS is the best way to understand the causes and mechanisms of DES failure, just as it was the best way to understand BMS failure. The most common mechanism is stent underexpansion. This is predictable; once IH is mostly suppressed, what is left is an underexpanded stent. However, strut fracture, inhomogeneous stent expansion, and incomplete lesion coverage have also been reported as causes of DES restenoses, especially in well-expanded

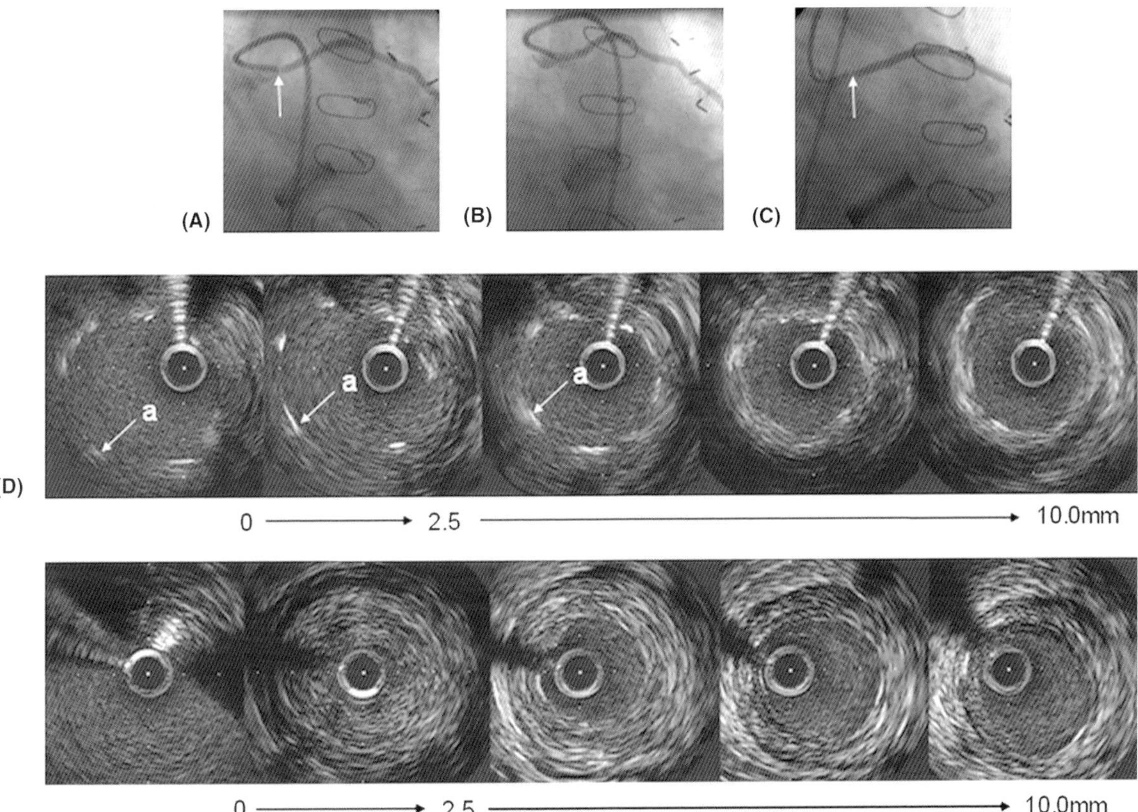

Figure 7 This ostial vein graft stenosis (*arrow* in **A**) was treated with cutting balloon angioplasty and implantation of an 8 mm long Cypher® stent. The final angiographic result is shown in (**B**). At 7 month follow-up, there was focal restenosis (*arrow* in **C**). (**D**) shows the final (post-stent implantation) IVUS; note that approximately half of the length of the stent (*a*) protrudes into the aorta. No stent is seen at follow-up (**E**); presumably, removal of the guiding catheter dislodged the stent. *Source*: From Mintz GS. Intracoronary ultrasound. London: Taylor and Francis Group; 2005, with permission.

stents. There may be other causes as well. For example, we have studied patients with supposed DES failure only to be surprised that there was no DES present (Fig. 7). Conversely, IVUS has been useful in eliminating purported mechanisms of DES failure including acute incomplete stent apposition, plaque composition (i.e., calcification), and stent asymmetry (42,43). The optimal treatment for DES failure is not clear. At the very least, underexpanded stents (the most common mechanism for DES failure) should be properly expanded. It is not clear whether LSM should be treated by additional stent expansion or whether these patients should just have continued dual antiplatelet therapy.

REFERENCES

1. Fujii K, Carlier SG, Mintz GS, et al. Stent underexpansion and residual reference segment stenosis are related to stent thrombosis after sirolimus-eluting stent implantation: An intravascular ultrasound study. J Am Coll Cardiol 2005; 45: 995–998.
2. Cook S, Wenaweser P, Togni M, et al. Intravascular ultrasound in very late DES-stent thrombosis. J Am Coll Cardiol 2006; 47:9B (abstract).
3. Hong M.-K, Mintz GS, Lee CW, et al. Late stent malapposition after drug-eluting stent implantation: An intravascular ultrasound analysis with long-term follow-up. Circulation 2006; 113: 414–419.

4. Ako J, Morino Y, Honda Y, et al. Late incomplete stent apposition after sirolimus-eluting stent implantation: A serial intravascular ultrasound analysis. J Am Coll Cardiol 2005; 46:1002–1005.
5. Degertekin M, Serruys PW, Tanabe K, et al. Long-term follow-up of incomplete stent apposition in patients who received sirolimus-eluting stent for de novo coronary lesions: An intravascular ultrasound analysis. Circulation 2003; 108: 2747–2750.
6. Tanabe K, Serruys PW, Degertekin M, et al. Incomplete stent apposition after implantation of paclitaxel-eluting stents or bare metal stents: Insights from the randomized TAXUS-II trial. Circulation 2005; 111:900–905.
7. Aoki J, Colombo A, Dudek D, et al. Peristent remodeling and neointimal suppression two years after polymer-based, paclitaxel-eluting stent implantation. Insights from serial intravascular ultrasound analysis in the TAXUS-II study. Circulation 2005; 112:3876–3883.
8. Weissman NJ, Koglin J, Cox DA, et al. Polymer-based paclitaxel-eluting stents reduce in-stent neointimal tissue proliferation: A serial volumetric intravascular ultrasound analysis from the TAXUS-IV trial. J Am Coll Cardiol 2005; 45:1201–1205.
9. Weissman NJ, Ellis SE, Mintz GS, et al. Insights on the effect of polymer-based paclitaxel-eluting stents in long lesions and overlapping stents: Final results from the TAXUS-V IVUS substudy. Circulation 2005; 112:II-769 (abstract).
10. Mintz GS, Weissman NJ, Dawkins K, et al. Frequency, predictors, and clinical outcomes of late-acquired incomplete stent apposition in patients treated with Taxus stents: A volumetric intravascular ultrasound meta-analysis from the TAXUS IV, V, and VI trials. J Am Coll Cardiol 2006; 47:26B. (abstract).
11. Sonoda S, Morino Y, Ako J, et al. Impact of final stent dimensions on long-term results following sirolimus-eluting stent implantation: Serial intravascular ultrasound analysis from the SIRIUS trial. J Am Coll Cardiol 2004; 43:1959–1963.
12. Hong M.-K, Mintz GS, Lee CW, et al. Intravascular ultrasound predictors of angiographic restenosis after sirolimus-eluting stent implantation. Eur Heart J 2006; 27:1305–1310.
13. Takebayashi H, Kobayashi Y, Mintz GS, et al. Intravascular ultrasound assessment of lesions with target vessel failure after sirolimus-eluting stent implantation. Am J Cardiol 2005; 95: 498–502.
14. Kim S.-W, Mintz GS, Escolar E, et al. An intravascular ultrasound analysis of the mechanisms of restenosis comparing drug-eluting stents with brachytherapy. Am J Cardiol 2006; 97:1292–8.
15. Sano K, Mintz GS, Carlier SG, et al. Volumetric intravascular ultrasound assessment of neointimal hyperplasia distribution in sirolimus-eluting stent restenosis. Am J Cardiol (in press).
16. Seung KB, Kim YH, Park DW, et al. Effectiveness of sirolimus-eluting stent implantation for the treatment of ostial left anterior descending artery stenosis with intravascular ultrasound guidance. J Am Coll Cardiol 2005; 46:787–792.
17. Lemos PA, Saia F, Ligthart JM, et al. Coronary restenosis after sirolimus-eluting stent implantation: Morphological description and mechanistic analysis from a consecutive series of cases. Circulation 2003; 108:257–260.
18. Takebayashi H, Mintz GS, Carlier SG, et al. Nonuniform strut distribution correlates with more neointimal hyperplasia after sirolimus-eluting stent implantation. Circulation 2004; 110:3430–3434.
19. Sakurai R, Ako J, Morino Y, et al. Predictors of edge stenosis following sirolimus-eluting stent deployment: A quantitative intravascular ultrasound analysis from the SIRIUS trial. Am J Cardiol 2005; 96:1251–1253.
20. Lemos PA, Serruys PW, van Domburg RT, et al. Unrestricted utilization of sirolimus-eluting stents compared with conventional bare stent implantation in the "real world": the Rapamycin-Eluting Stent Evaluated At Rotterdam Cardiology Hospital (RESEARCH) registry. Circulation 2004; 109:190–195.
21. Fujii K, Mintz GS, Kobayashi Y, et al. Contribution of stent underexpansion to recurrence after sirolimus-eluting stent implantation for in-stent restenosis. Circulation 2004; 109:1085–1088.
22. Iakovou I, Schmidt T, Bonizzoni E, et al. Incidence, predictors, and outcome of thrombosis after successful implantation of drug-eluting stents. JAMA 2005; 293:2126–2130.
23. Kuchulakanti PK, Chu WW, Torguson R, et al. Correlates and long-term outcomes of angiographically proven stent thrombosis with sirolimus- and paclitaxel-eluting stents. Circulation 2006; 113: 1108–1113.

24. Abizaid A, Mintz GS, Pichard AD, et al. Clinical, intravascular ultrasound, and quantitative angiographic determinants of the coronary flow reserve before and after percutaneous transluminal coronary angioplasty. Am J Cardiol 1998; 82: 423–428.
25. Nishioka T, Amanullah AM, Luo H, et al. Clinical validation of intravascular ultrasound imaging for assessment of coronary stenosis severity: Comparison with stress myocardial perfusion imaging. J Am Coll Cardiol 1999; 33:1870–1878.
26. Takagi A, Tsurumi Y, Ishii Y, et al. Clinical potential of intravascular ultrasound for physiological assessment of coronary stenosis: relationship between quantitative ultrasound tomography and pressure-derived fractional flow reserve. Circulation 1999; 100:250–255.
27. Abizaid AS, Mintz GS, Mehran R, et al. Long-term follow-up after percutaneous transluminal coronary angioplasty was not performed based on intravascular ultrasound findings: importance of lumen dimensions. Circulation 1999; 100: 256–261.
28. Moses JW, Stone GW, Nikolsky E, et al. Drug-eluting stents in the treatment of intermediate lesions: Pooled analysis from four randomized trials. J Am Coll Cardiol 2006; 47:2164–71.
29. Maehara A, Mintz GS, Bui AB, et al. Determinants of angiographically silent stenoses in patients with coronary artery disease. Am J Cardiol 2003; 91:1335–1338.
30. Zhou Y, Kassab GS, Molloi S. On the design of the coronary arterial tree: a generalization of Murray's law. Phys Med Biol 1999; 44:2929–2945.
31. Jasti V, Ivan E, Yalamanchili V, et al. Correlations between fractional flow reserve and intravascular ultrasound in patients with an ambiguous left main coronary artery stenosis. Circulation 2004; 110:2831–2836.
32. Abizaid AS, Mintz GS, Abizaid A, et al. One-year follow-up after intravascular ultrasound assessment of moderate left main coronary artery disease in patients with ambiguous angiograms. J Am Coll Cardiol 1999; 34:707–715.
33. Park S.-J, Kim Y.-H, Lee B.-K, et al. Sirolimus-eluting stent implantation for unprotected left main coronary artery stenosis: Comparison with bare metal stent implantation. J Am Coll Cardiol 2005; 45:351–356.
34. de Ribamar Costa JR, Mintz GS, Carlier SG, et al. Intravascular ultrasound assessment of drug-eluting stent expansion. Am Heart J (in press).
35. Shimada Y, Honda Y, Hongo Y, et al. Sirolimus-eluting stent implantation in small coronary arteries: Predictors of long-term stent patency and neointimal hyperplasia. Circulation 2005; 112:II-736 (abstract).
36. Kimura M, Mintz GS, Carlier SG, et al. Outcome after acute incomplete sirolimus-eluting stent apposition as assessed by serial intravascular ultrasound. Am J Cardiol 2006; 98:436–42.
37. Balakrishnan B, Tzafriri AR, Seifert P, et al. Strut position, blood flow, and drug deposition: implications for single and overlapping drug-eluting stents. Circulation 2005; 111:2958–65.
38. Sousa JE, Costa MA, Abizaid AC, et al. Sustained suppression of neointimal proliferation by sirolimus-eluting stents: One-year angiographic and intravascular ultrasound follow-up. Circulation 2001; 104:2007–2011.
39. Stone GW, Ellis SG, Cannon L, et al. Comparison of a polymer-based paclitaxel-eluting stent with a bare metal stent in patients with complex coronary artery disease: a randomized controlled trial. JAMA 2005; 294:1215–23.
40. Costa MA, Sabate M, Angiolillo DJ, et al. Intravascular ultrasound characterization of the "black hole" phenomenon after drug-eluting stent implantation. Am J Cardiol 2006; 97: 203–206.
41. Costa RA, Mintz GS, Carlier SG, et al. Bifurcation coronary lesions treated with the "crush" technique: An intravascular ultrasound analysis. J Am Coll Cardiol 2005; 46:599–605.
42. Shimada Y, Kataoka T, Courtney BK, et al. Influence of plaque calcium on neointimal hyperplasia following bare metal and drug-eluting stent implantation. Catheter Cardiovasc Interv. 2006; 67:866–9.
43. Kaneda H, Ako J, Honda Y, et al. Impact of asymmetric stent expansion on neointimal hyperplasia following sirolimus-eluting stent implantation. Am J Cardio. 2005; 96:1404–7.

15

MRI of ischemic heart disease: Perfusion, viability, and coronary artery imaging

Asu Rustemli and Steven D. Wolff

INTRODUCTION

A growing number of percutaneous coronary interventions (PCI) are performed each year to treat obstructive coronary artery disease (CAD). For many patients, the need for revascularization is determined by diagnostic imaging, such as stress perfusion imaging with single photon emission computed tomography (SPECT), stress function imaging with echocardiography, and/or myocardial viability assessment with positron emission tomography (PET). However, the accuracy of these techniques is limited. As a result, a substantial number of patients referred for diagnostic coronary catheterization have no significant disease or have disease in a coronary artery that is inconsistent with the imaging findings.

Over the last several years, advances in software and hardware have enabled magnetic resonance imaging (MRI) to assess patients with suspected ischemic heart disease. Some general advantages of MRI include a large unobstructed view of the heart, high spatial and temporal resolution, good image contrast, and an absence of ionizing radiation or nephrotoxic dye. Perhaps most compelling of all from a clinical perspective is MRI's ability to provide a comprehensive evaluation of the heart that includes assessment of myocardial function, perfusion, and viability, as well as flow quantification and coronary artery visualization, all in a single examination.

MYOCARDIAL VIABILITY IMAGING

Determining myocardial viability can be important for prognostic reasons. For example, in the setting of acute ischemia, regional wall-motion abnormalities are irreversible if the myocardium is infarcted, whereas if the myocardium is viable (i.e., stunned), it is likely to recover function within several weeks. Perhaps more significantly, the identification of viable myocardium can be important for therapeutic decision making. For example, in the setting of chronic ischemia, revascularization is likely to improve the systolic function of viable (i.e., hibernating) myocardium, whereas nonviable tissue will not improve function. Furthermore, patients with CAD and severe left ventricular (LV) dysfunction have better peri-operative and long-term outcomes when their management is guided by viability assessment prior to revascularization. Multiple studies using different noninvasive modalities such as PET, dobutamine echocardiography, and SPECT have demonstrated that there is a reduction in peri-operative morbidity and mortality when only patients with viable myocardium undergo revascularization (1–4).

Each of the above techniques has its limitations. For example, SPECT has relatively poor spatial resolution and often has soft tissue attenuation artifacts. Stress echocardiography cannot reliably visualize the entire myocardium and has pro-blems with image misregistration and intra- and inter-observer variability. Finally, PET, which for years has been considered the standard of reference for viability assessment, has poor spatial resolution and limited clinical availability.

There are two principal methods by which MRI can assess myocardial viability. In the first method, MRI assesses contractile reserve in a manner analogous to low-dose dobutamine echocardiography. The earliest studies evaluating contractile reserve by MRI showed that dobutamine-induced systolic wall thickening was a better predictor of viability than an end-diastolic wall thickness of >5.5 mm (5). Comparison of dobutamine MRI with dobutamine echocardiography (with FDG-PET as the gold standard) yielded similar results for the detection of viability with a slightly higher sensitivity and specificity for MRI; overall diagnostic accuracies were 84% and 88% for dobutamine echo and dobutamine MRI, respectively (6).

The second MRI method for viability assessment is based on gadolinium contrast enhancement. This technique has uniquely high spatial resolution, probably making it the new standard of reference for myocardial viability assessment. In this case, the determination of myocardial viability is based on the steady-state distribution of gadolinium contrast. In normal tissue, gadolinium contrast is restricted to a small fraction of the total tissue volume, namely the intravascular and extracellular spaces. However, with acute infarction and cell membrane lysis, the gadolinium contrast can partition into what was formerly the intracellular space. In this case, the volume of contrast distribution increases approximately fivefold compared to living tissue and therefore regions of acute infarction appear bright. In the case of chronic infarction, the dead myocytes are replaced by scar tissue. Because scar tissue also has a higher (approximately threefold) volume of distribution for gadolinium contrast, chronic infarcts are also detected by this technique.

Contrast-enhanced viability imaging has been well-validated in both animal models and clinical studies (7). Figure 1 is an example of an

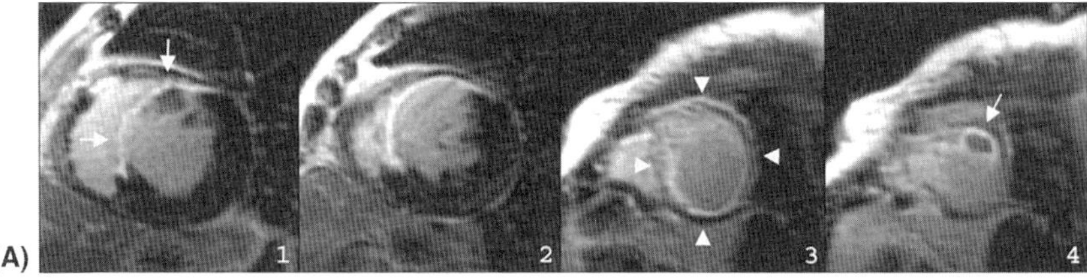

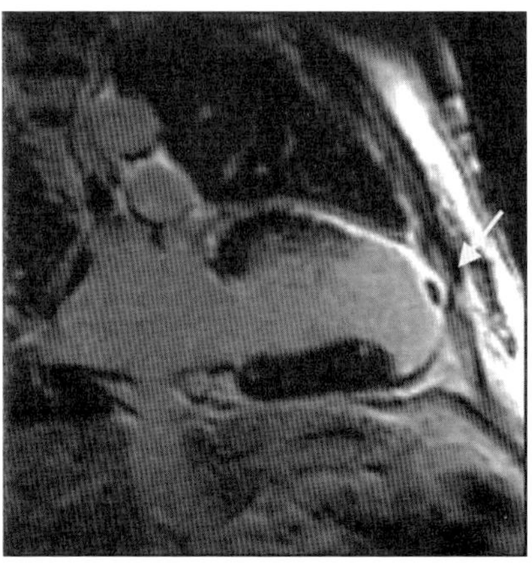

Figure 1 Anterior and apical infarct. (**A**) Short-axis contrast-enhanced delayed images of the left ventricle show a transmural infarct anteriorly, anteroseptally at the base (*arrows, image 1*) and at the mid-ventricle (*image 2*). The entire apex is infarcted (*images 3 and 4*) with a small apical thrombus (*arrow, image 4*). (**B**) 2-Chamber radial long-axis contrast-enhanced delayed image shows the anterior and apical infarct and the apical thrombus (*arrow*).

abnormal contrast-enhanced myocardial viability study. The normal myocardium has a dark homogeneous appearance, whereas the scar tissue involving the anterior wall, anteroseptum, and apex is bright. Contrast-enhanced images can also provide critical information regarding complications of myocardial infarction such as left ventricular thrombus (Fig. 1) or an aneurysm (Fig. 2).

An MRI examination to evaluate for the presence of hibernating myocardium typically includes an assessment of global and regional systolic left ventricular function by cine MRI as well as contrast-enhanced images to determine tissue viability. The functional images are generally acquired as sequential short–axis slices covering the entire left ventricle. Usually, 2-, 3-, and 4-chamber long-axis cine images of the left ventricle are also acquired. Viability imaging is typically performed 10–20 minutes after intravenous injection of 0.2 mmol/kg of gadolinium contrast. A 10-minute delay is recommended to give the contrast time to equilibrate within the various tissue compartments. Viability images are also acquired in short- and long-axis orientations to match the functional images. Hibernating myocardium is identified as regions of abnormal systolic function that exhibit little or no abnormal contrast enhancement. In addition to determining hibernating myocardium, these MRI studies provide other important functional and prognostic information such as LV ejection fraction, end-diastolic and end-systolic volumes, end-diastolic wall thickness, and LV mass.

There are a number of studies in the peer-reviewed literature documenting the efficacy of contrast-enhanced MRI for determining viability. In one study, 51 patients were imaged at the time of acute infarction and then 3 and 14 months later. Ninety-one percent of patients with 3-month-old infarcts and all patients with 14-month-old infarcts exhibited hyperenhancement (8). Klein et al. (9) also demonstrated an excellent correlation between contrast-enhanced MRI and FDG PET to identify and quantify scar tissue. It was shown that the likelihood of improvement in regional contractility after revascularization progressively decreased as the transmural extent of the hyperenhancement increased (9,10). For example, 77% of dysfunctional segments without any infarction showed improvement after revascularization, whereas only 5% of the dysfunctional segments with over 75% infarction showed improvement (9). This

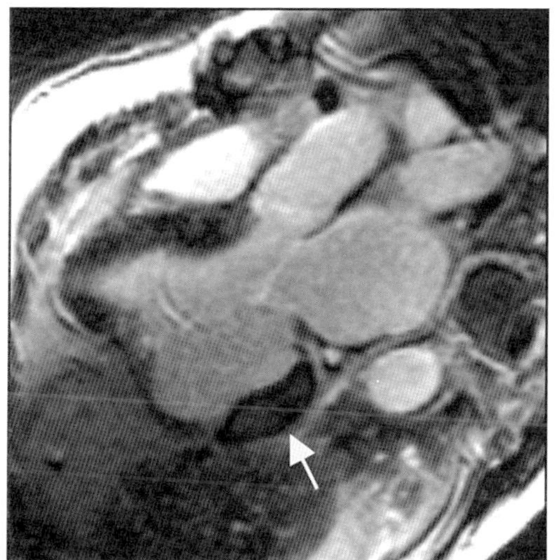

(A)

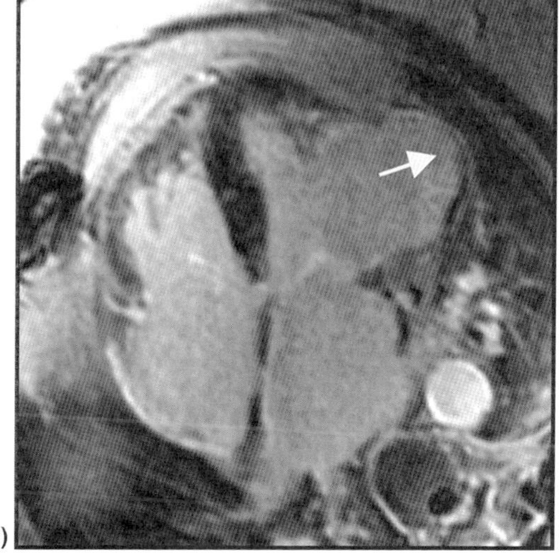

(B)

Figure 2 Left ventricular aneurysm and thrombus. (**A**) 3-Chamber contrast-enhanced radial image showing a large aneurysm secondary to a prior myocardial infarction. A layered thrombus is seen in the aneurysm (*arrow*). (**B**) 4-Chamber contrast-enhanced radial image showing the large inferolateral aneurysm of the left ventricle (*arrow*).

study nicely demonstrated that defining the transmural extent of viability was important in determining outcome. Figure 3 shows an example of how MRI can define the transmural extent of infarction. This patient with severe LV dysfunction had a prior myocardial infarction due to occlusion of the left anterior descending (LAD) coronary artery. The cine MRI study shows akinesis of the anterior wall at the midventricle and akinesis of the entire apex (Fig. 3A). Contrast-enhanced imaging shows a large anterior and apical infarct with little or no viable tissue in the LAD territory (Fig. 3B). The infarct is predominantly transmural with only a small region of subendocardial infarction at the midventricular anteroseptum. In this case, the information provided by the MRI study was important because it spared the patient an unnecessary revascularization. The patient was managed medically.

Figure 4 shows an example of how MRI can identify viable, hibernating myocardium. This patient presented with chest pain and had a prior SPECT perfusion study that showed a mostly "fixed" perfusion defect of the inferior wall with a small amount of peri-infarct ischemia (Fig. 4A). Further evaluation with cine MRI showed a thin (<3 mm), akinetic inferior wall (Fig. 4B) and a low-normal ejection fraction (52%). The contrast-enhanced MRI showed that the thin, akinetic inferior wall had no abnormal enhancement, suggesting it was entirely viable (Fig. 4B). Diagnostic coronary angiography showed severe stenoses of the ostial and proximal right coronary artery (RCA) (Fig. 4C). A repeat cardiac MRI performed 12 weeks following PCI of the RCA showed complete resolution of the wall motion abnormality and an improvement in the ejection fraction to 68% (Fig. 4D). The functional improvement following PCI exemplifies MRI's ability to assess for the presence of hibernating myocardium.

Contrast-enhanced MRI can detect subendocardial scar better than PET and SPECT (9,11).

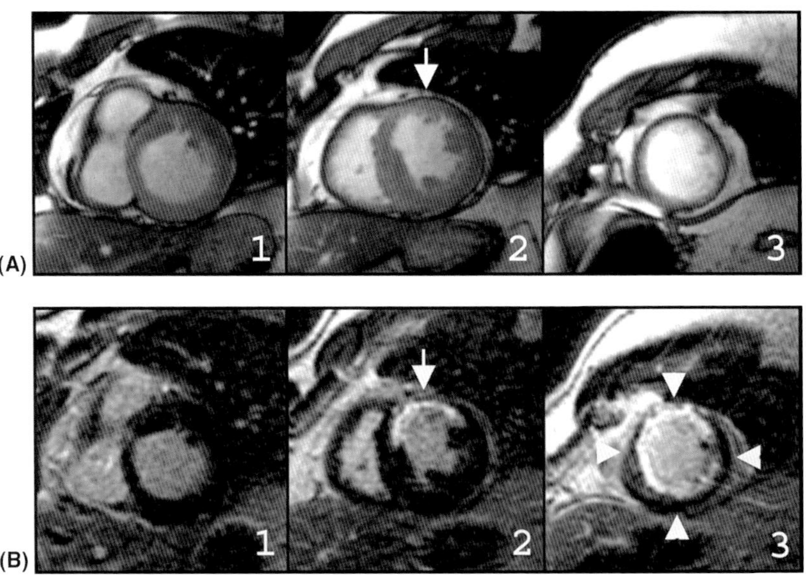

Figure 3 Nonviable myocardium. (**A**) Systolic frames of the short-axis cine images of the left ventricle show normal wall motion at the base (*image 1*), anterior and anteroseptal akinesis at the midventricle (*arrow, image 2*), and global akinesis at the apex (*image 3*). (**B**) Short-axis contrast–enhanced delayed images show an anterior and anteroseptal transmural infarct at the mid-ventricle (*arrow, image 2*) and the entire apex (*arrowheads, image 3*). These findings are consistent with absence of hibernating myocardium.

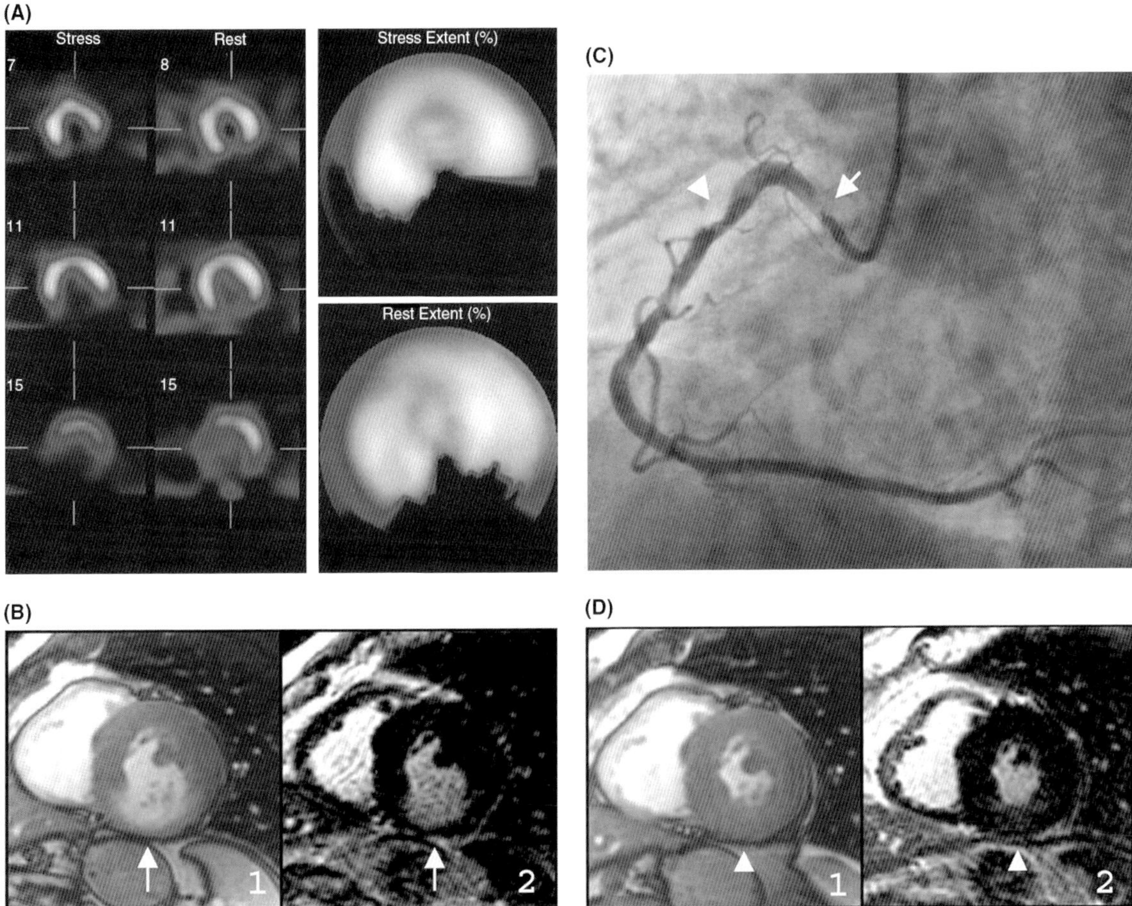

Figure 4 Hibernating myocardium. (**A**) A SPECT stress perfusion study showing an inferior infarct with mild peri-infarct ischemia. (*See color insert.*) (**B**) Cardiac MRI viability study prior to PCI of right coronary artery (RCA). Systolic frame of the cine image at the mid-ventricle shows a thin inferior wall and akinesis (*arrow, image 1*); a contrast-enhanced delayed image reveals a thin inferior wall without myocardial infarction (*arrow, image 2*). (**C**) Right coronary artery angiography shows severe stenosis of the ostial (*arrow*) and proximal RCA (*arrowhead*). (**D**) Normal systolic function of the inferior wall following PCI of RCA (*arrowhead, image 1*); a contrast-enhanced delayed image shows normal thickness of the inferior wall free of scar tissue (*arrowhead, image 2*).

In a study of 91 patients, 13% of the subjects with subendocardial infarcts visible by MRI had no evidence of infarction by SPECT (12). A possible reason for this lack of sensitivity is that the spatial resolution of SPECT images (with motional blurring) is comparable to the thickness of the heart wall. Thus, subendocardial infarcts, which by definition do not involve the entire heart wall, are essentially beyond the spatial resolution of SPECT. Conversely, breathheld MR viability images typically have a spatial resolution of 1–2 mm, making it possible to define the extent of subendocardial infarcts. Patients with radionuclide examination findings that are equivocal may benefit from contrast-enhanced MRI, particularly in the setting of a nontransmural infarct (13). Contrast-enhanced MRI is an essential tool in the management of patients with missed infarcts on other noninvasive modalities. Figure 5 shows an example of a small

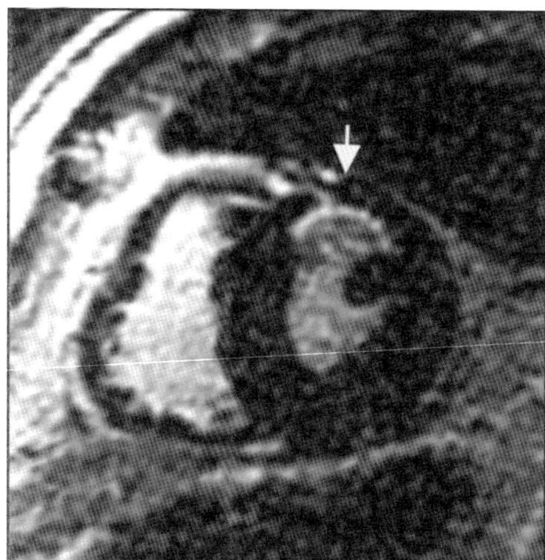

Figure 5 Subendocardial infarct. A single short-axis contrast-enhanced myocardial delayed image showing a thin rim of subendocardial infarct at the mid-ventricle level (*arrow*).

subendocardial infarct that was identified on a contrast-enhanced cardiac MRI study in a 65-year-old patient who had chest pain and a recent echocardiogram that showed normal regional wall motion. The thin rim of enhancement demonstrates an unsuspected anterior subendocardial infarction.

STRESS MYOCARDIAL PERFUSION MRI

Stress myocardial perfusion imaging identifies patients with obstructive CAD and provides information about the size and location of the ischemic burden. In clinical practice perfusion imaging is most commonly performed with SPECT. Its sensitivity and specificity for detecting significant coronary artery disease is 80% to 95% and 60% to 85%, respectively (14–17). An important limitation of SPECT is its intrinsically poor spatial resolution (approximately 10 mm), which is exacerbated by the respiratory motion that occurs during image acquisition (typically approximately 20 minutes). This limitation results in a diminished sensitivity for detecting small or subendocardial perfusion defects. In addition, SPECT suffers from soft tissue attenuation artifacts, which are common in obese individuals and women with large breasts or breast implants. These artifacts can simulate disease when none is present. Finally, because perfusion defects are detected by comparison to normally perfused portions of the heart, SPECT can be falsely negative in patients with global ischemia due to severe proximal three vessel disease, otherwise known as "balanced ischemia."

PET can also be used to assess myocardial perfusion. Although it does not have the disadvantages of SPECT with regard to soft tissue attenuation artifacts and balanced ischemia, it does have relatively poor spatial resolution that is exacerbated by respiratory motion. Its clinical use has been limited due to the necessity of having an on-site source of nuclear tracer and its higher cost.

MRI can also assess myocardial perfusion. It does so by imaging the first-pass of a gadolinium contrast bolus (18–20). The sub-second image acquisition techniques of cardiac MRI have substantially better spatial resolution than SPECT or PET (approximately 30 mm^3 vs. approximately 100 mm^3), leading to superior transmural evaluation of perfusion defects. Although MRI perfusion images are not artifact-free, they do not suffer from the soft-tissue attenuation artifacts that can limit SPECT studies. Stress perfusion imaging can also be accomplished much more quickly than SPECT. A comprehensive cardiac evaluation including stress perfusion, assessment of systolic function, and myocardial viability can be performed in 30 minutes, which can be very appealing in clinical practice.

The rationale for perfusion MRI is the same as that for nuclear techniques. Under resting conditions, patients with obstructive coronary artery disease often have normal perfusion because arterial resistance distal to a coronary artery stenosis decreases to maintain normal perfusion (autoregulation). The ability to detect diminished perfusion due to epicardial disease is enhanced during stress conditions. This is because during stress, normal arteries can dilate to augment blood flow three- to fivefold, whereas arteries distal to a significant stenosis cannot further dilate and therefore cannot further augment blood flow. Thus, hyperemic stress induces a relative heterogeneity of myocardial perfusion that is not present during resting conditions.

Most myocardial stress perfusion MRI studies are performed using pharmacologic agents because exercise often is not practical in the magnet. The agents that are most commonly used to induce coronary hyperemia are dipyridamole and adenosine (21,22). Dipyridamole is an indirect vasodilator that inhibits breakdown of adenosine. Adenosine is an endogenous substance that plays a role in regulation of blood flow in many organ beds, including the coronary circulation. Low doses of adenosine cause arterial vasodilatation and bronchial vasoconstriction. In higher doses, it can also cause bradycardia by acting on A_1 receptors in the sinus node and atrioventricular node. A low dose adenosine infusion typically causes a mild decrease in the systemic blood pressure and a mild reflex increase in the heart rate. A feeling of generalized warmth or flushing, chest pressure, and shortness of breath are common symptoms. These effects are short lasting due to its short half-life of approximately 10 seconds, and rapidly dissipate when the infusion is discontinued. Since adenosine is antagonized by caffeine, abstinence from caffeinated food and drinks for at least 12 hours prior to the perfusion test is essential. Second- or third-degree AV block, sick sinus syndrome, and active bronchoconstrictive lung disease (e.g., asthma) are contraindications to adenosine administration.

During a typical adenosine stress perfusion protocol, adenosine is infused for 2 minutes at a rate of 140 μg/kg/min under physician supervision. This is the same weight-based dose rate that has been validated for SPECT imaging and which has been shown to induce maximal coronary hyperemia (21, 23, 24). If there are no apparent physiologic effects from the adenosine (e.g., feeling of warmth, increased heart rate, etc.), the infusion may be extended for an additional minute. At peak vasodilatation, gadolinium contrast agent is administered as a rapid bolus (3–5 mL/sec) via an intravenous catheter in a separate extremity. Myocardial perfusion images are acquired during the first-pass of the gadolinium contrast bolus, usually for 30–60 seconds. Multiple short-axis slices of the left ventricle are usually obtained. After completion of the first pass of the contrast bolus, the adenosine infusion is terminated. The total duration of the adenosine infusion is typically 2.5–3.5 minutes.

There are a number of T1-weighted imaging sequences such as gradient-echo, echo-planar, and steady-state free precession sequences that have been used to image the first pass of the contrast bolus through the myocardium (25,26). Most of the techniques are based on qualitative evaluation of perfusion, where regions of diminished perfusion are visualized as areas of diminished signal intensity. Semi-quantitative assessment of myocardial perfusion often requires imaging with lower contrast doses that are less than optimal for the qualitative assessment of myocardial perfusion defects (27,28). Therefore, quantification of perfusion abnormalities is not commonly performed.

A normal perfusion study appears as homogeneous enhancement throughout the myocardium in all of the slices. Figure 6 is an example of a normal adenosine stress perfusion study acquired at peak vasodilatation. In this case, five short axis slices were acquired during the first-pass of the contrast bolus. Each slice shows homogeneous enhancement, indicating normal, homogeneous perfusion.

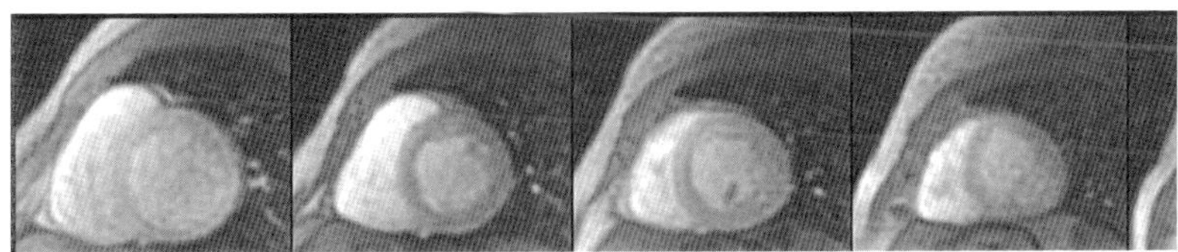

Figure 6 Normal adenosine stress perfusion MRI. Short-axis images from base (*image 1*) to apex (*image 5*) of the left ventricle acquired at peak vasodilation show homogeneous enhancement with gadolinium.

For nuclear myocardial perfusion imaging, a stress perfusion study is often accompanied by the acquisition of a resting perfusion study. This is usually done to distinguish scar (which shows perfusion defects both during stress and at rest) from reversible ischemia (which shows perfusion defects during stress but not at rest). The same rationale has been used for the MR assessment of myocardial perfusion by acquiring images both at stress and at rest. However, an alternative to acquiring rest perfusion images is acquisition of contrast-enhanced delayed images which also assess for myocardial scar. Figure 7 shows an example of a resting perfusion study and viability study in a patient with an anterior, septal, and apical infarct. The resting perfusion images show perfusion defects that appear as regions of diminished signal intensity in the anterior wall, septum, and apex. The contrast-enhanced images show these same regions to be bright, indicating the presence of scar. Since scar tissue is often shown with greater clarity in the contrast-enhanced viability images, many sites substitute these images for the resting perfusion images.

If there is no myocardial scar on the delayed images, then any perfusion defects seen on an adenosine stress perfusion study represent "reversible" ischemia. Figure 8 illustrates an abnormal adenosine stress perfusion study with perfusion defects involving multiple segments from base to the apex of the left ventricle (Fig. 8A). Since there is no myocardial scar seen on delayed images (Fig. 8B), the perfusion abnormalities represent "reversible" ischemia. In cases of matching perfusion defects and myocardial infarcts, the implication is that there is no ischemia that would benefit from revascularization (Fig. 9).

Another pharmacologic agent that is used in cardiac stress imaging is dobutamine. It causes an increase in oxygen demand by increasing the force of myocardial contraction. Therefore, myocardial regions that are supplied by a stenotic coronary artery reveal abnormal wall motion with increments of dobutamine dose. Abnormal LV contraction during dobutamine stress echocardiography (DSE) can detect inducible myocardial ischemia with sensitivities ranging from 55% to 96%, and specificities ranging from 60% to 100% (29). However, 10% to 15% of DSE are suboptimal or non-diagnostic (despite harmonic imaging) because of poor acoustic windows especially in patients with large body habitus, obstructive pulmonary disease, or cardiothoracic surgery (29,30). Dobutamine MRI offers several advantages compared with stress echocardiography such as reproducibility of good

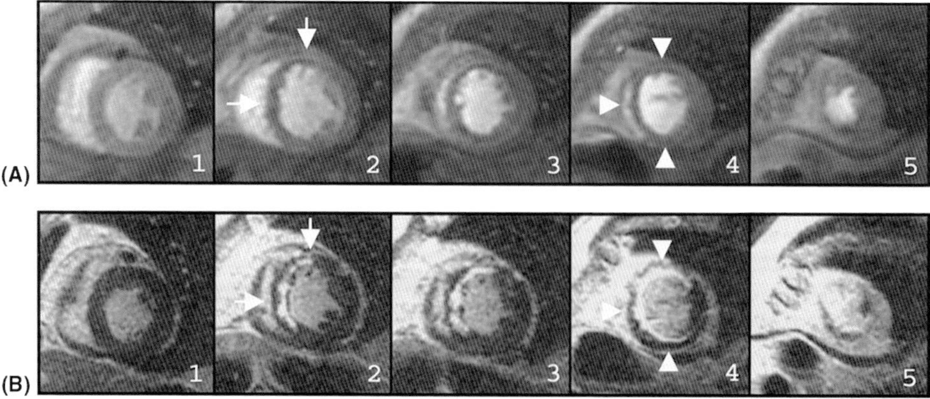

Figure 7 Rest perfusion and delayed enhancement study. (**A**) First-pass images acquired at resting state showing anterior and septal perfusion defects at the mid-ventricle (*arrows, images 2 and 3*) and apical perfusion defects (*arrowheads, images 4 and 5*). (**B**) Contrast-enhanced delayed images showing the areas of necrotic myocardium matching the regions of perfusion defects.

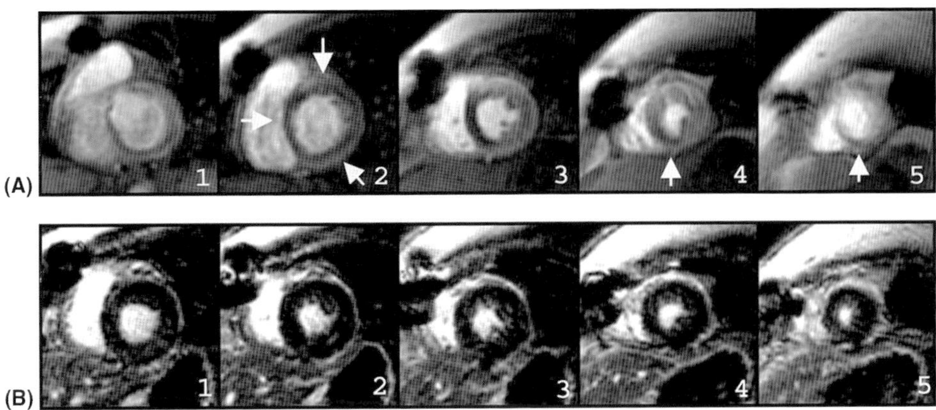

Figure 8 Abnormal adenosine stress perfusion MRI of a 70-year-old patient with chest pain and remote history of CABG surgery and multiple PCI procedures. (**A**) First-pass images during peak vasodilation show perfusion defects globally at the base (*arrows, images 1 and 2*), septally and inferiorly at the mid-ventricle (*arrows, images 3 and 4*), and inferiorly at the apex (*arrow, image 5*). Consequent cardiac catheterization revealed severe stenosis of the native coronaries, as well as occlusion of two of the vein grafts supplying the right posterior descending artery and obtuse marginal artery. (**B**) The short-axis contrast-enhanced delayed images of the left ventricle show no hyperenhancement to suggest a prior myocardial infarction.

quality cine images independent of patient's condition or the examiner at different dobutamine levels. Dobutamine MRI has been shown to be an accurate diagnostic tool for the detection of myocardial ischemia in patients who are poor candidates for stress echocardiography with a sensitivity and specificity for detecting a ≥50% luminal diameter narrowing of 83% and 83%, respectively (31). In another study, investigators compared DSE directly to dobutamine MRI. The data showed MRI to be superior to DSE for detecting significant CAD (defined as ≥50%

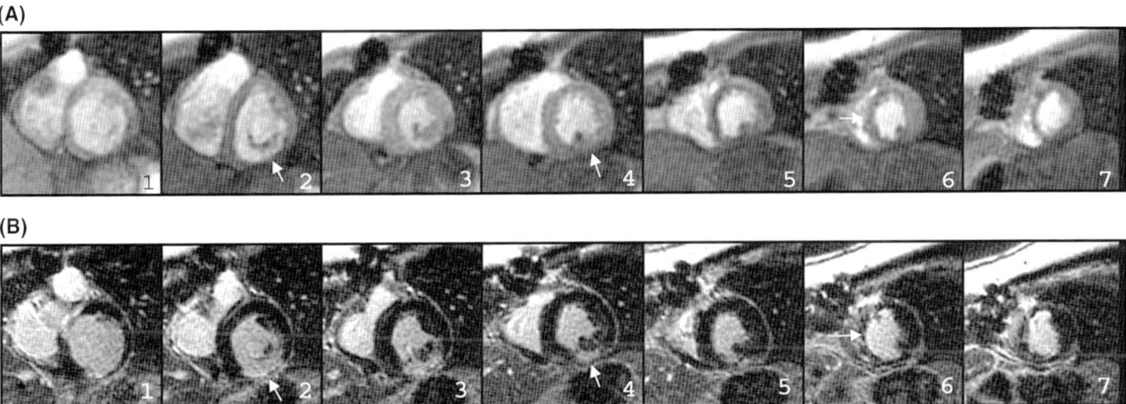

Figure 9 Matched perfusion defects and myocardial infarction. (**A**) Abnormal adenosine stress myocardial perfusion study showing perfusion defects inferolaterally at the base (*arrows, images 1 and 2*), the mid-ventricle (*arrows, images 3, 4, and 5*) and at the apex (*arrows, images 6 and 7*). (**B**) Contrast-enhanced delayed images showing mostly transmural infarct involving the regions of perfusion defects indicating absence of ischemia.

diameter stenosis on coronary angiography). Compared to DSE, dobutamine MRI showed higher sensitivity (86% vs. 74%), specificity (86% vs. 70%), and accuracy (86% vs. 73%) (32). The higher diagnostic accuracy of dobutamine MRI was mainly attributed to the improved image quality. The duration of a dobutamine stress MRI examination is determined by the time taken to reach the target heart rate and is similar to the DSE. However, the procedure time is substantially longer than that of adenosine stress perfusion MRI examination. Because the two tests yield similar information, we prefer to perform adenosine perfusion MRI and reserve dobutamine stress MRI for those patients with a contraindication to adenosine, such as asthma.

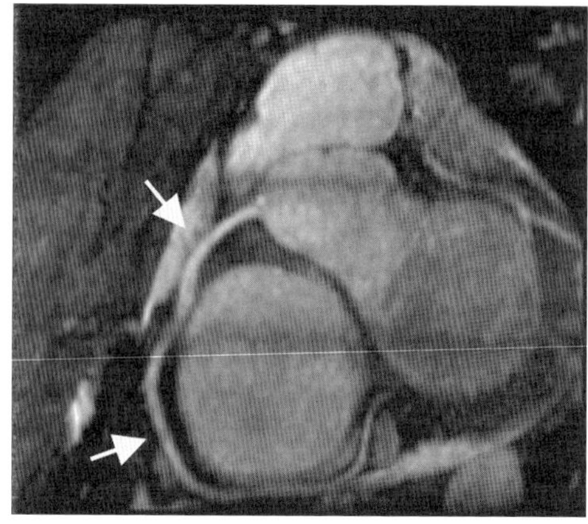

Figure 10 MRA of a right coronary artery illustrating its normal course (*arrows*) without any stenosis.

CORONARY ARTERY MR IMAGING

Conventional X-ray coronary angiography is the gold standard for identifying the presence and the severity of epicardial coronary artery stenoses. Although much progress has been made over the past decade, MRI of the coronary arteries is still limited mainly due to small caliber of the epicardial vessels and artifacts from cardiac and respiratory motion. Typically, a coronary MR angiogram has an in-plane spatial resolution of approximately 1 mm. This is substantially worse than X-ray coronary angiography, which has a spatial resolution of 0.3 mm and coronary computed tomography (CT) angiography, which can have a spatial resolution of < 0.6 mm. Nevertheless, there have been several studies looking at the accuracy of coronary MRI to assess obstructive (i.e., a ⩾ 50% stenosis) coronary artery disease. Sensitivities and specificities for identification of significant coronary artery stenoses have been reported to be 70% to 93% and 85% to 95%, respectively. However, these numbers are artificially elevated because investigators only assessed "evaluable" proximal and mid coronary artery segments (33–36). Currently, CT's advantage in spatial resolution probably makes it a better less-invasive alternative to X-ray angiography for evaluating coronary artery stenosis.

MRI's spatial resolution is more than adequate to accurately assess the course of anomalous coronary arteries, and it can do so without the need for iodinated dye or ionizing radiation (Fig. 10). It is particularly helpful for determining whether the artery has a "malignant" course (i.e., traveling between the aorta and main pulmonary artery) (37,38). Figure 11 is an example of a left main coronary artery that has an anomalous origin from the right coronary cusp and travels between the aorta and the pulmonary artery. Cardiac MRI can often provide additional pertinent information during the exam, such as assessing for the clinical significance of the anomaly in terms of myocardial infarction or ischemia, as well as identifying any associated congenital cardiac abnormalities.

CONCLUSION

Cardiac MRI is an excellent test for assessing the patient with suspected ischemic disease. A single examination provides information about cardiac structure and function, stress perfusion, myocardial viability and coronary artery anatomy. MRI can assess ischemic burden and myocardial viability prior to PCI and can help the interventional cardiologist plan the revascularization procedure. In many ways, cardiac MRI is complementary to coronary CT angio-graphy. While coronary CT angiography is principally used to

(A)

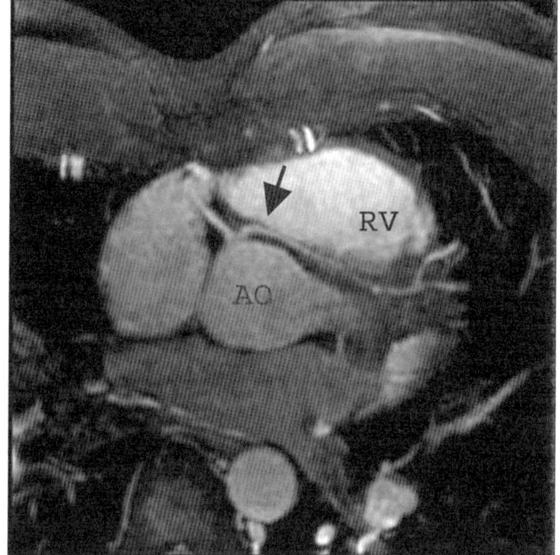

(B)

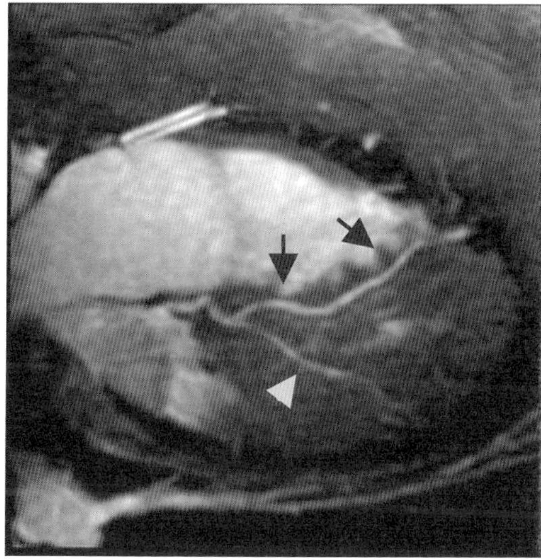

Figure 11 Anomalous origin of left main (LM) coronary artery. (**A**) Coronary MRA showing LM originating from the right coronary cusp, traveling anterior to the aorta (*arrow*). (**B**) Coronary MRA clearly showing the course of the mid to distal left anterior descending (LAD) coronary artery (*arrows*) and a diagonal branch of the LAD (*arrowhead*). *Abbreviations*: Ao, aorta; RV, right ventricle.

assess the coronary lumen, MRI's strength is in evaluating all other aspects of the heart. As more multicenter trials are performed documenting its efficacy, cardiac MRI will become an increasingly routine test over the next several years.

REFERENCES

1. Beanlands RS, deKemp RA, Smith S, Johansen H, Ruddy TD. F-18-fluorodeoxyglucose PET imaging alters clinical decision making in patients with impaired ventricular function. Am J Cardiol 1997; 79:1092–1095.
2. Schinkel AFL, Poldermans D, Vanoverschelde JLJ, et al. Incidence of recovery of contractile function following revascularization in patients with ischemic left ventricular dysfunction. Am J Cardiol 2004; 93:14–17.
3. Allman KC, Shaw LJ, Hachamovitch R, Udelson JE. Myocardial viability testing and impact of revascularization on prognosis in patients with coronary artery disease and left ventricular dysfunction: a meta-analysis. J Am Coll Cardiol 2002; 39:1151–1158.
4. Rizello V, Poldermans D, Biagini E, et al. Benefits of coronary revascularisation in diabetic and non-diabetic patients with ischaemic cardiomyopathy: Role of myocardial viability. Eur J Heart Fail 2006; 8:314–320.
5. Baer FM, Voth E, Schneider CA, Theissen P, Schicha H, Sechtem U. Comparison of low-dose dobutamine-gradient-echo magnetic resonance imaging and positron emission tomography with [18F]fluorodeoxyglucose in patients with chronic coronary artery disease. A functional and morphological approach to the detection of residual myocardial viability. Circulation 1995; 91:1006–1015.
6. Baer FM, Voth E, LaRosee K, et al. Comparison of dobutamine transesophageal echocardiography and dobutamine magnetic resonance imaging for detection of residual myocardial viability. Am J Cardiol 1996; 78:415–419.
7. Kim RJ, Fieno DS, Parrish TB, et al. Relationship of MRI delayed contrast enhancement to irreversible injury, infarct age, and contractile function. Circulation 1999; 100:1992–2002.
8. Wu E, Judd RM, Vargas JD, Klocke FJ, Bonow RO, Kim RJ. Visualisation of presence, location, and transmural extent of healed Q-wave and non-Q-wave myocardial infarction. Lancet 2001; 357:21–28.
9. Klein C, Nekolla SG, Bengel Fm, et al. Assessment of myocardial viability with contrast-enhanced magnetic resonance imaging: comparison with positron emission tomography. Circulation 2002; 105:162–167.

10. Kim RJ, Wu E, Rafael A, et al. The use contrast-enhanced magnetic resonance imaging to identify reversible myocardial dysfunction. N Engl J Med 2000; 343:1445–1453.
11. Wagner A, Mahrholdt H, Holly TA, et al. Contrast-enhanced MRI and routine single photon emission computed tomography (SPECT) perfusion imaging for detection of subendocardial myocardial infarcts: an imaging study. Lancet 2003; 361:374–379.
12. Choi KM, Kim RJ, Gubernikoff G, Vargas JD, Parker M, Judd RM. Transmural extent of acute myocardial infarction predicts long-term improvement in contractile function. Circulation 2002; 104:1101–1107.
13. Lee VS, Resnick D, Tiu SS. MR imaging evaluation of myocardial viability in the setting of equivocal SPECT results with (99 m) Tc sestamibi. Radiology 2004; 230:191–197.
14. Go RT, Marwick TH, MacIntyre WJ, et al. A prospective comparison of rubidium 82 PET and thallium 201 SPECT myocardial perfusion imaging utilizing a single dipyridamole stress in the diagnosis of coronary artery disease. J Nucl Med 1990; 31:1899–1905.
15. Hachamovitch R, Hayes SW, Friedman JD, et al. Stress myocardial perfusion single-photon emission computed tomography is clinically effective and cost effective in risk stratification of patients with a high likelihood of coronary artery disease (CAD) but no known CAD. J Am Coll Cardiol 2004; 43:200–208.
16. Nishimura S, Mahmarian JJ, Boyce TM, et al. Quantitative thallium-201 single-photon emission computed tomography during maximal pharmacologic coronary vasodilation with adenosine for assessing coronary artery disease. J Am Coll Cardiol 1991; 18:736–745.
17. Van Train KF, Maddahi J, Berman DS, et al. Quantitative analysis of tomographic stress thallium-201 myocardial scintigrams: A multicenter trial. J Nucl Med 1990; 31:1168–1179.
18. Wilke N, Kroll K, Merkle H, et al. Regional myocardial blood volume and flow: first-pass MR imaging with polylysine-Gd-DTPA. J Magn Reson Imaging 1995; 5:227–237.
19. Lauerma K, Virtanen KS, Sipila LM, et al. Multislice MRI in assessment of myocardial perfusion in patients with single-vessel proximal left anterior descending coronary artery disease before and after revascularization. Circulation 1997; 96:2859–2867.
20. Wagner A, Mahrholdt H, Holly TA, et al Contrast-enhanced MRI and routine single photon emission computed tomography (SPECT) perfusion imaging for detection of subendocardial myocardial infarcts: an imaging study. Lancet 2003; 361:374–379.
21. Nishimura S, Mahmarian JJ, Boyce TM, et al. Quantitative thallium-201 single-photon emission computed tomography during maximal pharmacologic coronary vasodilation with adenosine for assessing coronary artery disease. J Am Coll Cardiol 1991; 18:736–745.
22. Takase B, Nagata M, Kihara T, et al. Whole-heart dipyridamole stress first-pass myocardial perfusion MRI for the detection of coronary artery disease. Jpn Heart J 2004; 45:475–486.
23. Miller DD. Pharmacologic stressors in coronary artery disease. In: Dilsizian V, Narula J, Braunwald E, eds. Atlas of Nuclear Cardiology. Philadelphia: Current Medicine, 2003:47–62.
24. Hachamovitch R, Hayes SW, Friedman JD, et al. A prognostic score for prediction of cardiac mortality risk after adenosine stress myocardial perfusion scintigraphy. J Am Coll Cardiol 2005; 45:722–729.
25. Wang Y, Moin K, Akinboboye O, et al. Myocardial first pass perfusion: Steady-state free precession versus spoiled gradient echo and segmented echo planar imaging. Magn Reson Med 2005; 54:1123–1129.
26. Fenchel M, Helber U, Kramer U. Detection of regional myocardial perfusion deficit using rest and stress perfusion MRI: a feasibility study. AJR 2005; 185:627–635.
27. Wolff SD, Schwitter J, Coulden R. et al. Myocardial first-pass perfusion magnetic resonance imaging; a multicenter dose-ranging study. Circulation 2004; 110:732–737.
28. Slavin S, Wolff SD, Gupta SN, et al. First-pass myocardial perfusion MR imaging with interleaved notched saturation: feasibility study. Radiology 2001; 219:258–263.
29. Geleijnse ML, Fioretti PM, Roelandt JR. Methodology, feasibility, safety and diagnostic accuracy of dobutamine stress echocardiography. J Am Coll Cardiol 1997; 30:595–606.
30. Thomas JD, Rudin DN. Tissue harmonic imaging: why does it work? J Am Soc Echocardiogr 1998; 11:803–808.

31. Hundley WG, Hamilton CA, Thomas MS, et al. Utility of fast cine magnetic resonance imaging and display for the detection of myocardial ischemia in patients not well suited for second harmonic stress echocardiography. Circulation 1999; 100:1697–1702.
32. Nagel E, Lehmkuhl HB, Bocksch W, et al. Noninvasive diagnosis of ischemia-induced wall motion abnormalities with the use of high-dose dobutamine stress MRI: comparison with dobutamine stress echocardiography. Circulation 1999; 99:763–770.
33. Botnar RM, Stuber M, Danias PG, et al. Improved coronary artery definition with T2-weighted free breathing 3D-coronary MRA. Circulation 1999; 3139–3148.
34. Sandstede JJ, Pabst T, Beer M, et al. Three-dimensional MR coronary angiography using the navigator technique compared with conventional coronary angiography. Am J Roentgenol 1999; 172:135–139.
35. Kim WY, Danias PG, Stuber M, et al. Coronary magnetic resonance angiography for the detection of coronary stenoses. N Engl J Med 2001; 345:1863–1869.
36. So NM, Lam WW, Li D, Chan AK, Sanderson JE, Metreweli C. Magnetic resonance angiography of coronary arteries with a 3-dimensional magnetization-prepared true fast imaging with steady-state precession sequence compared with conventional coronary angiography. Am Heart J 2005; 150:530–535.
37. Bunce NH, Lorenz CH, Keegan J, et al. Coronary artery anomalies: assessment with free-breathing three-dimensional coronary MR angiography. Radiology 2003; 227:201–208.
38. Post JC, van Rossum AC, Bronzwaer JG, et al. Magnetic resonance angiography of anomalous coronary arteries. A new gold standard for delineating the proximal course? Circulation 1995; 92:3163–3171.

16

Tips and tricks for endovascular carotid interventions

B. Reimers, Jennifer Sugita, and Horst Sievert

INTRODUCTION

Stroke is the third most frequent cause of death in developed countries. Nearly 50% of the patients suffer from significant intellectual or physical disorders after their stroke.

Ischemic events are the cause of the vast majority of strokes (80–85%). Nearly one-third of all ischemic strokes are caused by carotid artery disease. In carotid stenoses more than 80% of clinical symptoms are due to embolism originating from the arteriosclerotic plaque. In 20%, strokes occur because of hemodynamic impairment of the cerebral circulation (1,2).

The intention of the interventional or surgical treatment of the carotid artery stenosis is therefore firstly focused on plaque covering or removal in order to minimize the risk of debris dislodgment and distal embolization. Secondly, significant hemodynamic vessel lumen narrowing can also be repaired and normal flow can be restored.

In the past several years, carotid stenting has rapidly developed to be a successful alternative to surgery and is increasingly the preferred method in surgically high-risk patients (3–6). Additionally, many patients tend to favor stenting to surgery because it is less invasive, does not cause a scar, and requires only a short hospital stay (under 24 hours). Other advantages of the interventional approach over carotid surgery include the ability to diagnose and treat embolic complications immediately. Furthermore, the fact that the patient can be awake allows close neurologic monitoring during the entire procedure. Complications like distal embolization can be recognized and treated immediately.

Several large randomized trials of carotid surgery have proven the advantage of surgery in symptomatic patients compared to medical treatment alone. In 1991, the North American and European carotid surgical trials (NASCET and ECST trials) demonstrated the long-term benefit for symptomatic patients who experienced a non-disabling stroke or TIA within the last 6 months and had a degree of carotid stenosis exceeding 50% (7–9). However, among patients who suffered from carotid artery disease without any neurological symptoms, the balance between surgical or interventional risk and long-term benefits of the procedure was indistinct and remained very controversial for many years.

Results from the Veterans Affairs Asymptomatic Carotid Endarterectomy Trial (VA trial) in 1993 and Asymptomatic Carotid Artherosclerosis Study (ACAS) in 1995 were promising, showing a significant reduction in the incidence of TIA and minor stroke. However, the reduction of the incidence of fatal or major stroke was not significantly beneficial compared to medical treatment (10,11).

In 2004, the ACST trial examined asymptomatic patients and established beneficial results when the patient was younger than 75 years and had a stenosis exceeding 70% measured in duplex scan (12). The risk of stroke or death within 30 days of surgery was 3.1%. Immediate carotid endarterectomy could lower the net five-year stroke risk of 12% by half to only 6%. Half of this five-year benefit involved disabling or fatal strokes.

It was proven that surgery of asymptomatic lesions is justified because the risk of suffering a stroke in patients with adequate history under medical treatment alone is higher than the operative risk. The more comorbidities, the higher the stroke and death rates but the greater the benefit from surgery within mid- and long-term course. The results of the ACST trial are an important extension of the results of earlier trials of asymptomatic carotid artery disease because they also proved the prevention of disabling and fatal strokes in women.

Currently, the indications for intervention with carotid stenting are considered to be similar to those for carotid surgery. Therefore, the guidelines for surgery are applied to carotid stenting as well. Carotid stenting should be recommended for symptomatic lesions of $\geq$ 50% and asymptomatic lesions $\geq$ 70%.

When a significant carotid stenosis is assumed, a carotid duplex scan or an MRI should be performed. The diameter of the stenosis measured either by duplex scan or MRI often shows a false positive result or overestimates the degree of the lesion. To avoid unnecessary additional invasive tests, the decision whether or not to stent is usually made during the intervention after angiographic measurement of the minimal diameter of stenosis.

We discuss the technical aspects of carotid stenting and different approaches to treatment that may reduce the risk of periprocedural complications. Furthermore the initial clinical results of CAS with cerebral protection are presented and discussed.

THE CAROTID ARTERY STENT PROCEDURE

Patient preparation

Continuous ECG monitoring is mandatory to control eventual bradycardia, and direct pressure monitoring through the guiding catheter or through the introducer sheath is highly recommended to observe the hemodynamics of the patient. Before the carotid artery stenting procedure, we administer aspirin (100–325 mg) and ticlopidine (250 mg, two times a day, starting at least 5 days before the procedure) or clopidogrel (75 mg once a day for 5 days before the procedure or 600 mg if administered immediately before the procedure). If there is uncertainty regarding exact timing about the starting of thienopyridine treatment we still give a loading dose. During the procedure, heparin (70–100 IU/Kg) is administered, maintaining ACT between 250 and 300 seconds. At the end of the procedure it is advisable to repeat an ACT evaluation particularly in elderly patients, patients with high blood pressure, and patients in whom flow in the internal carotid artery was impaired before the procedure. In these patients with increased risk of hyperfusion syndrome (ACT values >250 sec) heparin can be neutralized using protamine sulphate. Just before the post-dilatation, we suggest, administering 1 mg of atropine intravenously to prevent or attenuate possible bradycardia or asystole. During the procedure an infusion pump of dopamine is prepared ready for use in case of prolonged hypotension. Keeping the systolic blood pressure at adequate values is particularly important in patients with an occluded carotid artery and those in whom a proximal occlusion device is going to be used.

After the procedure aspirin therapy is continued indefinitely and ticlopidine or clopidogrel therapy is continued for one month. In the increasingly frequent cases of CAS preceding the aortocoronary bypass intervention, we have reduced the post-stent anti-platelet therapy to only aspirin without any problems. The use of drugs inhibiting glycoprotein IIb/IIIa is not recommended during the procedures of carotid artery stenting (13,14).

Vascular access

Access from the femoral artery that allows easy access of the common carotid arteries is preferred. Only if the femoral arteries are occluded or if access of the common carotid artery from the femoral artery is unsuccessful, the brachial access is used. The right brachial artery appears favorable for the treatment of both the right and left carotid artery (Figs. 1 and 2).

Diagnostic angiography

The selective cannulation of the common carotid artery by a diagnostic catheter is necessary to achieve adequate angiographic images, which allow visualization and exact evaluation of the severity of the lesion. Usually right curve-type Judkins catheters are used. Suitable alternative catheters include the right Amplatz, Headhunter, Vitek, Berenstein, and Simoons catheters, which allow, after a brief training session, stable cannulation of the anatomically difficult carotid arteries because their curve can be positioned in the ascendant aorta. The dimensions of the diagnostic catheters range from 4 to 6 French. With a slightly traumatic 4 French catheter selectively positioned in the carotid artery, it is possible to achieve good quality carotid angiography. With a the exception of very simple cases it is preferable to manipulate the catheter forward using soft, hydrophilic, 0.035 in. wires. We usually use wires that are very soft and slightly traumatic. However these guides must not move forward beyond the carotid bifurcation. Carotid angiography is an integral element of the CAS intervention and care must be taken to minimize the incidence of thromboembolic complications. It has been shown that using NMR, cerebral focal lesions have been demonstrated in more than 25% of diagnostic cerebral angiographies (15,16). After selective angiography of the carotid bifurcation, we suggest to perform an intracranial angiography in anteroposterior and lateral projection, through the carotid artery as well.

Many operators perform a pigtail injection in the carotid arch at the very beginning of the angiographic procedure in order to detect possible lesions at the ostium of the common carotid and/or anonymous trunk, and to better assess the baseline anatomy to facilitate selective access.

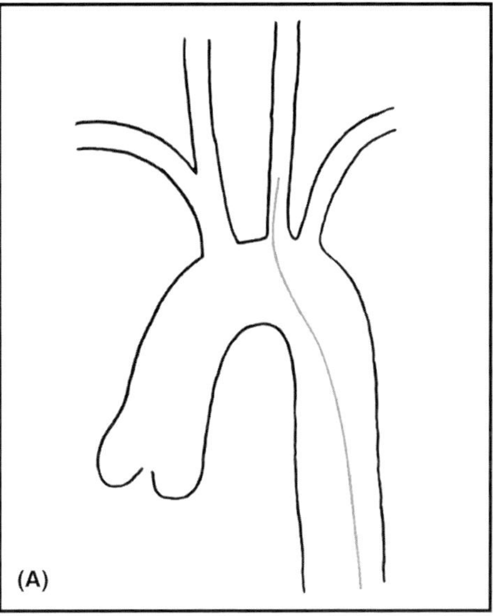

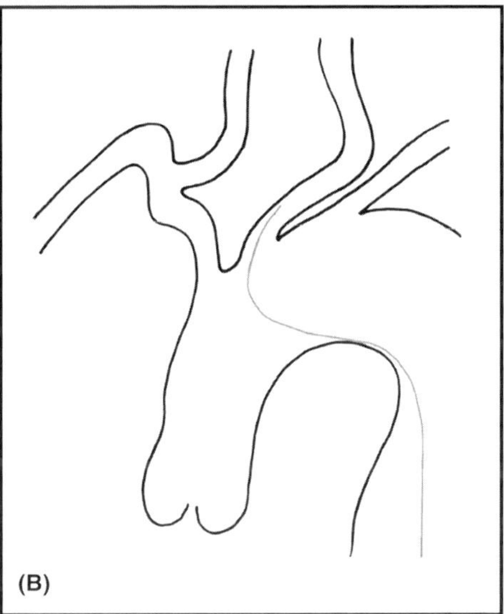

Figure 1 Variations of the aortic arch. With vessels like that in (**A**), the access can be performed without complications. In (**B**) the access is more difficult as a catheter might tend to prolapse into the ascending aorta.

Access with sheaths or guiding catheters into the common carotid artery

A pivotal factor in obtaining technical success in a CAS procedure is the ability to gain access to the common carotid artery. The principal reason for procedural failure is the inability to advance an introducer or a guide catheter in the common carotid artery due to a difficult take-off from the anonymous trunk or from the aortic arch, or due to important kinking or coiling of the common

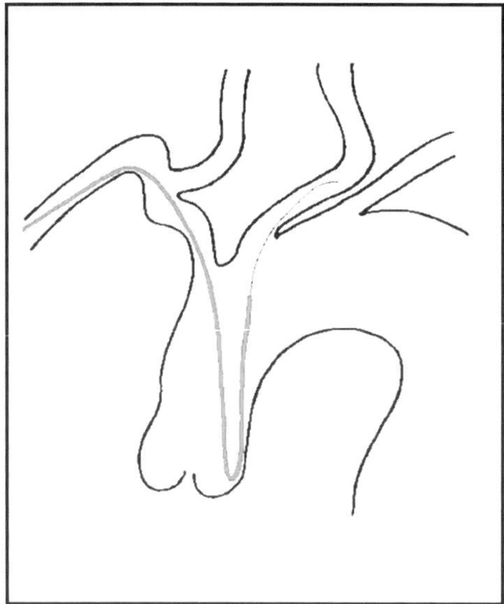

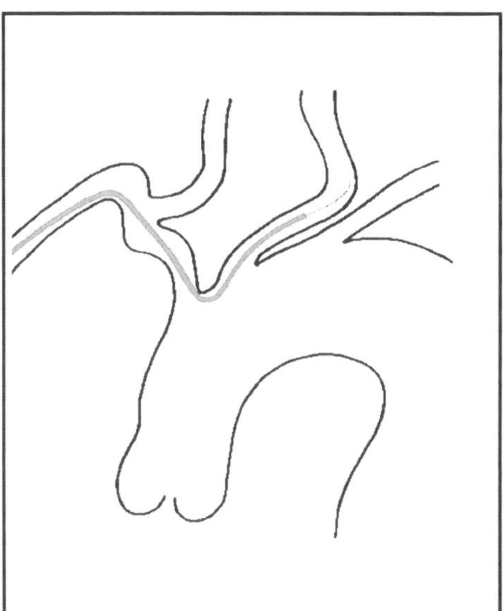

Figure 2 Transbrachial access.

carotid itself. Baseline images of the arch obtained angiographically or with MRI are very helpful in planning the procedure and selecting the best of the following strategies.

The long introducer of 6 or 7 French is the preferred instrument to obtain the cannulation of the common carotid artery by the Roubin's school. This involves positioning of a diagnostic catheter relatively distally in the common carotid artery or in the proximal part of the external carotid artery. To move the catheter forward into the vessel, the technique of very slow "push and pull" of the catheter on the 0.035 in. or 0.038 in. floppy, hydrophilic wire can be used. Following this the floppy wire is retracted and a long (220–260 cm) high support-floppy tip wire of 0.035 in. (e.g. Supracore™, Guidant Corp., St. Paul, MN) is positioned in the external carotid artery through the diagnostic catheter (Fig. 3). During this procedure the angiographic application of the "road mapping" may be useful. Once the guide has been positioned into the external carotid artery the diagnostic catheter is removed and the introducer with its inner dilator is advanced into the common carotid artery close to the bifurcation, and then the dilator and the guide are removed. Armed introducers, 80–100 cm long, are used providing both an acceptable flexibility and sufficient stability so that they do not bend after removal of the dilator. Recently hydrophilic coated introducers became available that are particularly suitable in complex anatomies. Alternatively, some operators may prefer to use the coaxial (or telescope) technique to position the sheath (in contrast to the previously described sequential technique). In this case a long (>120 cm), 4–5 French diagnostic catheter is preloaded into a long sheath. Using the hydrophilic wire the common carotid artery is engaged with the diagnostic catheter. Subsequently the sheath is advanced on the wire and the diagnostic catheter into the common carotid artery. Only in rare cases a support wire is needed to advance the sheath into the common carotid artery.

Another system to access the common carotid artery is guiding catheters. Most protection and filter systems require 8 French catheters; some can be used with 7 French and few with 6 French catheters. Coronary catheters such as right Judkins-type for both carotid arteries, the multipurpose for the right carotid artery, and the hockey-stick type for a mammary artery, or even a left or right Amplatz catheter for the left carotid artery may be used.

Usually the guide catheters are carefully rotated in the aortic arch until they engage the common carotid artery or the anonymous trunk. The coronary guide catheters are parked in the

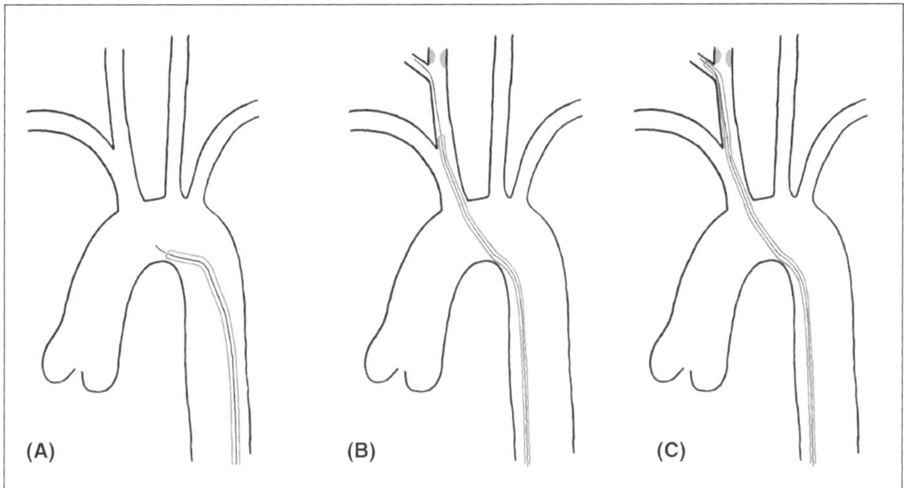

Figure 3 Over-the-wire technique: The wire is advanced into the common (**B**) and later into the external (**C**) carotid artery, followed by the catheter.

aortic arch without deep intubation into the common carotid artery. Despite that fact, they usually give sufficient support to the angioplasty execution due to the low profile stents and to the system of protection available. There are specific guide catheters with a very soft tip and a distal segment of 5 cm that allow a more distal advancing of the catheter into the common carotid artery.

It is not easy to choose between the long introducer and the guide catheter as to which is the best technique. The introducer technique, which comprises a diagnostic catheter, the cannulation of the external carotid artery with a support guide switch-type, and the introducer itself, is surely more complex and more expensive. The most important advantage is the advancing of the introducer in a very controlled way from the aorta into the common carotid artery using the introducer tip tapered by the dilator or by the diagnostic catheter, reducing the risk of dislocation of the plaque with a possible embolization to the brain. Furthermore, the introducer positioned into the common carotid artery assures a high support to complete the stenting procedure.

The guide catheter technique is simpler and less expensive but potentially has a theoretical increase of embolization risk in case of an aortic arch with severe atheromatous alterations. The recent possibility of using smaller and potentially less traumatic 7 or even 6 French guiding catheters because of the reduced (<5 French) of stent systems is very appealing.

If the access to the common carotid artery is difficult, we suggest stopping the attempts after 30 minutes and reconsidering the surgical therapy because, experience tells, major complications may occur after prolonged maneuvers with catheters in the aortic arch.

Protection systems

Actually, three different approaches for cerebral protection are used: two systems of distal protection such as distal occlusive balloons and filters, and proximal protection using the occlusion of the common and external carotid arteries (Fig. 4).

Distal occlusion balloons

Distal occlusion balloons constitute the first system of protection used on a large scale. They consist of a 0.014 in. guide-wire with a balloon on the distal portion that may be inflated and deflated through a very small channel contained in the guide itself (Percusurge/Guardwire; Medtronic, Minneapolis, MN). The lesion is crossed with the guide, thereby positioning the balloon distally to the stenosis where it is

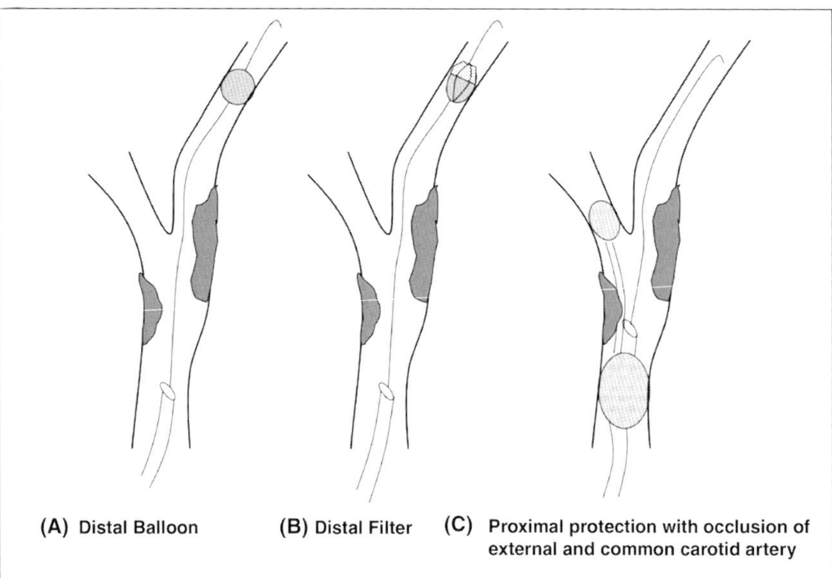

Figure 4 Cerebral protection systems: (**A**) Distal balloon, (**B**) distal filter; (**C**) proximal protection with occlusion of external and common carotid artery.

inflated until the blood flow in the internal carotid artery is blocked. Following this, the angioplasty and stenting procedure is carried out. On completion of the procedure, a catheter is advanced up to the distal balloon and the column of blood contained in the occluded internal carotid artery is aspirated. In this way debris dislodged incidentally during the stent procedure is eliminated. Afterward the balloon is deflated and the guide is removed.

The advantages of distal occlusion balloons are the small diameter (2.2 French) and the good maneuverability and flexibility of the system. Possible disadvantages are that the occlusion is not tolerated by 6–10% of patients (17,18) and it is not possible to image the vessel with contrast medium during the inflation.

Distal filters

The protection filters consist of a metallic structure (or skeleton) coated by a membrane of polyethylene or a net of nitinol wires that contain holes 80–200 μm in diameter (Fig. 4) (19,20). The filters are usually positioned at the distal portion of a 0.014 in. guide. During the procedure the filters are enveloped into a delivery catheter with which they are advanced distally to the stenosis. After the lesion is crossed, the filter is opened by removing the delivery sheath. At the end of the stenting procedure the filter is closed with a retrieval catheter and is removed from the carotid artery.

In the presence of sharp stenoses from calcified or very fibrous plaques, the passage of the closed filter may be impossible. Usually, following the use of a 0.014 in. "buddy wire" or careful predilatation with 2–2.5 mm diameter balloons, it becomes possible to cross the stenosis with the filter.

A great number of protection filters of second or third generation exist. The technical characteristics of a good protection filter consist of a low profile (<3 French), adequate torqueability to cross even tortuous vessels, and, when open, adequate apposition to the wall to ensure the best possible protection. Filter systems with a "free wire" that allow positioning of the wire followed by the advancement of the filter itself are now available and may be useful in patients with internal carotid arteries with important tortuousity.

Proximal protection

Distal protection devices (occlusive balloons or filters) have the disadvantage that they must cross the lesion before they are inflated or opened (21). This passage (or crossing) carries the risk of embolization during this "unprotected" step of the procedure. The proximal protection systems, in contrast, provide cerebral protection before the passage of any type of device through the stenoses. These systems consist of a long introducer sheath with a balloon that is inflated in the common carotid artery. A second balloon, inflated in the external carotid artery, assures the total blockade of the antegrade blood flow in the internal carotid artery. The proximal protection systems use the cerebral vascular connections of the Willis circuit. After the occlusion of the common and external carotid artery, the collateral flow through the Willis circuit will create so-called "back-pressure," which will prevent antegrade flow in the internal carotid artery. After stent positioning, and before the deflation of the balloons in the common and external carotid artery, the blood present in the internal carotid artery, possibly containing dislodged debris, is aspirated and removed.

The advantage of the proximal protection system is that the entire procedure is carried out under protection and, if correctly applied, should completely avoid any type of embolization. The disadvantages of the proximal protection system are that it is not tolerated by all patients and that the two systems actually available (Parodi, Arteria, San Francisco, CA; Mo.Ma, Invatec, Roncadelle, Italy) require 10 or 9 French introducer sheaths.

The stent implantation

With the exception of treatment of in-stent restenoses, every carotid angioplasty procedure requires the use of stent implantation. Direct stenting without predilation is performed in the majority of lesions. In cases of very severe (>90%) calcified lesions, or fibrotic post-surgical restenotic lesions that may cause a difficult passage or a difficult stent expansion, predilatation using coronary balloons (diameter 3.5–4.00 mm) is performed. Usually stents of a diameter from 6 to 9 mm are used, and the diameter of the distal common carotid artery is used as a reference. In the rare cases where the stent is positioned only into the internal carotid artery without covering the bifurcation, the endoprosthesis dimensions are selected in accordance to the diameter of the internal carotid artery. Relatively long stents that allow covering and sealing the entire lesion are used. The stent length generally ranges from 30 to 40 mm and, contrary to what was demonstrated for coronary stenting, there are no data demonstrating a relationship between the length of the stent and the incidence of restenosis. The stent is positioned as far proximal as possible ensuring the coverage of the complete lesion. Generally, the stent is positioned covering the bifurcation. Rare cases of occlusions of the external carotid are described, which, however, clinically remained silent.

Self-expandable stents are used almost exclusively in the carotid artery because they have a lower risk of deformation or fracture compared to balloon-expandable stents, in case of sharp movements or neck trauma. There are two different kinds of self-expanding stents. The first are "mesh wire" stents (Fig. 5) consisting of braided alloy wires that open like a spring to adapt to the vessel diameter (Carotid Wallstent; Boston Scientific, Natick, MA). Advantages of this stent are: the very low profile (5.5 French) with a flexible shaft, the rapid exchange feature that allows the use of short guide-wires and the excellent deliverability. The possibility of re-closing a half-released stent allows repositioning of the stent's distal edge. Possible drawbacks are the important foreshortening at upon stent release and vessel straightening leading to possible distal kinking. More recently self-expandable Nitinol stents have been introduced, which are characterized by a higher radial strength and by a higher adaptability to tortuous vessels and to the differences of diameter between the internal and the common carotid (Fig. 6). These stents open to a given diameter because of their thermal memory. Some nitinol stents are made in a conic way (tapered stents) and have a lower diameter at the distal portion to be positioned in the internal carotid, and a larger diameter at the proximal portion to be positioned in the common carotid artery (Fig. 7). Nitinol stents with open cell design are thought to adapt better to vessel tortuosities, whereas closed cell nitinol stents are more rigid but thought to provide better plaque coverage. At present it is impossible to decide which design and which stent material gets the best results in the long term because comparative studies between the different types of stents are not available.

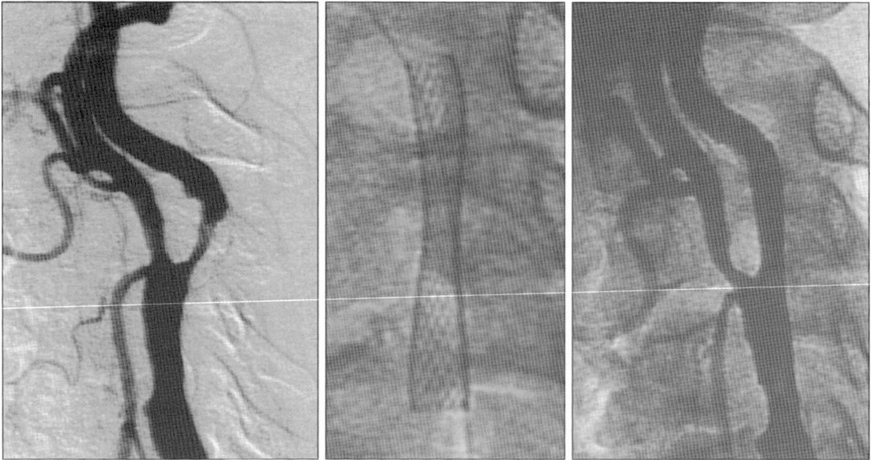

Figure 5 Mesh-wire stent.

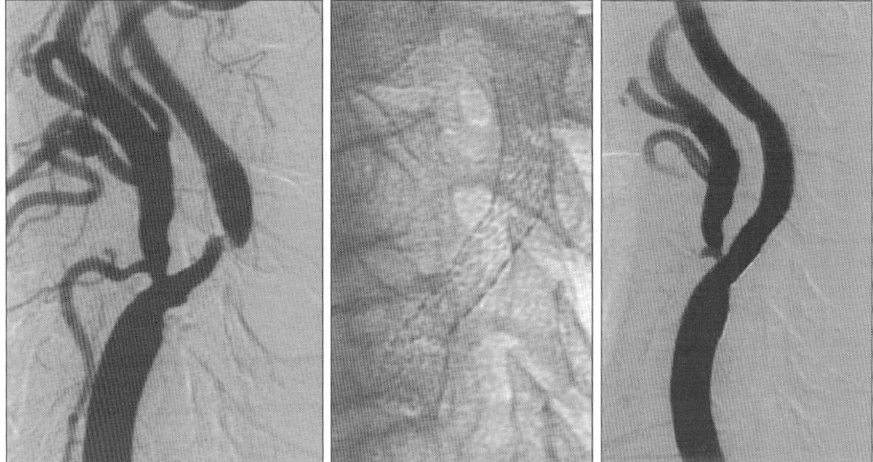

Figure 6 Nitinol stent.

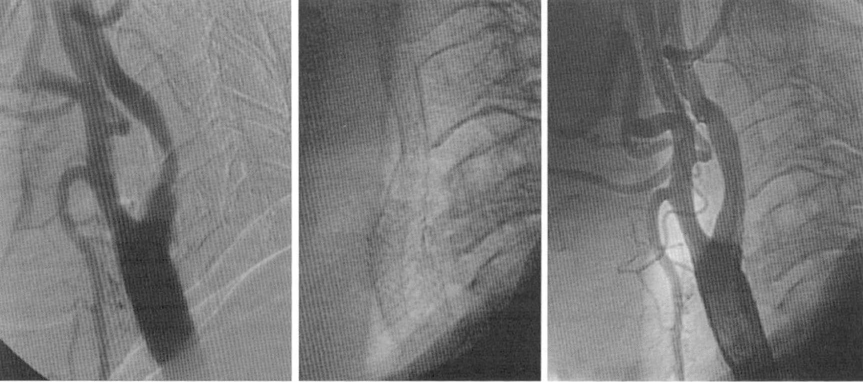

Figure 7 Tapered stent.

Balloon post-dilatation of the stent

Due to the risk of embolization we recommend, even if protection systems are used, the use of undersized diameter balloons in respect to the vessel diameter and inflation pressures not higher than 10 atmospheres. Unlike coronary stenting, during carotid stenting, it is not necessary to obtain a residual stenosis close to 0%. Angiographic results showing a residual stenosis up to 50%, obtained without an excessive embolization risk, assure very good clinical and echographic results post-procedurally and at long term.

EDITORS' COMMENTS

An open debate and question is: which is the best protection system to be used?

In general the operator faces several dilemmas: the easy and user-friendly nature of filters, the theoretical more powerful protection of proximal or distal occlusive systems, and the lack of any specific data to demonstrate any advantage of occlusive devices versus filters.

Even if there are no specific studies addressing this issue some operators will use proximal or distal protection systems in high-risk patients or lesions evaluated by clinical history (old age, prior ischemic events) or sonography data (soft plaque).

Among the two occlusive systems currently available we think that, whenever possible, usage of proximal protection devices is better.

Despite any attempt to use the best protection device or approach, we should never forget that 100% safety does not exist and the operator should always trade risks versus benefits. Most probably careful performance of the baseline study and ability to resist optimal postdilatation are very useful caveats.

When should a filter be used?

In general I use a filter in a medium- or low-risk situation. A typical case is a patient under 70 years old, asymptomatic with 80% or less stenosis and no specific echo evidence of soft plaque or angiographic evidence of ulcerated plaque, or any patient who cannot tolerate a temporary occlusion. If the patient is high risk, surgery should be considered.

When should distal occlusive protection (Percusurge, Medtronic, Natick, MA) be used?

Use distal occlusive protection for high-risk patients with at least one of the following: older than 70 years, prior history of stroke, ulcerated or soft plaque, or more than 90% stenosis when a proximal protection device cannot be used.

When it is very difficult to access the common carotid or when there is a total occlusion of the external carotid preventing placement of a SupraCore wire in this vessel, do not use a proximal protection device. The general rule is that if you can place a SupraCore wire in the external carotid you will be able to advance a proximal protection device in the common carotid.

When should a proximal protection device be used?

In a patient who meets all the following criteria: the external carotid is patent and accessible with a SupraCore wire; the patient is high risk as defined above; and the patient is able to tolerate temporary occlusion. Of course the answer to this question is only obtainable after having placed the device. In case the patient is not able to tolerate occlusion we can switch to a filter if we consider the risk of suboptimal protection acceptable in a high risk patient or lesion, otherwise the procedure needs to be stopped and the patient will be referred to surgery.

Which type of stent should be used?

Unless the lesion is localized only to the internal carotid we prefer to cover the bifurcation and almost always use a tapered (conical) stent with the most frequently used length of 40 mm. In situations where the lesion is confined to the internal or common carotid and there is no need to cover the bifurcation, we use a standard stent. We prefer to cover the bifurcation if there are doubts regarding extension of the disease.

What about stents with dense struts?

Stents such as Abbott, Invatec and Wallstent have more coverage of the plaque but are less flexible. Many prefer to use these types of stents in soft plaque to minimize prolapse. No clear data are available to support this rationale. Despite this limitation we think that if the anatomy is not particularly tortuous and the lesion does not involve a sharp bend, the usage of a stent with high plaque coverage in a high-risk lesion is very acceptable. In all the other situations we use a more flexible and more open cells stent.

When should we not implant a stent?
When I treat in-stent restenosis and I get a good result following balloon dilatation I will not implant another stent.

What happens if a stent cannot be advanced and predilation has already been done?
The first approach is always to place a buddy wire, which may be high support such as the Ironman wire (Guidant, Abbott). If we are working without a proximal protection device, switching to this more supportive system can be considered. If the result is optimal, a stent may not need to be placed. What we should not do is try to optimize the result with a balloon when we know we cannot advance a stent at a later point if needed. Never forget that carotid surgery is still a viable option.

REFERENCES

1. American Heart Association. Heart Disease and Stroke Statistics—2004 Update. http://americanheart.org
2. Wolf PA, Kannel WB, McGee PC. Epidemiology of strokes in North America. In: Barnet HJM, Stein BM, Mohr JP, Yatsu FM, eds. Stroke: Pathophysiology, Diagnosis and Management Vol. 1. (New York: Churchill Livingstone, 1986: 1929.
3. Mathias K, Perkutane transluminale Katheterbehandlung supraaortaler Arterienobstruktionen, Angio 1981; 3:47–50.
4. Roubin SG, New G, Iyer SS, et al. Immediate and late clinical outcomes of carotid artery stenting in patients with symptomatic and asymptomatic carotid artery stenosis. A 5-year prospective analysis. Circulation 2001; 103:532–537.
5. Endovascular versus surgical treatment in patients with carotid stenosis in the carotid and vertebral artery transluminal angioplasty study (CAVATAS): a randomised trial. Lancet 2001; 357:1729–1737.
6. Yadav JS, Wholey MH, Kuntz RE, et al. Protected carotid-artery stenting versus endarterectomy in high-risk patients (the SAPPHIRE study). N Engl J Med 2004; 351:1493–1501.
7. North American Symptomatic Carotid Endarterectomy Trial Collaborators: Beneficial effect of carotid endarterectomy in symptomatic patients with high grade carotid stenosis. N Engl J Med 1991; 32: 445–453.
8. European Carotid Surgery Trialists' Collaborative Group. Randomised trial of endarterectomy for recently symptomatic carotid stenosis: final results of the MRC European Carotid Surgery Trial (ECST). Lancet 1998; 351:1379–1387.
9. Mayberg MR, Wilson SE, Yatsu F, et al. Carotid endarterectomy and prevention of cerebral ischemia in symptomatic carotid stenosis. Veterans Affairs Cooperative Studies Program 309 Trialist Group. JAMA 1991; 266:3289–3294.
10. Executive Committee for the asymptomatic carotid arteriosclerosis study. Endarterectomy for the asymptomatic carotid artery stenosis. JAMA 1995; 273:1421–1428.
11. Hobson RW, Weiss DG, Fields ES, et al. Efficacy of carotid endarterectomy for asymptomatic stenosis: The veterans affairs cooperative study group. N Engl J Med 1993; 328:221–227.
12. MRC Asymptomatic Carotid Surgery Trial (ACST) Collaborative Group. Prevention of disabling and fatal strokes by successful carotid endarterectomy in patients without recent neurological symptoms: randomised controlled trial. Lancet 2004; 363: 1491–1502.
13. Hofmann R, Kerschner K, Steinwender C, et al. Abciximab bolus injection does not reduce cerebral ischemic complications of elective carotid artery stenting: a randomized study. Stroke. 2002; 33:725–727.
14. Qureshi AI, Saad M, Zaidat OO, et al. Intracerebral hemorrhages associated with neurointerventional procedures using a combination of antithrombotic agents including abciximab. Stroke 2002; 33: 1916–1919.
15. Schlüter M, Tübler T, Steffens JC, Mathey DG, Schofer J. Focal Ischemia of the brain after neuroprotected carotid artery stenting. J Am Coll Cardiol 2003; 42:1007–1013.
16. Crawley F, Clifton A, Buckenham T, et al. Comparison of hemodynamic cerebral ischemia and

microembolic signals detected during carotid endarterectomy and carotid angioplasty. Stroke 1997; 28:2460–2464.

17. Al-Mubarak N, Roubin GS, Vitek JJ, et al. Effect of the distal-balloon protection system on microembolization during carotid stenting. Circulation 2001; 104:1999–2002.
18. Tübler T, Schlüter M, Dirsch O, et al. Balloon-protected carotid artery stenting: relationship of periprocedural neurological complications with the size of particulate debris. Circulation 2001; 104:2791–2796.
19. Reimers B, Corvaja N, Moshiri S, et al. Cerebral protection with filter devices during carotid artery stenting. Circulation 2001; 104: 12–15.
20. Al-Mubarak N, Colombo A, Gaines PA, et al. Multicenter evaluation of carotid artery stenting with a filter protection system. J Am Coll Cardiol 2002; 39:841–846.
21. Adami CA, Scuro A, Spinamano L, et al. Use of the Parodi anti-embolism system in carotid stenting: Italian trial results. J Endovasc Ther 2002; 9:147–154.

17

Transseptal puncture

Ted Feldman and Westby G. Fisher

INTRODUCTION

The technique of transseptal puncture was developed to gain access to the left atrium (LA) for pressure measurement. Methods to measure left atrial pressure prior to the transseptal approach included direct left atrial puncture through the anterior chest wall, and transbronchial puncture via the left mainstem bronchus (1–8). These methods had obvious limitations. The transseptal approach was first described by Cope in 1959, using a 17-gauge solid needle introduced through polyethylene tubing via the right femoral vein (9). He employed the procedure in two patients and described left atrial and ventricular pressure measurement and angiography. In 1958 Ross et al., while working at the National Institutes of Health, were catheterizing the LA in patients with atrial septal defects. Ross was a fellow at the time. A visiting physician observed this procedure and asked whether Ross had considered using a needle to puncture the intact septum. This rapidly led to the development of a needle device for transseptal puncture via femoral cutdown in the animal laboratory (10). A few years later, when the Seldinger technique was introduced, a surgical resident working with Braunwald designed a catheter, the Brockenbrough catheter, through which the Ross needle could be placed percutaneously (11–13). The substitution of the Mullins sheath for the Brockenbrough catheter was the last major advance in the basic procedure. Subsequently, the transseptal puncture procedure has undergone only minor modifications (Fig. 1) (14,15).

Due to the technical challenges and the risks involved with transseptal puncture, pulmonary wedge pressure (PCW) measurement has been accepted as a surrogate for left atrial pressure assessment (16). PCW measurement remains the most common approach for estimation of the left atrial pressure in patients with heart failure and valvular heart disease. There are clear limitations to PCW, especially among patients with pulmonary hypertension (17–21). In the setting of pulmonary hypertension, elevated pulmonary artery pressure may "contaminate" the wedge pressure waveform and result in a significant overestimation of the PCW. Similarly, over-wedging may yield an underestimation.

Methods for retrograde catheterization of the LA via the left ventricle have been developed using specialized catheter shapes (22–24). Shirey and Sones described a multipurpose-type catheter that could be folded in the left ventricular apex and introduced into the left atrium (22). This approach is complicated by frequent ventricular ectopy, ventricular perforation, and inconsistent ability to cannulate the left atrium. Stefanadis et al. developed a guide catheter with a pull wire to flex the catheter tip backward from

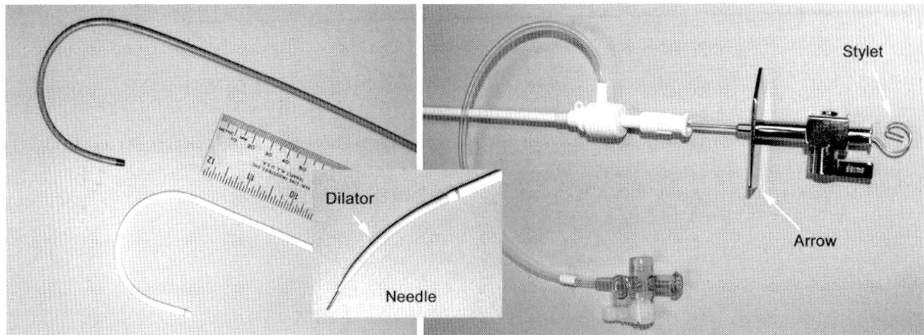

Figure 1 Mullins sheath and transseptal needle. The left panel shows 2 brands of 8-French Mullins sheaths. The curve helps direct the tip of the sheath toward the left ventricle after placement in the left atrium. The inset shows the tip of the transseptal needle protruding from the end of the dilator-sheath assembly. The right panel shows the hub of the dilator, sheath, and needle assembly. The large metal arrow indicates the orientation of the curve of the tip of the needle. A stylet is placed within the needle as the needle is passed through the dilator initially, to keep the tip of the needle from catching or perforating the transseptal dilator and sheath during insertion of the needle.

the left ventricle toward the LA, which allows introduction of a wire consistently and reliably into the left atrium (25). This device is not available in the United States and has not gained wide popularity for diagnostic purposes, being used only for retrograde, transarterial mitral balloon valvuloplasty.

Thus, transseptal puncture remains the gold standard for left atrial pressure assessment. It has clearly become more important in both electrophysiology and interventional cardiology as therapeutic procedures that require left atrial access become more common (21).

TECHNIQUE

The basic technique involves right femoral vein access. A 0.032 in. small guide wire is passed into the superior vena cava. A pigtail catheter is placed in the aortic root to better define the location of the aortic valve. A Mullins sheath and dilator are tracked over the wire into the superior vena cava and ideally angulated toward the left subclavian vein (Fig. 2). The wire is removed. A transseptal needle is introduced into the dilator. The needle contains a stylette that keeps the tip of the needle from catching on the body of the transseptal sheath dilator as the needle is advanced. The stylette must be withdrawn from the needle before the needle gets too close to the distal end of the transseptal dilator. The needle is positioned with its tip a few millimeters proximal to the distal end of the Mullins dilator, connected to a manifold and flushed (Fig. 2, inset). Right

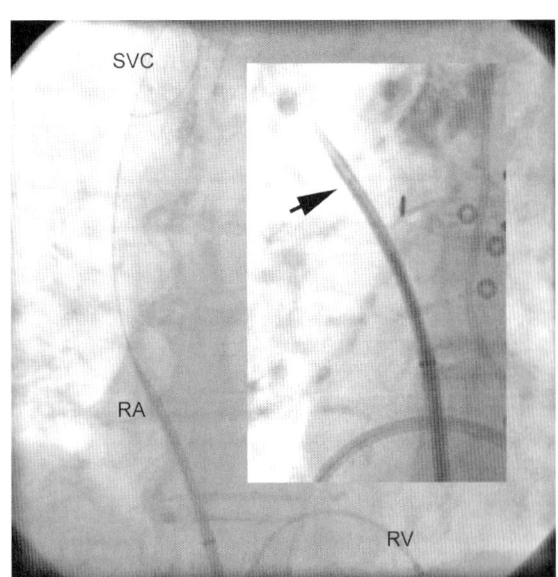

Figure 2 The initial step in the transseptal procedure is placement of the dilator and sheath in the superior vena cava (SVC). A 0.025 in. or 0.032 in. wire is placed in the SVC. The inset shows the tip of the transseptal needle placed just within the end of the dilator (*arrow*). *Abbreviations*: RA, right atrium; RV, right ventricle; SVC, superior vena cava.

atrial pressure is recorded from the tip of the needle. The needle and sheath/dilator assembly are pulled caudally through the superior vena cava (SVC) toward the right atrium (RA) as a unit. There is an indicator arrow on the hub of the needle that shows the direction of the angle of the needle. As the entire apparatus is pulled inferiorly from the SCV, the needle and Mullins sheath are rotated as a unit clockwise until the indicator arrow points inferiorly to between the 4 o'clock and 6 o'clock position (Fig. 3). The degree of rotation is less in structurally normal hearts, and progressively more in aortic stenosis and mitral valve disease. The fossa ovalis lies in the posterior aspect of the intra-atrial septum and is bounded superiorly by the limbus, an arch shaped outer muscular rim. Classic descriptions note two rightward movements as the needle is withdrawn from the SVC to the RA. The needle can be felt to move over the aortic knob, and then drop into the fossa ovalis (Fig. 4). The first movement over the aortic knob is often difficult to appreciate or absent. When the needle and dilator are in place on the fossa ovalis, it usually appears that the curve of the Mullins sheath will directly puncture the aorta. If the image intensifier is moved from an anteroposterior view to either a right or far left anterior oblique, it is possible to see that the needle is pointing posterior to the aorta (Fig. 5). A slight forward pressure on the needle will engage or catch on the limbus of the fossa ovalis. In many cases, the dilator will cross the intraatrial septum spontaneously at that point and the left atrial pressure will be seen. If this is not the case, pressure will damp as the needle tip contacts the interatrial septum. The transseptal needle is advanced out from the tip of the transseptal dilator. The needle must be advanced forcefully to avoid simply pushing the fossa away in front of it. The fossa ovalis comprises roughly 25% to 30% of the total septal area and is usually the thinnest portion of the septum. The diameter of the fossa can vary dramatically from patient to patient. This membrane consistency varies, however, usually becoming thicker and more fibrotic with age. The fossa may extremely thickened after prior cardiac surgery. When the needle enters the LA, left atrial pressure is recorded, and the dilator can be advanced into the LA and the needle withdrawn. Perforation of the LA posteriorly or anteriorly *with the needle alone* has rarely resulted in significant cardiac complications. It is typically the dilation with the sheath dilator or sheath itself that can cause significant cardiac compromise. If there is aortic or pericardial staining following what is presumed to be transseptal puncture, the needle must be removed and the dilator withdrawn and then the 0.032 in. J wire repositioned to the SVC and the process repeated. When the needle is clearly in the LA, the sheath can be advanced over the dilator and needle to secure access in the LA. Free back-bleeding of arterial blood should be noted from the hub of the Mullins dilator. Any air bubbles must be

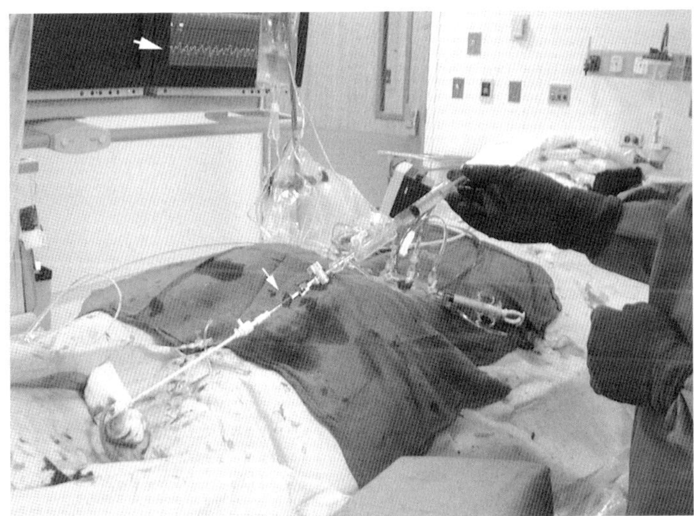

Figure 3 The arrow indicator (*lower arrow*) on the transseptal needle is oriented toward about 4 or 5 o'clock, relative to the patient. The patient's head is on the left side of the picture, and the feet are on the right. The transseptal needle is shown attached to a manifold for pressure measurement. In the upper left corner of the picture, *a second white arrow* shows the right atrial pressure, displayed on the monitor.

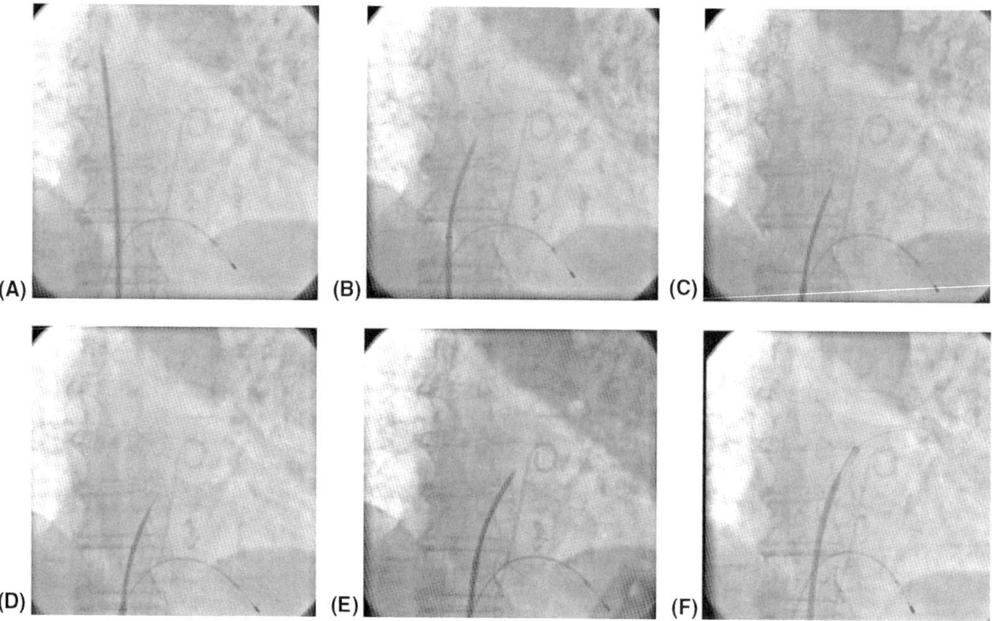

Figure 4 The basic steps in the transseptal procedure. (**A**) The sheath, dilator, and needle have been placed in the superior vena cava. (**B**) The sheath, dilator, and needle are pulled down inferiorly over the bulge of the aorta. (**C**) The assembly has engaged the fossa ovalis. The indicator arrow is rotated to between 4 and 6 o'clock relative to the patient. (**D**) The needle has been extended out of the dilator, through the fossa ovalis into the left atrium. Left atrial pressure should be seen on the monitor. (**E**) The dilator has been advanced over the needle into the left atrium. (**F**) A wire is advanced into the left upper lobe pulmonary vein, and the sheath advanced over the dilator. The sheath and wire are carefully removed to avoid aspiration of air, and the sheath system flushed. Heparin is administered at that point.

aspirated. Contrast injection can be used to verify the position of the Mullins sheath within the LA (Fig. 6). It is useful to pass a guidewire through the dilator just after the needle has been removed to stabilize forward advancement of both the dilator and the sheath. One of the disappointing modes of failure for this procedure is to successfully puncture the septum, but then have the tip of the dilator jump forward and perforate the left atrial free wall. Using a wire to help pass the dilator and sheath across the intra-atrial septum thus makes advancing the dilator safer. After successful puncture of the intra-atrial septum, heparin is given. The heparin dose depends on the purpose of the procedure. For a diagnostic procedure where the catheter time in the LA would be very brief, an arbitrary small dose of heparin might be used. For procedures such as valvuloplasty, activated clotting time between 200 and 300 seconds is desirable, depending on the procedure. Percutaneous mitral valve repair or longer electrophysiology procedures require activated clotting times ⩾ 300 seconds.

The left femoral vein is usually not a successful approach, since the angulation of the left iliac vein as it joins the inferior vena cava will force the transseptal needle to move away from the intra-atrial septum. Only in patients who are very narrow hipped with a steep angle between the iliac vein and the inferior vena cava may left femoral access be likely to succeed.

Measurement of pressure through the transseptal needle is not a uniform practice. In our opinion, it is essential for the safest method for accessing the LA. If the needle is advanced and LA pressure is not detected, a number of possibilities exist. The needle may be buried in the tissue of the septum, having taken a tangential through the septum. It is possible that the free wall of the roof of the RA or the inferior

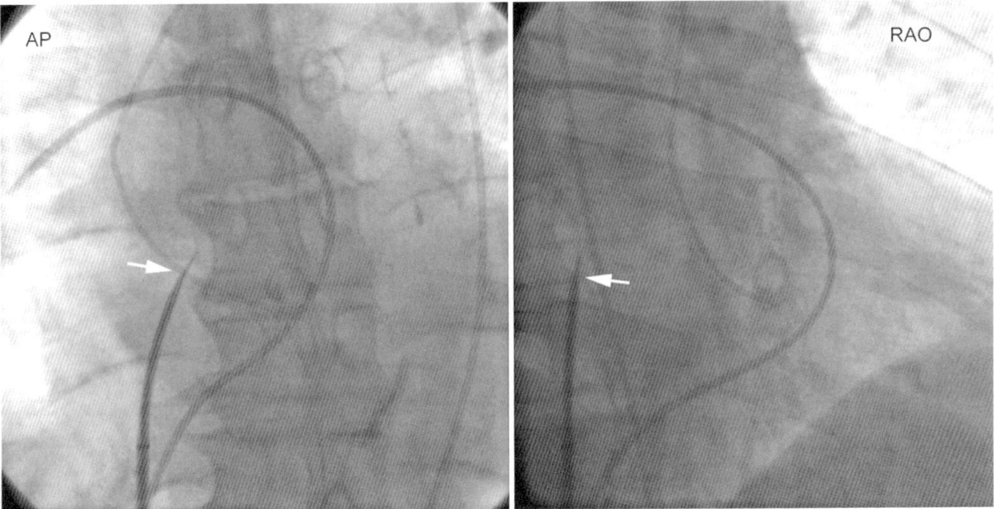

Figure 5 The *left panel* shows an anteroposterior (AP) view. The *arrow* points at the tip of the dilator, from which the needle is extended into the left atrium. The *right panel* shows a right anterior oblique (RAO) view. The *arrow* again indicates the tip of the dilator, from which the needle extends. The pigtail catheter is resting against the aortic valve. On the AP view it appears that the needle has transected the aorta, while on the 30° right anterior oblique view it is clear that the needle overlies the spine, and is thus posterior to the aorta and pigtail.

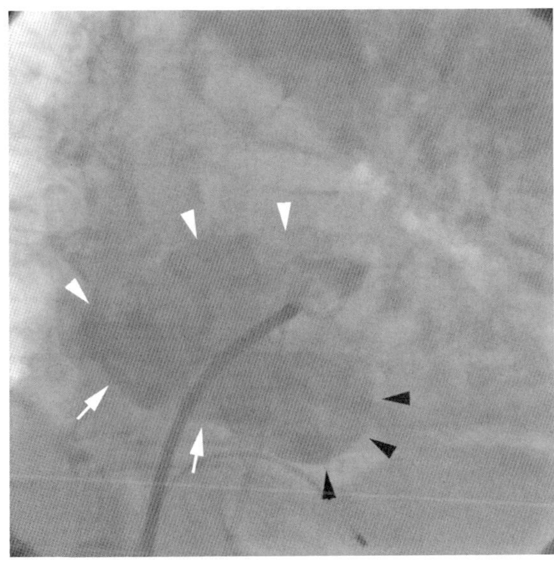

Figure 6 Contrast injection after successful transseptal puncture. The *white arrowheads* mark the upper border of the left atrium; the *white arrows* mark the intra-atrial septum; the *black arrowheads* show the mitral valve, closed in this angiographic frame.

border of the RA or LA has been perforated. It is also possible that the LA has been entered, but that a small thrombus has occluded the pressure lumen of the needle. In any of these eventualities, as long as the needle is withdrawn and the 8-French sheath is not advanced, and as long as the patient is not anticoagulated, the potential for pericardial tamponade is small. As long as the incorrect position of the needle is recognized and the attempt abandoned at that point, complications from needle perforations are infrequent. This emphasizes the need to have patients off of coumadin or heparin anticoagulation prior to beginning a transseptal puncture procedure.

FLUOROSCOPIC AND INTRA-CARDIAC ECHOCARDIOGRAPHY GUIDANCE

Since fluoroscopy only allows indirect assessment of the location of the fossa ovalis without good visual representation of these critical anatomic landmarks, advancement of the transseptal needle using only fluoroscopically-guided techniques can be frequently associated with unpredictable outcomes. The introduction of intracardiac echocardiography has added greatly to the safety and appreciation of the anatomic variability and location of fossa ovalis. Some centers routinely perform transesophageal echocardiography to facilitate transseptal catheterization. Transesophageal echocardiography can readily image the fossa ovalis and needle assembly, but requires a second operator, greater degrees of sedation, and is not practical for long procedures. More recently, intracardiac echocardiography has been employed to facilitate transseptal catheterization. With the introduction of this technology, a single operator can perform this procedure painlessly and continuously without sedation. Intracardiac echocardiography has permitted less experienced transseptal operators to adopt the procedure.

The classic approach to transseptal puncture uses fluoroscopic guidance coupled with tactile feedback from the dilator. The location of the puncture is "guestimated" based on the location of the aortic root as marked by a pigtail combined with bony landmarks. The variability of the puncture location is extreme. The classic fluoroscopic landmark for the puncture site is in the center of the spine, at the level of the aortic root. Depending on the patient's age, the relative amounts of right and left atrial dilatation, and spinal deformities, the puncture site may frequently be to the left or right of the center of the spine, sometimes by many centimeters. Tactile feedback from the transseptal needle is one of the most important descriptors of the location of the puncture. As the dilator is withdrawn from the SVC and felt to catch on the lumbus with a slight forward motion, a pulsatile motion can be felt in some cases. If fluoroscopy shows the needle pointing posterior and away from the aorta, the pulsatility represents the atrial "septal bounce," whereas if the needle is pointing at the aorta, it is the aorta that is being felt. Advancement of the needle will yield a left atrial pressure tracing, which confirms the left atrial location.

A variety of methods can be used to determine the location of the center of the intra-atrial septum. One of the simplest is right atrial contrast injection with filming of the levo phase. Contrast of 20 or 30 mL can be given as a bolus in the RA. A long acquisition time is required to be able to see the left atrial filling on the levo phase.

More recently, intravascular ultrasound has become the method of choice to clearly visualize the atrial septum to assist in transseptal puncture (26-31). Intracardiac echo (ICE) is widely available. A relatively simple ICE catheter is available which uses a single rotating crystal ultrasound transducer based on either 9-French 9 MHz rotating crystal or a 6.5-French 12.5 MHz ultrasound crystal (CVIS®, Boston Scientific, Sunnyvale, CA). This has the advantages of being compatible with standard coronary intravascular ultrasound consoles, and it is relatively inexpensive, costing about the same as a coronary IVUS catheter. It has the disadvantages of a limited depth of field, and it provides no more than a planar 2-dimensional view of the atrial septum. Nonetheless, in many cases it is adequate to demonstrate contact of the transseptal needle with the fossa ovalis. Accuson, a 64-element phased-array ultrasound system using a 10-French 9 MHz transducer (AcuNav®, Seimens Acuson, Mountain View, CA) that images in a sector field oriented in the plane of the catheter rather than a circumferential field of view intracardiac echo, requires a Siemens echo machine console, and the catheters are significantly more expensive than the simple Boston Scientific ultrasound. They have the advantage of a greater depth of field, image quality that appears basically equivalent to transesophageal echocardiography, and the availability of color Doppler as well. Accuson ICE is used widely in conjunction electrophysiology ablation procedures and with shunt closure procedures, because in addition to verifying catheter placement, it aids with device placement and assessment of post-procedure shunting.

When the transseptal dilator engages the fossa, it causes a pushing or tenting of the fossa from the RA into the LA (Fig. 7). It is important to note that the tip of the transseptal needle itself is often echolucent and tenting is the only reliable sign of proper engagement of the fossa ovalis. Simply seeing the echo shadow of the catheter close to the septum can be highly deceptive, since the body of the transseptal catheter may be transected by the plane of the ultrasound beam even when the tip of the needle is far away from the septum.

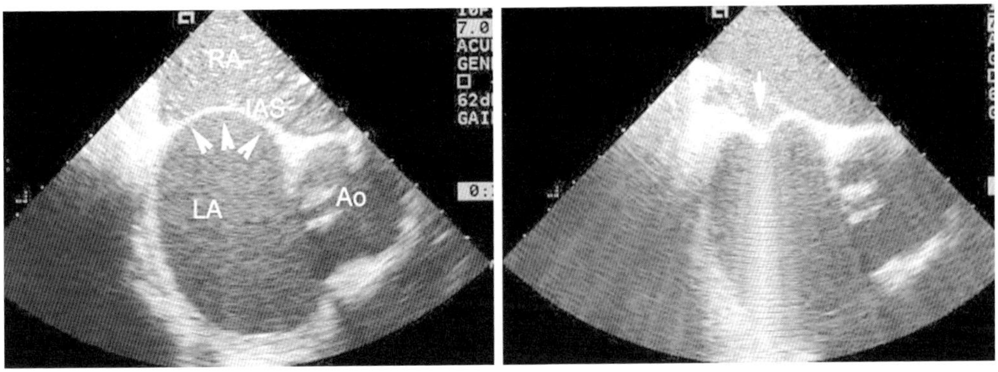

Figure 7 Intracardiac echo guidance for transseptal puncture. The left panel shows a baseline image. The arrowheads show the intra-atrial septum (IAS). In the *right hand panel* the transseptal needle has been engaged in the foramen ovale; the *arrow* shows tenting of the intra-atrial septum into the LA caused by forward pressure of the transseptal dilator. There is considerable shadowing in the left atrium from the transseptal apparatus. It is notable that the needle itself is not visible, but that the tenting is well displayed. The needle is either out of plane or, because of its relatively thin structure, is in this frame echolucent. *Abbreviations*: RA, right atrium; AO, aorta; LA, left atrium.

The electrophysiology approach

A totally venous access approach to transseptal procedures is now commonly utilized in experienced electrophysiology (EP) laboratories. Because EP catheters are placed in strategic anatomic locations defined by their recorded electrograms, EP recording equipment is required. It is our practice to begin by placing a His bundle and coronary sinus catheter to provide anatomic landmarks fluoroscopically (Fig. 8). A His bundle catheter *that is recording a His bundle* always identifies the most inferior aspect of the non-coronary cusp of the aorta. This obviates the need for an arterial puncture to place a pigtail catheter in the ascending aorta. A coronary sinus catheter properly placed along the artereovenous groove demarcates the widest portion of the LA parallel and just posterior to the mitral annulus. One must ensure that the coronary sinus catheter courses near the mitral annulus by seeing equal-amplitude atrial and ventricular electrograms exist throughout the course of the catheter. If not, the catheter may have inadvertently been placed in a posterolateral branch of the coronary sinus and should be repositioned prior to performing transseptal catheterization.

The fluoroscopic views are adjusted so the His bundle catheter is pointing directly at the image intensifier of the fluoroscopic camera. The right anterior oblique angulation is adjusted so the coronary sinus catheter intersects the His bundle catheter and its midpoint. Careful evaluation of the His bundle recording should be maintained to ensure an accurate anatomic reference relative to the inferior aspect of the aorta. The transseptal needle and sheath assembly are withdrawn in the LAO view as a *single unit* maintaining the position of the needle to the dilator from the SVC position to the RA with the needle usually oriented in the 4 o'clock psosition. If the coronary sinus catheter has been placed from a superior approach, care must be utilized to ensure that, during torquing of the sheath, the coronary sinus catheter is not twisted around the sheath and needle assembly.

As the needle/sheath assembly is withdrawn, an initial slight leftward jump of the assembly is noted as it enters the RA, and then a second movement leftward occurs as the catheter tip approaches the level of the His bundle catheter, which is below the superior limbus of the fossa ovalis. At this level the RAO view confirms that the catheter tip is posterior to the site of the His bundle recording and angled posterior and parallel to the projection of the coronary sinus

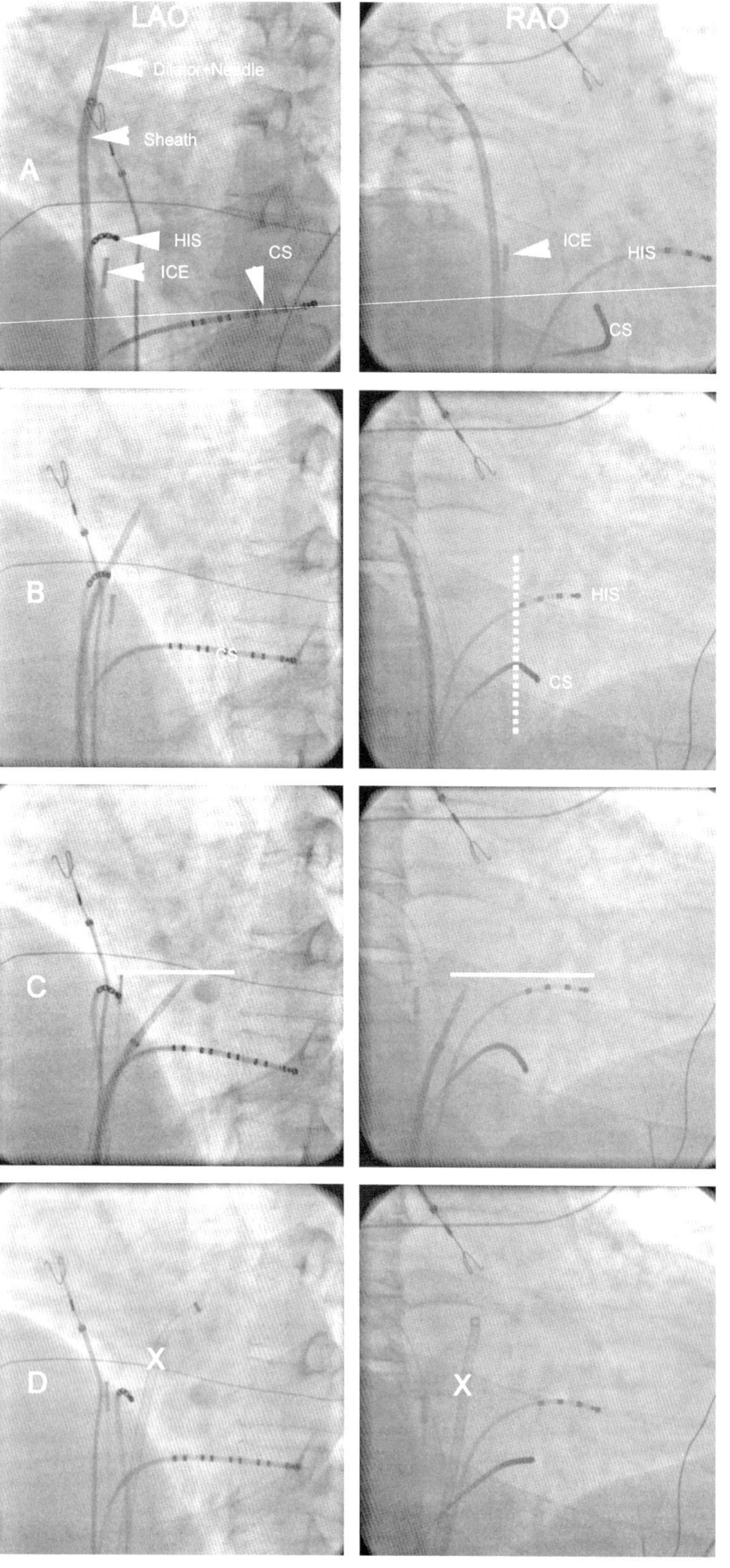

Figure 8 (**A**) RAO 40 and LAO 40 fluoroscopic images of the sheath, dilator, needle assembly positioned in the superior vena cava. Note the position of the His bundle catheter (His), coronary sinus catheter (CS), and intracardiac echocardiography catheter (ICE). (**B**) Angulation of the RAO camera is adjusted to 30 degrees so the proximal electrode of the His catheter is in the same vertical plane as the CS catheter (dashed white line in RAO view). Withdrawal of the sheath/dilator/needle (SDN) has entered the right atrium. Note the assembly is positioned too posteriorally in the RAO 30-degree view despite having the needle torqued to approximately a 4 o'clock position. (**C**) Proper positioning of the SDN position prior to transseptal puncture. Note the SDN assembly is oriented posterior to the His bundle catheter in the RAO view. Note that the electrograms of the His bundle must be seen to be able to use this catheter as a reliable anatomic landmark. Typically, the tip of the dilator is at the same level as the His bundle catheter (*solid white line*) and well to the left (posterior) of the His bundle catheter in the LAO view, and oriented posterior and parallel to the CS catheter in the RAO view. (**D**) Sheath position following transseptal crossing. Following transseptal puncture the dilator is advanced over the needle and dilator assembly into the left atrium. Only after the sheath is advanced into the left atrium should the needle and dilator be removed, because they provide support for the sheath to pass into the left atrium. The point of transseptal crossing is marked by an "x".

catheter. This angle ensures that the assembly is not pointing too posteriorally, in which case the needle may perforate the posterior wall of the LA, and not pointing too anteriorally, at which point the needle might enter the ascending aorta. Adjustments of angulation between 3 o'clock and 6 o'clock may be necessary, with enlarged left atria often requiring a more posterior (or 5 to 6 o'clock) angulation and vertically oriented hearts requiring a more anterior (3 to 4 o'clock) angulation of the needle.

When the angulation of the needle is confirmed, transseptal crossing is done in the LAO projection. The assembly is withdrawn. 25–.5 cm farther and then advanced to engage the limbus of the fossa ovalis. Patients with patent foramen ovale will have the dilator move toward the left atrium. If hemodynamics are utilized, the left atrial pressure recording can be recorded from the transseptal needle or the needle location can be confirmed by ICE or contrast injection. More commonly, however, the dilator does not pass spontaneously into the left atrium. Pressure measurements are usually damped when the needle and dilator are juxtaposed to the intra-atrial septum. When the transseptal needle is advanced to enter the LA, a tactile "pop" is felt. This can be confirmed by contrast injection or pressure recording from the tip of the needle. The dilator is then advanced over the needle assembly to enter the LA and, with the support of the needle, the sheath is advanced over the dilator into the LA. If there is any question about the location of the needle the dilator should not be advanced. Once the sheath is in the LA and has been flushed, heparin is given.

Thickened atrial septum

A septum thick enough to make puncture difficult may be encountered in older patients with lipomatous hypertrophy and after prior open heart surgery (31–36). Patients with prior valve surgery may develop endocardial thickening, and in some cases the fossa is sutured to prevent air embolism. Puncture may also be performed after atrial septal patching or repair for congenital heart disease. In all of these situations ICE is extremely helpful and puncture is often unsuccessful without ICE guidance (Fig. 9). The needle may be advanced tangentially into the septal tissue, so that even if the puncture location is correct, it is not possible to reach the LA. When the transseptal needle causes "tenting" of the septum, more force than is otherwise acceptable can be used to advance into the LA. Another method to cross a tough or thick septum is with radiofrequency perforation (37). This requires specialized equipment, and is best performed with ICE.

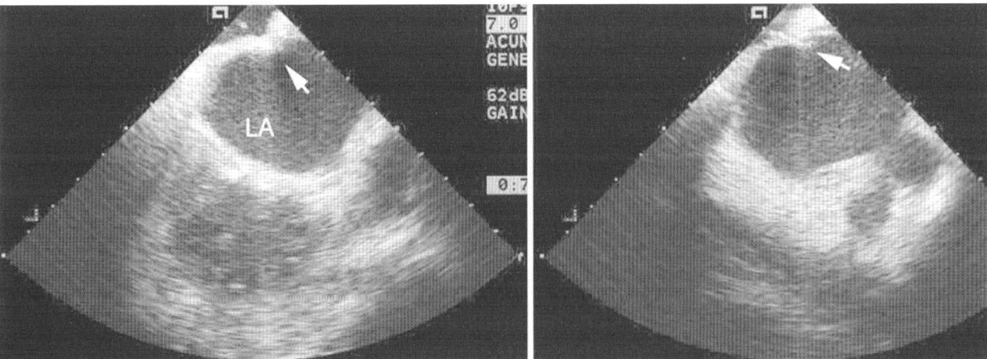

Figure 9 Intracardiac echo images from a patient with a markedly thickened intra-atrial septum. This patient had undergone prior resection of a right atrial myxoma from the right atrial free wall. The septum is almost 1-cm thick. The *left panel* shows tenting of the septum from a transseptal dilator marked by the *arrow*. With full extension of the needle, the left atrium could not adequately be entered. Forward pressure on the needle, more extreme than would be possible without echo guidance, was necessary to force the needle into the left atrium, and ultimately record left atrial pressure via the needle before advancing the dilator. The *right panel* shows the needle across the septum, marked by the *arrowhead*. *Abbreviation*: LA, left atrium.

Indications, contraindications, and complications

Indications

Indications for transseptal procedures include a variety of diagnostic uses, and an increasing array of therapeutic procedures (35–39). Diagnostic assessment of mitral and aortic valve disease, congenital lesions, and hypertrophic cardiomyopathy are the most frequent situations in which transseptal puncture is employed. Mitral stenosis is, of course, the most classic, and catheter-based mitral valve repair the most recent (39). Direct measurement of left atrial pressure combined with retrograde left ventricular pressure yields accurate assessment of the transmitral pressure gradient. It is also possible to pass a French Mullins sheath into the LA, and through this float a 7-French balloon tip catheter into the left ventricle (Fig. 10). Thus simultaneous left atrial and left ventricular pressure can be obtained via a single venous puncture without the need for arterial catheterization or retrograde crossing of the aortic valve. Similarly, this approach for left ventricular pressure measurement can be coupled with retrograde placement of a catheter in the central aorta for accurate assessment of the transaortic valve pressure gradient in aortic stenosis or hypertrophic cardiomyopathy. This method yields pressures recorded directly from either side of the valve and avoids all of the artifacts of pressure amplification and damping that are common in peripheral arterial sheath substitution for the central aortic pressure when assessing aortic valve stenosis.

In rare instances, the transseptal approach has been used to pass a catheter into the aortic root

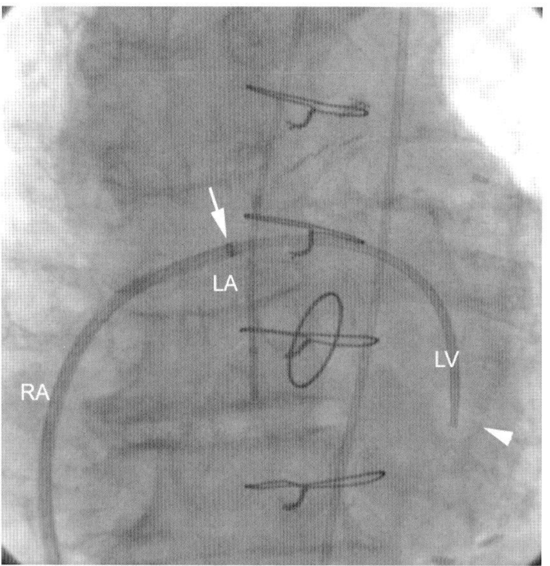

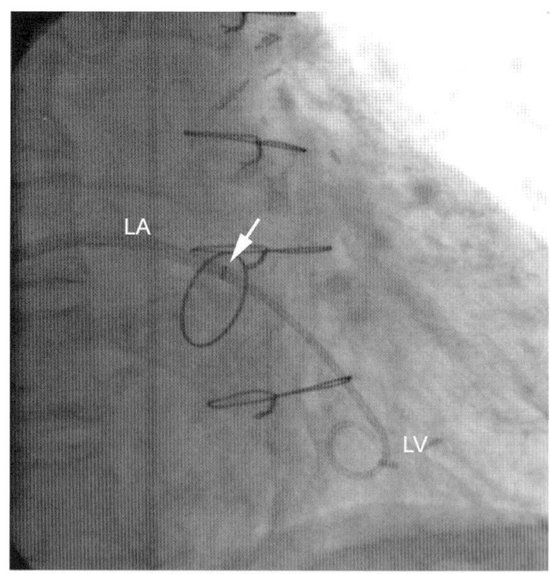

Figure 10 Catheterization of the left ventricle via the mitral valve after transseptal puncture. This is an excellent method to record a transaortic or transmitral valve pressure gradient. In this case, the patient has a Hancock bioprosthetic aortic valve replacement. A pigtail catheter sits in the sinus of Valsalva adjacent to the valve in the *left panel* (AP view). The *arrow* marks the tip of the Mullins sheath. A 7-French single lumen balloon catheter has been floated across the mitral valve into the left ventricle. The inflated balloon is marked by the *arrowhead*. In the *right hand panel* in a right anterior oblique view, a pigtail catheter has been substituted for the single lumen balloon catheter for ventriculography. Simultaneous recording of the left atrial and left ventricular pressures for evaluation of mitral stenosis, and of the left ventricular and aortic pressures for evaluation of the transaortic valve pressure gradient can be easily accomplished. A central aortic pigtail catheter is just visible in the upper left corner of this frame. *Abbreviations*: RA, right atrium; LA, Left atrium; LV, left ventricle.

for coronary arteriography. This can be accomplished in patients with limited access from the extremities. It, of course, requires a great deal of catheter manipulation and time to achieve selective or semiselective coronary arteriography.

The method for access of the aorta via the transseptal route is used increasingly for therapeutic procedures but also has diagnostic utility. A 8-French transseptal sheath is placed in the LA. A 7-French balloon catheter is floated into the left ventricle. The catheter can be curved in the left ventricular apex, or a curved wire can be introduced into the catheter to help it make the turn around the apex, and then the balloon catheter is floated across the aortic valve into the aortic root. This allows measurement sequentially of the entire right and left heart circulations, or passage of a guidewire from the RA, across the septum into the LA, through the left ventricle, into the aorta, and sometimes out through a femoral arterial sheath. This transcirculatory wire loop is sometimes called "flossing" the circulation (Fig. 11) (21,36).

Therapeutic uses for transseptal catheterization are increasing rapidly. Catheter ablation for left sided accessory pathways and atrial fibrillation in electrophysiology have become common procedures. Antegrade valvuloplasty of the mitral valve, and also of the aortic valve is accomplished using transseptal access. Paravalvular leak closure also frequently requires transseptal access either for delivery of a closure device, or for wire passage to ultimately allow retrograde delivery catheter placement. The variety of new percutaneous valve repair and replacement therapies require transseptal puncture as well. Mitral valve repair is predicated on left atrial access via the transseptal route. The E-valve procedure uses a 24-French venous cannula to access the LA, and then place a clip directly on the mitral leaflets. A great advantage of the transseptal route is the ability to place large catheters in the femoral vein, and then achieve left heart access. The obviates the need for large bore atrial sheaths in many instances. Antegrade aortic balloon valvuloplasty is accomplished using a 14-French venous sheath. This bears the challenges of arterial access and hemostasis using sheaths of that caliber via the arterial route, necessary of course for retrograde aortic valvuloplasty.

Contraindications

The most important contraindications to transseptal puncture include atrial thrombus or mass. Right atrial thrombus may form on pacemaker leads or inferior vena cava filters. It is unusual for right atrial thrombus to directly preclude transseptal puncture. Left atrial appendage thrombus is a more common problem (Fig. 12). In mitral stenosis patients who have not been on coumadin, left atrial appendage thrombi will often resolve in 2 to 4 months with coumadin therapy. For patients who have been on coumadin, the addition of antiplatelet therapy and more intense coumadin therapy is sometimes successful. Smoke, or spontaneous echo contrast, in the LA is not a contraindication to transseptal puncture. Rare cases of atrial septal thrombus are encountered and represent an important contraindication to transseptal puncture. In cases where left atrial appendage thrombus is seen on a baseline echo, and then appears in a stable concave, echo-dense (organized) configuration on a follow-up echo after prolonged anticoagulation therapy, it is sometimes safe to proceed with transseptal puncture. If the atrial appendage thrombus is well organized, there is little risk of embolization. Unfortunately it is prospectively very difficult to tell whether any fresh or mobile thrombus might exist on the surface of an echo-dense organized thrombus. Thus, left atrial appendage thrombus remains an important relative contraindication to this procedure.

Another strong relative contraindication to transseptal puncture is in patients who have abnormal coagulation or thrombocytopenia. Many patients present for transseptal catheterization having been on coumadin. Coumadin is typically discontinued 3 or 4 days before the catheterization procedure. A bridge using heparin or Lovenox® (Aventis, Bridgewater, NJ) is commonly employed. It is my practice to proceed with transseptal puncture only if the international normalized ratio (INR) is less than or equal to 1.7. After a hiatus off of coumadin therapy, patients will occasionally appear with an elevated INR and the procedure must be delayed. Platelet counts of 50,000 to 100,000 represent a degree of thrombocytopenia that imposes an important risk for tamponade if an

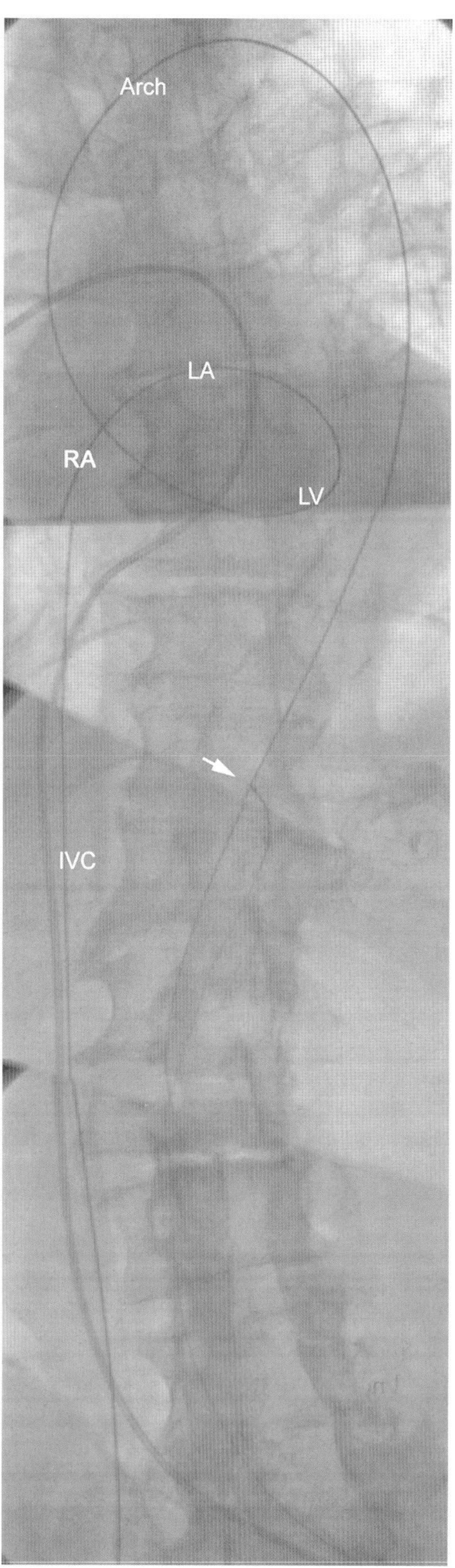

Figure 11 A guidewire has been placed via the transseptal route throughout the whole circulation. This is sometimes called "flossing" the circulation. The course of the wire involves introduction through a transseptal sheath via the inferior vena cava (IVC), right atrium (RA), left atrium (LA), across the mitral valve and into the left ventricle (LV), then out into the aortic arch and the descending aorta. In this example the wire has been snared in the descending aorta (*arrow*). The snare has been closed on the wire to provide stability for antegrade aortic balloon valvuloplasty. It is also possible to snare the wire and exteriorize it, which allows introduction of devices from either the arterial or venous limbs of the same wire. Importantly, when a wire loop like this is removed from the circulation it is critical to cover it with a diagnostic catheter so that friction of the wire does not lacerate the heart valves.

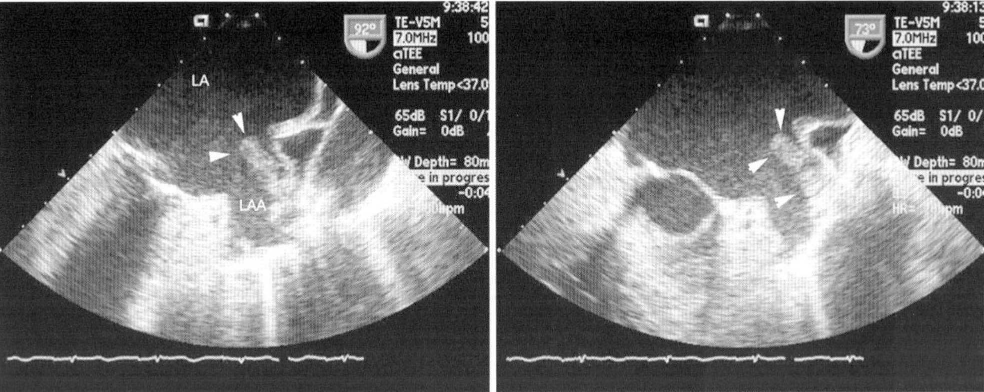

Figure 12 Transesophageal echocardiographic images showing left atrial thrombus. Atrial appendage thrombus is one of the most important contraindications to transseptal procedures. In the *left panel*, the arrowheads show a large thrombus. In the *right panel* in a second frame, the thrombus is seen to have a lobular or globular appearance. The thrombus extends out of the left atrial appendage (LAA) into the body of the left atrium (LA). Echocardiographic smoke is seen in the appendage and extending out into the body of the left atrium.

errant puncture results from the procedure. A platelet count over 100,000 can generally be regarded as acceptable for proceeding with a transseptal puncture.

Complications

Thromboemboli from the catheter, needle, or cardiac chambers may occur. Extreme care to flush and wipe the transseptal system frequently is needed to avoid thrombus formation on the transseptal needle. The stainless steel needle is metal and highly thrombogenic. In most reported series cardiac tamponade occurs in 0.5–2%, and stroke in <1% (41). Both cardiac perforation and thromboembolism can be fatal.

The vast majority of complications that arise from transseptal catheterization occur from inadvertent puncture of adjacent structures to the interatrial septum and fossa ovalis. Thus, anticoagulation is not given until the LA has been safely entered. The interatrial septum is bounded posteriorly by the pericardium. The aortic root lies superior and anterior to the fossa ovalis while the coronary sinus ostium lies inferior to the fossa ovalis and posterior to the tricuspid valve orifice. In pathologic hearts there is frequent distortion of the atrial and interatrial septum anatomy, which can significantly alter the proximity of these structures. The septum tends to lie more horizontal in patients with left atrial enlargement and can be more vertical in patients with aortic valve disease or a dilated aortic root. Varying degrees of kyphoscoliosis can also alter intrathoracic cardiac rotation. Also, prior open heart surgery can result in a thickened fossa ovalis because surgeons occasionally must over-sew the fossa in patients with a patent foramen ovale to ensure evacuation of air from the LA before coming off cardiopulmonary bypass. Cardiac perforation may result from perforation of the RA, perforation of the LA after successful transseptal puncture, and also by perforation through the inferior border of the RA across the transverse pericardial sinus and then into the LA. This latter route for perforation may not be recognized until the conclusion of the procedure, since the catheter will exit the RA and very quickly enter the LA, yielding a good left atrial pressure wave form. It is not until the catheter is removed that the puncture through the space between the RA and LA at the lower border can be recognized. After balloon mitral valvotomy procedures, it is my practice to leave the wire across the transseptal puncture after the catheters have been removed for about 5 minutes with continuous arterial pressure monitoring. This allows re-access to the puncture site and LA if a puncture across the transverse pericardial sinus has occurred.

The performance of transseptal puncture cannot reasonably be undertaken without readiness also to perform pericardiocentesis (42). When hypotension occurs during a transseptal procedure, it is fair to assume that it is due to cardiac perforation until proven otherwise. Pleuritic chest pain, shoulder pain, or new atrial fibrillation should also raise suspicion regarding potential perforation. The ready availability of echocardiography to help with both the confirmation of the diagnosis and the performance of pericardiocentesis is helpful. In the event that pericardiocentesis is necessary, it can almost always be accomplished using equipment already available on the catheterization table without a special pericardiocentesis set. A standard 18-gauge thin wall needle is adequate to reach the pericardial space in the vast majority of patients. While the traditional approach for pericardiocentesis involves directing the needle from the left subxiphoid angle toward the left shoulder, in the setting of acute pericardial tamponade, it is common for the effusions to be much smaller and a more vertical pathway is needed to reach the pericardial space. It is my usual practice when echocardiographic guidance is not available, to make a first pass with the needle angulated toward the mid part of the left clavicle. A standard pigtail catheter of any French size can be used for initial pericardial drainage. Once the blood pressure is stabilized, the pigtail catheter can be exchanged for a multihole pericardial drainage catheter. Generally, the drain should be left overnight, since continued bleeding from a perforation may occur. It is disappointing to create a perforation during a transseptal procedure, successfully drain the pericardium, and then have the patient tamponade some hours later from recurrent bleeding if the drain has been removed prematurely. The drain can be discontinued when there is less than 100 mL of drainage in a 24-hour period.

If perforation is recognized after administration of heparin, protamine should be used to reverse the anticoagulation. Protamine sulfate is itself a mild anticoagulant, but when given with heparin (which is strongly acidic) a stable, non-coagulating salt is created and inactivates the anticoagulant effect of heparin. On average 1 mg of protamine will reverse approximately 90 USP units heparin derived from beef lung or 115 USP units of heparin derived from porcine intestinal mucosa. Usually it is advised that no more than 50 mg of protamine be given over 10 minutes. Rapid administration of protamine can result in severe hypotension, anaphylactoid reactions, and respiratory compromise. In practice, administration of 5–10 mg of protamine at one time with frequent reassessment of the ACT will achieve reversal of anticoagulation with a minimum of complications. Typically no more than 100 mg of protamine should be administered acutely. Because protamine sulfate can cause anaphylaxis, medications should also be available to deal with this emergency as well. Anaphylactoid reactions are more common in diabetic patients who have taken NPH insulin, which contains protamine and sensitizes some of them to protamine.

REFERENCES

1. Facquet J, Lemoine J, Alhomme P, Lefeboie J. La mesure de la pression auriculaire gauche por voie transbronchque. Arch Mal Coeur 1952; 8:741.
2. Aluson PR, Linden RJ. The bronchoscopic measurement of left auricular pressure. Circulation 1953; 7:669.
3. Bjork VO, Malmstrom G, Uoola LG. Left auricular pressure measurements in man. Ann Surg 1953; 138:718.
4. Radner S. Suprasternal puncture of the left atrium for flow studies. Acta Med Scandinav 1954; 148:57.
5. Brock R, Milstein BB, Ross DH. Percutaneous left ventricular puncture in the assessment of aortic stenosis. Thorax 1956; 11:163.
6. Lehman JS, Musser BG, Lykens HD. Cardiac ventriculography: Direct transthoracic needle puncture opacification of the left (or right) ventricle. Am J Roentgenol 1957; 77:207.
7. Levy MJ, Amplatz K, Lillehei CW. Transthoracic left heart catheterization and angiocardiography for combined assessment of mitral and aortic valves. Radiology 1962; 78:638.
8. Levy MJ, Lillehei CW. Percutaneous direct catheterization-a new method, with results in 122 patients. New England J Med 1964; 271:273.
9. Cope C. Technique for the transseptal catheterization of the left atrium: preliminary report. J Thorac Surg 1959; 37:482–486.

10. Ross J, Braunwald E, Morrow AG. Transseptal left atrial puncture: new technique for the measurement of left atrial pressures. Am J Cardiol 1959; 3:653–655.
11. Brockenbrough EC, Braunwald E, Ross J Jr. Transseptal left heart catheterization: a review of 450 studies and description of an improved technique. Circulation 1962; 25:15–21.
12. Ross J Jr. Considerations regarding the technique for transseptal left heart catheterization. Circulation 1966; 34(3):391–399.
13. Braunwald E. Transseptal left heart catheterization. Circulation 1968; 37(suppl 3):74–79 .
14. Laskey WK, Kusiak V, Untereker WJ, Hirshfeld JW Jr. Transseptal left heart catheterization: utility of a sheath technique. Catheter Cardiovasc Diagn 1982; 8(5):535–542.
15. Mullins CE. Transseptal left heart catheterization: Experience with a new technique in 520 pediatric and adult patients. Pediatr Cardiol 1983; 4:239–245.
16. Swan HJ, Ganz W, Forrester J, Marcus H, Diamond G, Chonette D. Catheterization of the heart in man with use of a flow directed balloon-tipped catheter. N Engl J Med 1970; 283:447–451.
17. Schoenfeld MH, Palacios IF, Hutter AM Jr, Jacoby SS, Block PC. Underestimation of prosthetic mitral valve areas: role of transseptal catheterization in avoiding unnecessary repeat mitral valve surgery. J Am Coll Cardiol 1985; 5(6):1387–1392.
18. Marzocchi A, Piovaccari G, Zimarino M, Branzi A, Magnani B. Adjustment of pulmonary capillary wedge pressure for wave delay increases the accuracy of mitral valve area measurement. J Heart Valve Dis 1995; 4(3):242–246.
19. Haskell RJ, French WJ. Accuracy of left atrial and pulmonary artery wedge pressure in pure mitral regurgitation in predicting left ventricular end-diastolic pressure. Am J Cardiol 1988; 61(1): 136–141.
20. Kane PB, Askanazi J, Neville JF Jr, Mon RL, Hanson EL, Webb WR. Artifacts in the measurement of pulmonary artery wedge pressure. Crit Care Med 1978; 6(1):36–38.
21. Syed Z, Salinger MH, Feldman T. Alterations in left atrial pressure and compliance during balloon mitral valvuloplasty. Catheter Cardiovasc Interv 2004; 61:571–579.
22. Shirey EK, Sones FM Jr. Retrograde transaortic and mitral valve catheterization. Physiologic and morphologic evaluation of aortic and mitral valve lesions. Am J Cardiol 1966; 18(5):745–753.
23. Freeman DJ. New performed catheter and method for retrograde left atrial or complete left heart catheterization. Catheter Cardiovasc Diagn 1978; 4(3):305–310.
24. Freeman DJ. New family of preformed left atrial-coronary catheters for retrograde left atrial catheterization and coronary and/or aortocoronary bypass angiography via brachial artery cutdown. Catheter Cardiovasc Diagn 1981; 7(3):321–326.
25. Stefanadis CI, Stratos CG, Lambrou SG, et al. Retrograde nontransseptal balloon mitral valvuloplasty: immediate results and intermediate long-term outcome in 441 cases—a multicenter experience. J Am Coll Cardiol 1998; 32(4):1009–1016.
26. Hung JS, Fu M, Yeh KH, Wu CJ, Wong P. Usefulness of intracardiac echocardiography in complex transseptal catheterization during percutaneous transvenous commisurotomy. Mayo Clin Proc 1996; 71:134–140.
27. Daoud EG, Kalbfleisch SJ, Hummel JD. Intracardiac echocardiography to guide transseptal catheterization for radiofrequency catheter ablation. J Cardiovasc Electrophysiol 1999; 10: 358–363.
28. Epstein LM, Smith T, TenHoff H. Nonfluoroscopic transseptal catheterization: safety and efficacy of intracardiac echocardiographic guidance. J Cardiovasc Electrophys 1998; 9:625–630.
29. Sethi KK, Mohan JC. Transseptal catheterization for the electrophysiologist: modification with a "view". J Intervent Card Electrophys 2001; 5: 97–99.
30. Gonzalez MD, Otomo K, Shah N, et al. Transseptal left heart catheterization for cardiac ablation procedures. J Interv Cardiac Electrophys 2001; 5: 89–95.
31. Green NE, Hansgen AR, Carroll JD. Initial clinical experience with intracardiac echocardiography in guiding balloon mitral valvuloplasty: technique, safety, utility, and limitations. Catheter Cardiovasc Interv 2004; 63(3):385–394.
32. El-Said HG, Ing FF, Grifka RG, et al. 18-year Experience with transseptal procedures through baffles, conduits, and other intra-atrial patches. Catheter Cardiovasc Interv 2000; 50: 434–439.
33. Koenig P, Hijazi ZM. Transseptal puncture through an artificial material: a safe technique. Catheter Cardiovasc Interv 2000; 50:440.

34. Schneider MBE, Zartner PA, Magee AG. Transseptal approach in children after patch occlusion of atrial septal defect: first experience with cutting balloon. Catheter Cardiovasc Interv 1999; 48: 378–381.
35. Sakata Y, Feldman T. Transcatheter creation of atrial septal perforation using radio frequency transseptal system: novel approach as an alternative to transseptal needle puncture. Catheter Cardiovasc Interv 2005; 64:327–332.
36. Feldman T. Transseptal antegrade access for aortic valvuloplasty. Catheter Cardiovasc Intervent 2000; 50:492–494.
37. Sakata Y, Sayed Y, Salinger MH, Feldman T. Percutaneous balloon aortic valvuloplasty: antegrade transseptal vs. conventional retrograde transarterial approach. Catheter Cardiovasc Interv 2005; 64:314–321.
38. Feldman T, Herrmann HC, Inoue K. The technique of percutaneous transvenous mitral commissurotomy using the Inoue balloon catheter. Catheter Cardiovasc Diagn 1994; (supp 2):26–34.
39. Feldman T. Core Curriculum for interventional cardiology: Percutaneous valvuloplasty. Catheter Cardiovasc Interv 2003; 60:48–56.
40. Feldman T, Wasserman HS, Herrmann HC, et al. Percutaneous mitral valve repair using the edge-to-edge technique: 6 month results of the EVEREST Phase I Clinical Trial. J Am Coll Cardiol 2005; 46:2134–2140.
41. Roelke M, Smith AJ, Palacios IF. The technique and safety of transseptal left heart catheterization: the Massachusetts General Hospital experience with 1,279 procedures. Catheter Cardiovasc Diagn 1994; 32(4):332–339.
42. Feldman T, Sandborn T, Ziskind AA, Kern MJ. Pericardiocentesis, balloon pericardiotomy and special techniques. In: Kern MJ, ed. Interventional Cardiac Catheterization Handbook. 2nd ed. Mosby-Year Book, St. Louis, MO, 2004: 481–499.

18

Patent foramen ovale, cryptogenic stroke, and migraine headaches

Jonathan Tobis and Babak Azarbal

INTRODUCTION

The association among intracardiac shunts, cryptogenic stroke, and migraine headaches represents a potential groundbreaking area in medicine that could have significant implications for millions of people and could open up new areas of research that will improve our understanding of both stroke and migraine. This represents a paradigm shift in our concepts about migraine, a neurovascular disorder that afflicts 12% of all people. Paradigm shifts in medicine are revealing because they demonstrate how cautious we must be about preconceived notions. Several examples will serve to demonstrate the necessity for having an open mind about the etiology of cryptogenic stroke, migraine headaches, and the possible role of intracardiac shunts in these conditions.

1. For thousands of years it was assumed that the only function of the kidney was to make urine... until the discovery of erythropoietin revealed that the kidney provided hormonal control over the hematopoietic tissues.
2. Since the development of psychoanalysis, it was believed that bleeding ulcers were due to emotional stress. In addition to antacids, patients were subjected to years of introspective therapy as well as vagotomy and pyloroplasty... until the discovery that a bacterial infection due to *Helicobacter pylori* was the cause of most ulcers.
3. In cardiology, it was taught that acute myocardial infarction was not due to a coronary thrombus but that the thrombus was a secondary phenomenon due to slow flow following the infarction... until angiography performed within hours of an acute myocardial infarction revealed the presence of intracoronary thrombus.
4. Similarly, generations of physicians have been told that migraine headache was due to intense arterial spasm, which was then followed by cerebral arterial dilatation which produced the throbbing headache... until recent observations, to be described in this chapter, suggest that the mechanism

of migraine is more complicated and the initiating factors are more fascinating than had been previously conceived.

ANATOMY OF PATENT FORAMEN OVALE (PFO)

All mammals have a patent foramen ovale in utero. Since the fetus cannot breathe, oxygen is obtained from maternal transfer through the placenta. The oxygen saturation of umbilical cord blood is 63% and umbilical arterial cord blood is only 27%. If the placental blood were to pass through the right side of the heart and the un-oxygenated pulmonary circulation before it got to the left side of the heart, there would be even less oxygen available for the brain. If this blood were to pass through the right side of the heart and the un-oxygenated pulmonary circulation before it got to the left side of the heart, there would be even less oxygen available for the brain. Mammals therefore have evolved a mechanism for providing a direct shunt of blood from the inferior vena cava across the atrial septum to the left atrium. The PFO is not a hole or empty space such as an atrial septal defect (ASD). The PFO is a passageway with a flap, like a one-way trap door opening into the left atrium. Post partum, after the lungs expand, the left atrial pressure exceeds the right atrial pressure, pressing the septum primum against the septum secundum, and right to left shunting ceases. In the majority of people, the septum primum and the septum secundum fuse during the first year of life and the foramen ovale is closed permanently. Lack of post natal tissue fusion results in a patent foramen ovale (Fig. 1).

The foramen ovale remains patent in about 25% of adults (1–3). The incidence of PFO is inversely related to age, suggesting that some patients with PFO have spontaneous closure of their PFO with time. However, an alternative explanation could be that PFO predisposes to stroke and a higher mortality as we get older. In one autopsy study the prevalence of PFO progressively declined with increasing age from 34.3% during the first three decades of life to 25.4% during the 4th through 8th decades, and to 20.2% during the 9th and 10th decades. Older patients with a PFO tend to have larger PFOs compared to younger patients (2).

(A)
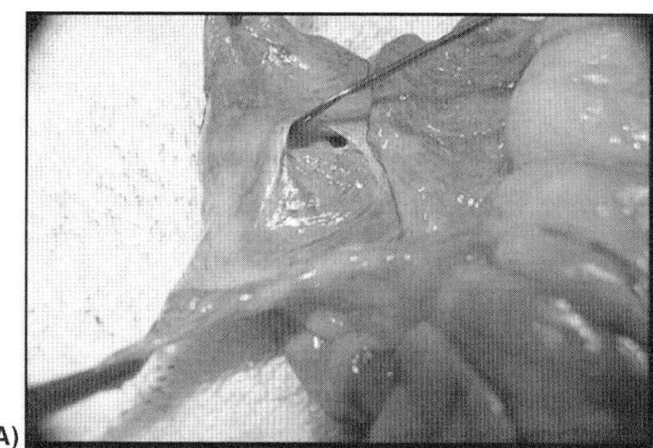

(B)
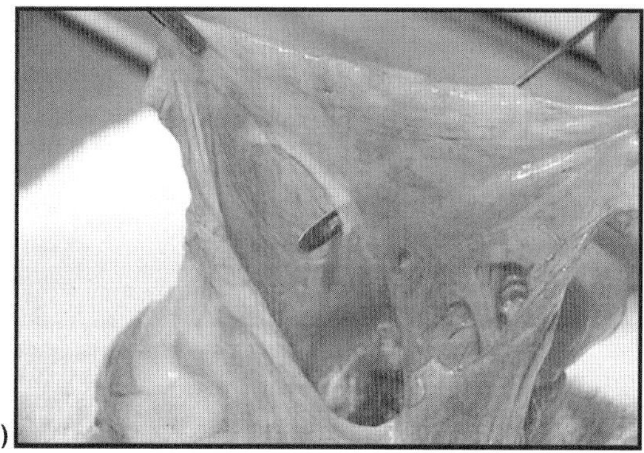

Figure 1 (**A**) Right atrial and (**B**) left atrial images of the patent foramen ovale flap.

CRYPTOGENIC STROKE AND PFO

Although the patent foramen ovale has been described anatomically for centuries, no one believed that it was of any clinical consequence since the degree of shunting was considered too small to be of hemodynamic importance. With the advent of echocardiography, isolated examples were seen of large clots that were trapped in the foramen ovale straddling the atrial septum (Fig. 2).

These large clots ordinarily would have passed to the pulmonary circulation to produce a pulmonary embolus. Based on these observations, it was reasoned that smaller venous emboli could potentially pass from the right atrium to the left atrium through the patent foramen ovale and proceed to the brain where they could produce much more devastating impact. The same small

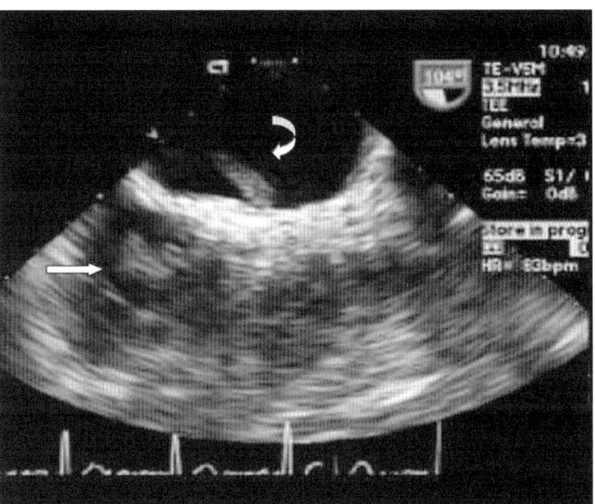

Figure 2 Large vermiform thrombus straddling the interatrial septum.

emboli, perhaps 1–3 mm in diameter, ordinarily would pass to the pulmonary circulation if no PFO were present. The pulmonary vasculature is so large that these small emboli would have no clinical impact.

There are two necessary conditions required for this hypothetical etiology of paradoxical embolism. The first is the presence of a small venous thrombus. In most cases of cryptogenic stroke, there is no obvious source of venous thrombosis, but our ability to image the venous circulation is limited to a macroscopic scale. The incidence of finding deep venous thrombosis post cryptogenic stroke is less than 10% by phlebography (4); however, a recent study utilizing magnetic resonance imaging (MRI) venography of the pelvis in patients who had suffered a cryptogenic stroke demonstrated a 20% incidence of pelvic deep vein thrombosis (5). Any woman who has been pregnant potentially has enough venous varicosities to harbor multiple small emboli. In addition, with increasing age, venous varicosities become more prevalent in men and women. Thus, the potential sources for formation of small venous emboli are quite prevalent and increase with age.

The second necessary condition for paradoxical embolism is that right to left shunting must occur through the PFO. Using transesophageal and intracardiac ultrasound imaging, it is possible to demonstrate with Doppler flow that the predominant direction of blood flow is left to right through a PFO. However, patients with a PFO also have intermittent right to left shunting, which may occur with normal respiratory cycles and may become pronounced when right atrial pressure exceeds left atrial pressure during valsalva maneuver or whenever the patient strains.

The hypothesis that cryptogenic stroke is caused by paradoxical embolism of a small venous thrombus through a PFO is impossible to prove directly through any medical imaging test. However, a large body of observational clinical studies has demonstrated a high incidence of PFO in patients with cryptogenic stroke. In one study of 60 patients with ischemic stroke who were more than 55 years old and had no evidence of cardiac disease, the prevalence of PFO was higher (40% vs. 10%, $p < 0.001$) compared to a control group of 100 patients without stroke (6). In this study, the prevalence of PFO was 54% in patients with no identifiable cause of stroke, 40% in patients with no identifiable cause of stroke but with a risk factor for stroke, and 21% in patients with an identifiable cause of stroke ($p < 0.10$).

In a meta-analysis by Overell et al. (7) in patients older than 55 years who suffered a stroke, the odds ratio for stroke was 3.1 if a PFO were present, 6.1 for an atrial septal aneurysm, and 15.6 for the presence of a PFO plus atrial septal aneurysm compared to controls. In patients of any age who were determined to have had a cryptogenic stroke, the odds ratio for stroke was 3.1 for PFO (22 studies), 3.7 for atrial septal aneurysm (5 studies), and 23.3 for PFO plus atrial septal aneurysm (2 studies). In patients younger than age 55 years who were also determined to have had a cryptogenic stroke, the risk for stroke was 6.0 times higher in patients with versus without a PFO.

CLINICAL PRESENTATION OF CRYPTOGENIC STROKE AND PFO

The usual clinical setting where a paradoxical embolism is considered to be the etiology for stroke is when a young person (less than 60 years old) without any obvious predisposing risk factors for stroke presents with the sudden onset of neurologic deficit and an MRI pattern indicating an isolated recent stroke. In 10–20% of cases there may be multiple abnormalities on the MRI, suggesting that previous embolic phenomena have occurred, some of which may have been clinically silent. The diagnosis of cryptogenic stroke is a diagnosis of exclusion. There must be no other structural abnormalities on the MRI that could account for the neurologic findings. In addition, there must be no other potential causes of embolic phenomena such as atrial fibrillation, mitral stenosis, or significant atherosclerotic disease of the ascending aorta, carotid, or cerebral vessels. As part of this evaluation, it is routine to perform a transesophageal echo to rule out any potential cardiac source of emboli. During these studies, the atrial septum is evaluated both at rest with Doppler flow as well as with an agitated saline injection to determine the presence of right to left shunting across the atrial septum.

A minority of patients (around 5%) report that their stroke occurred shortly after predisposing conditions for venous stasis, such as extended airplane or automobile rides. Another 10% of patients associate the onset of the stroke with physical straining such as going to the bathroom or lifting a heavy object. In our series of 120 patients with cryptogenic stroke and documented PFO, there were 3 patients who were pregnant. Not only does the pregnancy predispose to venous thrombosis, but the choice of medical therapy and timing of any interventional procedure must be carefully considered. Our recommendation is to close the PFO in the third trimester to decrease the risk of radiation exposure to the fetus, but prior to delivery when the patient will be straining and therefore increasing the risk of recurrent stroke due to the greater amount of right to left shunting through the PFO.

HYPERCOAGULABLE STATES AND CRYPTOGENIC STROKE

All patients with cryptogenic stroke should be evaluated with a panel of blood tests that can determine whether they have a hypercoagulable state. The most prevalent condition predisposing to hypercoagulability is pharmacologic use of estrogen containing birth control pills or hormone replacement therapy. In our series, excluding pregnancy or administration of estrogen, the incidence of one or more predisposing hypercoagulable conditions is 10%. The most common condition is the antiphospholipid syndrome, followed by a variety of abnormal coagulation conditions outlined below. The blood tests that we use to screen for hypercoagulability are:

- Protein C
- Protein S
- Factor 5 Leiden
- Factor 8
- Phospholipid antibodies
- Cardiolipin antibodies
- Diluted Russell viper venom test (DRVVT)
- Beta 2-glycoprotein antibodies
- Prothrombin 20210A
- Antithrombin deficiency

If possible, estrogen therapy should be stopped. Appropriate therapy with coumadin should be determined by a hematologist. The potential risks or benefits of percutaneous closure of the PFO in addition to anticoagulation is being analyzed in the RESPECT trial registry, which is enrolling patients with hypercoagulable states to receive anticoagulation plus the Amplatzer PFO occluder device in a nonrandomized fashion.

NEUROLOGICAL DECOMPRESSION ILLNESS IN SCUBA DIVERS

Neurologic decompression illness is due to formation of free nitrogen gas bubbles coalescing in the vasculature from tissues as the diver ascends to the surface (8). The free gas bubbles can block venous or arterial flow, or lead to activation of inflammatory and/or clotting cascades. Symptoms may be mild and include fatigue, malaise, sense of foreboding, arthralgias, lymphadenopathy, and pruritis (Type I decompression sickness). Patients with more extensive decompression illness (Type II) may develop neurological and pulmonary manifestations. The neurologic insult may involve the spinal cord (especially the lower thoracic spinal cord) or the cerebrum. Neurologic symptoms can include parasthesias, paraplegia, urinary and bowel incontinence, ataxia, memory loss, speech and visual disturbances, and change in personality. The pulmonary manifestations include dyspnea, wheezing, chest pain, and pharyngeal irritation. The condition can result in death if untreated.

The incidence of PFO appears increased in patients with neurological decompression illness (9,10). Conversely, the risk for neurologic decompression illness is much higher in individuals with PFO compared to controls (11). In one study, the presence of a PFO increased the risk for decompression illness events in divers by 4.5-fold ($p = 0.03$) compared to divers without a PFO (11). Almost twice as many ischemic brain lesions were seen in divers with PFO than in those without PFO ($p = 0.07$). In another study of sport divers, multiple brain lesions were associated with presence of a large PFO even in asymptomatic individuals (12). Transcatheter closure of patent foramen ovale has been successful in prevention of the recurrence of neurological decompression sickness in divers (13).

PLATYPNEA-ORTHODEOXIA SYNDROME

Platypnea-orthodeoxia is a rare and poorly understood syndrome where patients develop dyspnea and arterial desaturation in the upright position (14–16). The disorder is due to orthostatic accentuation of a right to left shunt across an interatrial communication, usually a PFO. The syndrome is most commonly recognized in patients with a history of a major pulmonary disorder such as pneumonectomy, recurrent pulmonary emboli, or chronic lung disease. Pulmonary artery pressures are typically normal. The physiologic mechanism is unknown (14). Transcatheter closure of the interatrial communication has resulted in increased arterial saturation and improved respiratory symptoms (16–18).

Not all patients who have arterial desaturation associated with a PFO have the complete syndrome with desaturation only in the upright position. Some patients have desaturation whether they are supine or upright. Desaturation may be exacerbated in the presence of pulmonary hypertension and tricuspid regurgitation. Although some patients demonstrate improved arterial oxygenation and obtain symptomatic relief when the PFO is closed, we have observed other patients who remain symptomatic despite PFO closure, suggesting a primary pulmonary etiology for the arterial desaturation. In those patients who have pulmonary hypertension, the PFO may function as a "pop-off" valve that releases right atrial pressure and prevents the development of right-sided heart failure. In these cases, our recommendation is to place an occlusive balloon across the PFO temporarily and measure the right atrial pressure. If there is more than a 5 mmHg increase in right atrial pressure, then the PFO should not be closed.

Other clinical conditions in which a PFO has been implicated is fat embolization associated with orthopedic surgical procedures or air embolization during neurosurgery. In these conditions, the fat or air could enter the venous system due to the trauma of the surgical procedure. This material would be sequestered in the lungs without causing any clinical sequelae unless the volume of fat or air were extremely large. However, if a PFO were present, then the adipose tissue or air could embolize to the brain producing the neurologic sequelae that are associated with these clinical scenarios.

ARE ONLY CRYPTOGENIC STROKES "PARADOXICAL"?

The definition of cryptogenic stroke has been limited to people who are less than 55 to 60 years old because it is assumed that any stroke in older patients must be due to atherosclerotic disease. There is an interesting observational study that raises significant questions about the potential role of PFO in the elderly population. In a substudy analysis from the Warfarin Aspirin Recurrent Stroke Study (WARSS), Homma et al. looked at 250 patients who had a cryptogenic stroke in which a transesophageal echo was performed. The patients were separated according to whether a PFO was present and then were compared in three age-matched groups. In patients less than 55 years old, there was no difference in the incidence of recurrent stroke or death in the subsequent two years whether a PFO was present (2%) or not (9%) ($p = 0.15$). In the age group of 55–64 years, there was also no significant difference (10% vs. 14%, $p = 0.7$). However, in patients 65–85 years old, there was a threefold increased risk of recurrent stroke or death if a PFO were present compared to the group without a PFO (38% vs. 14.5%, $p = 0.01$). This increased risk was independent of traditional risk factors for atherosclerosis such as hypertension, diabetes, or hypercholesterolemia. In addition, this was not associated with larger PFOs, which were actually less prevalent with increasing age.

These observations suggest that the presence of a PFO may be more important than concurrent atheroma in elderly patients with an embolic stroke. In other words, just because a 70-year-old patient with a stroke has mild atheroma in the carotid or aortic arch, does not necessarily mean that the stroke came from the atherosclerotic disease. It may be more likely that the stroke was due to a paradoxical embolism through the PFO. The authors hypothesized that the risk for paradoxical embolism may increase with age due to the increased risk of venous emboli and decreased right ventricular compliance, which in turn could increase right atrial pressure. This hypothesis needs to be tested in a prospective randomized trial in elderly patients who have a stroke as well as a PFO. It may well be that elderly stroke patients need to receive therapy both to reduce atherosclerosis as well as to close the pathway for paradoxical embolism through the heart.

DETECTION OF INTERATRIAL COMMUNICATIONS

Detection of interatrial communications can be accomplished using several imaging modalities. These include transthoracic echocardiography, transesophageal echocardiography (TEE), and transcranial Doppler assessment of the middle cerebral arteries with intravenous microbubble injections. While the transthoracic echocardiogram with agitated saline echocontrast injection is easy to perform and relatively inexpensive, it has poor sensitivity for detection of interatrial communications compared to either TEE or transcranial Doppler (TCD) (19–20).

TEE provides a reliable method for visualization of the interatrial septum and possible interatrial communications, as well as evaluating other cardiac sources of potential emboli such as atrial appendage thrombus, left ventricular thrombus, valvular vegetation/endocarditis, or presence of intracardiac tumors (20). The disadvantage of TEE is that it can be associated with significant patient discomfort. Patients often need to be sedated during this procedure, which may limit their ability to provide an adequate valsalva maneuver. Critics of TEE as a screening modality argue that some patients with PFO will be missed due to their inability to cooperate while the echo probe is sitting in their esophagus.

TCD is a non-invasive method for detection of right to left shunting. Several studies have demonstrated that TCD is at least as sensitive in detection of intracardiac shunts as TEE (21,22). However, the TCD does not identify the etiology of the shunt and does not provide any information on cardiac structure or function including other possible cardiac sources of embolization. Intrapulmonary right to left shunts will also yield a positive TCD examination. All positive transcranial Doppler studies need to be eventually followed by a TEE or intracardiac echocardiogram (ICE) to define the cause of the right to left shunting.

PERCUTANEOUS CLOSURE OF PFO

Although surgical closure of PFOs can be performed, the procedure has been applied to only a limited population due to the inherent risks and morbidity associated with open heart surgery. After many years of development, several devices are currently available for percutaneous closure of PFOs. The two most common devices are the CardioSEAL® (NMT Medical, Boston, MA) and the Amplatzer PFO occluder device (AGA Medical Corp., Golden Valley, MN).

Device descriptions

The Amplatzer septal occluder device is a self-expandable, double-disk device with connecting waist made from a nitinol wire mesh (0.004–0.0075 in.). Dacron patches are sewn within each disk and the connecting waist, which serve to occlude blood flow through the device (4). The Amplatzer septal occluder device is available in sizes measured by the diameter of the connecting waist ranging from 4 to 40 mm. The Amplatzer

(A)

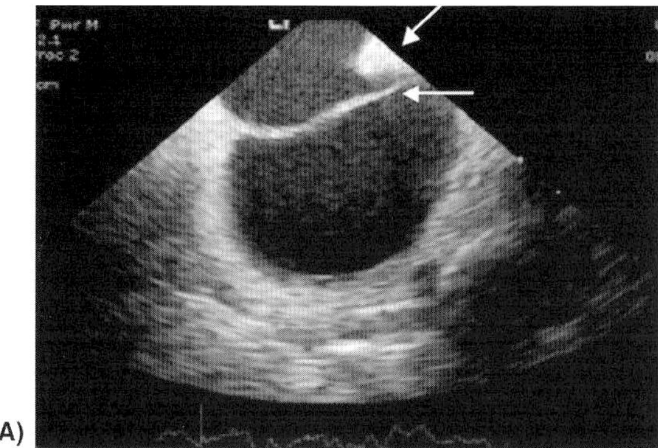

(B)

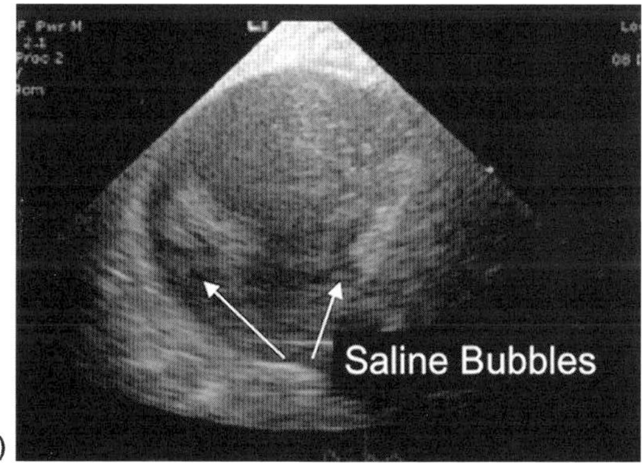

Figure 3 (**A**) Intracardiac echocardiography. An AcuNav™ (Seimens Medical Solutions, Malvern, PA) 10 French imaging catheter is passed from the femoral vein to the right atrium. The thin septum primum overlaps the thick septum secundum on the left atrial side. (**B**) Intracardiac echocardiography with injection of agitated saline into the femoral vein. The microbubbles pass from the right atrium across the PFO and swirl within the left atrium.

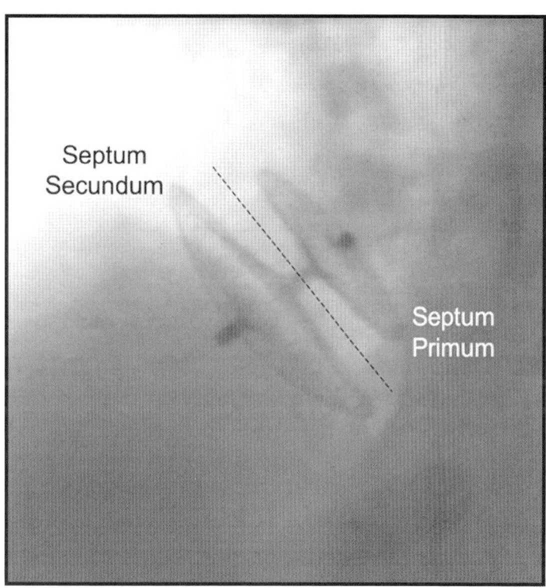

Figure 4 X-ray image of an Amplatzer PFO occluder in the LAO cranial angulation. The plane of the interatrial septum is shown by the dotted line.

PFO occluder device comes in three sizes (18 mm, 25 mm, and 35 mm), which describe the diameter of the larger right atrial disk. The CardioSEAL device is also a self-expanding device, which consists of two square "umbrellas" made by Dacron cloth that are attached to each other in the center[5]. Each umbrella is supported by four stainless steel spring arms radiating from the center of the device. The CardioSEAL device sizes, measured by the length of the diagonal of an umbrella, are 17, 23, 28, 33, and 40 mm.

Although there are different techniques and variations for percutaneous closure, PFO closure is usually performed as an outpatient procedure. Our preference is to use mild sedation with intravenous VERSED® (Roche, Basel, Swetzerland) and fentanyl. We prefer to use ICE because it is better tolerated than the transesophageal approach. This also decreases the likelihood that general anesthesia will be necessary. Since the Food and Drug Administration (FDA) has now approved the use of resterilized ICE catheters, the cost of these devices has decreased by approximately two-thirds. The procedure usually takes 30–45 minutes to perform. We use prophylactic antibiotics intravenously because this is a permanent implanted device, although there are no data to demonstrate this is necessary. We prescribe aspirin for three months and clopidogrel 75 mg per day for one month following implantation. Our protocol includes obtaining a follow-up TEE at one month to ensure absence of thrombus formation on the device and to document proper positioning of the closure device. We recommend standard endocarditis prophylaxis with antibiotics for one year following device implantation, although no randomized trials exist to prove the necessity of endocarditis prophylaxis in this population.

In 2000, Meier et al. published their five-year experience with a variety of transcatheter devices in 80 patients who had cryptogenic stroke. All patients were treated with aspirin alone for six months following the procedure. Although there were no recurrent strokes, the incidence of recurrent TIA was 2.5% and peripheral embolus occurred in 0.9% (23). Their more recent update describes 250 patients with an embolic recurrence rate of 1.6%. This group does not use echocardiographic guidance during the implantation of the device, which could shorten the procedure but may also lead to incomplete closure depending on the type of device. In our experience at UCLA, in 120 patients who have had PFO closure for cryptogenic stroke, the embolic, TIA, or stroke recurrence rate over five years has been 0%.

POTENTIAL COMPLICATIONS OF PERCUTANEOUS PFO CLOSURE DEVICES

Although the procedure of percutaneous PFO closure is relatively simple to perform and is well tolerated by patients, there are potential acute and chronic complications that operators and patients need to be aware of. During the procedure, meticulous care must be given to prevent air from being introduced through the guiding catheter into the left atrium. As with any interventional procedure, there is a learning curve to implanting these devices so that closure of the PFO is optimized. Following device implantation, there are two major complications that have been described. With the CardioSEAL device, we found a high incidence of thrombus on the left atrial surface. TEE was performed in 70 patients at one month post implantation. In 23 patients who received the CardioSEAL, there were 5 (22%) cases of thrombus, whereas we have never observed any thrombus formation on any of the ASD or PFO Amplatzer occluding devices. In one of these CardioSEAL cases, the large mass of mobile echoes on the left atrial side convinced us to prophylactically remove the device. The transesophageal image and the anatomic specimen found at open-heart surgery is shown in Figure 5. Because we removed the device prophylactically, it is impossible to know whether these thrombi would have embolized or perhaps this was just a normal variant of scar tissue formation. However, we suspect that the small incidence of recurrent emboli in some series of percutaneous PFO closure may be due to formation of thrombus on the left atrial side on some of the devices.

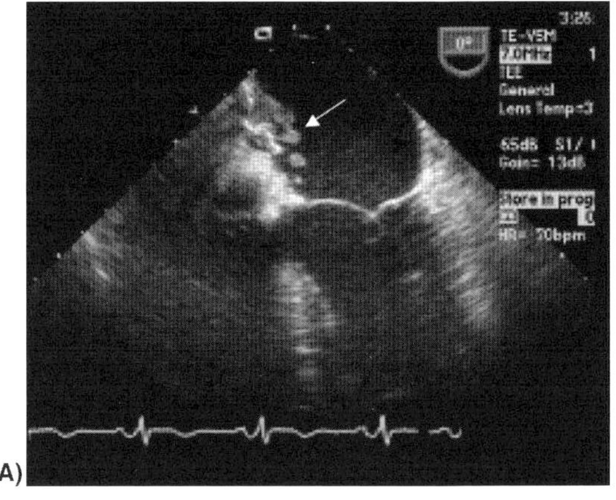

(A)

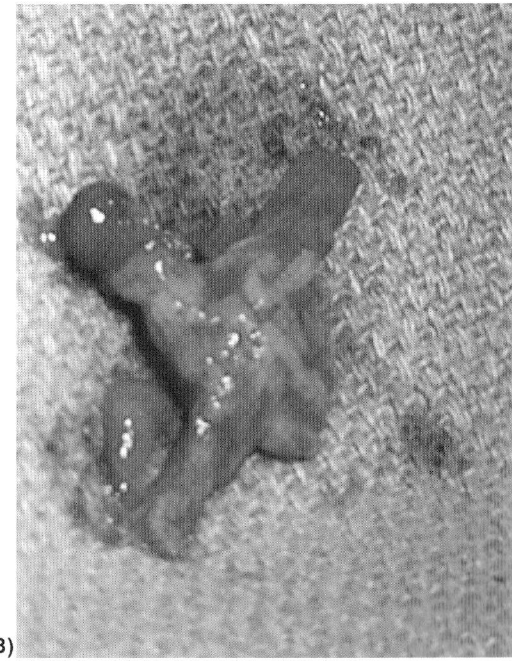
(B)

Figure 5 (**A**) Transesophageal echocardiogram (TEE) demonstrating multilobular echoes in the left atrium extending from the surface of the CardioSEAL® device. (**B**) Surgical specimen removed from the left atrial side of the CardioSEAL reveals a multilobular structure consisting of organizing thrombus and fibrous tissue.

Although we and others (Sievert et al.) have not observed any thrombus formation on the Amplatzer device, it has a different yet very serious potential complication. Erosion of the superior aspect of the atrial wall or aorta has been reported with the Amplatzer devices. Twenty-five of these cases occurred with Amplatzer ASD occluding devices and are believed to be associated with oversizing the device, which puts excessive pressure on the atrial walls. There have been three reported cases of erosion associated with the PFO Amplatzer occluder out of approximately 20,000 procedures. Emergency surgery is required to remove the device and deaths have been reported.

Both of these types of complications, although rare, need to be considered before recommending implantation of these permanent devices. Only a randomized prospective trial can determine the relative benefit versus risk of percutaneous closure of PFO. There are currently two randomized trials to determine whether percutaneous closure of a PFO is preferable to medical therapy in patients who present with cryptogenic stroke. The CLOSURE trial is investigating the CardioSEAL device, and the RESPECT trial is assessing the Amplatzer PFO occluder versus medical therapy to prevent recurrent cryptogenic stroke. Unfortunately, physicians and patients have been able to circumvent enrolling patients into these randomized trials because other devices have been used off-label. With continued persistence, it is hoped that enough patients will be enrolled in these clinical trials to obtain the necessary information that will permit a more rational use of these devices.

In addition to these two serious potential complications, approximately 10% of patients complain of some palpitations following implantation of these devices, and 5% of patients describe some mild chest discomfort. With the Amplatzer device, 5% of patients complain of increased or new onset of migraine headaches or visual aura. All of these symptoms tend to dissipate within 3–6 months. We believe this is consistent with an inflammatory reaction to the foreign materials, which resolves as part of the process of scar formation.

THE CONNECTION BETWEEN PFO AND MIGRAINE HEADACHES

Despite medical advances in the treatment of migraine headache (HA), many patients suffer frequent and disabling episodes of migraine. Migraine affects approximately 12% of the population (18% of women and 6% of men). The economic burden in terms of cost of labor lost to migraine disability is estimated between $5.6 and $17.2 billion annually (24,25). Migraines are also a risk factor for development of stroke in young people, especially in women on oral contraceptives.

Sztajel et al. investigated the association between PFOs and migraine headache in patients with cryptogenic stroke. Among patients where PFO was thought to play a causal role in the stroke, 52% had migraine with aura, compared to 16% of patients in whom PFO was considered unrelated. Among patients with PFO who had migraine with aura, 7 of 15 (48%) had complete suppression of their aura attacks after surgical closure or anticoagulant treatment (26). In another study, transcatheter closure of the PFO in 27 patients with migraine and large shunts as assessed by transcranial Doppler, resulted in improvement or disappearance of migraine headaches in 21 of 27 (77%) patients (27). Of those patients who had migraine with aura, the aura disappeared in 10 of 14 (71%) patients. Morandi et al. demonstrated that transcatheter closure of PFO in 17 patients with migraine headaches (8 with migraine and aura) resulted in resolution of migraine in 5 of 17 (29%) patients, and substantial improvement in another 10 patients (total of 88% with improvement) (28).

Wilmshurst et al. (29) retrospectively examined patients who underwent PFO closure because of decompression illness. Among 37 patients, 45% reported no further migrainous attacks following PFO closure. The largest epidemiological study of cryptogenic stroke, PFO, and migraine was published in 2002 by Lamy et al. (30). In 500 patients with cryptogenic stroke, 46% were found to have a PFO, and migraine was twice as common among patients with PFO (28%) as in those without (14%).

The Migraine Intervention with STARFlex Technology (MIST) trial in Great Britain is a randomized blinded trial evaluating the efficacy of PFO closure compared to standard medical therapy for treatment of migraine headache. In the patient enrollment phase of this trial, right to left shunts were found in 60% of people with migraine and 40% of patients enrolled had a large atrial shunt (as opposed to 27% and 7% in the general population, respectively) (31).

These observations along with demonstration of platelet hyperaggregability (32) and reduction in migraines for some patients treated with warfarin (33) suggest that right to left intracardiac shunts with microemboli may play an important role in the etiology of migraine. Another hypothesis is that the PFO permits right to left shunting of chemicals that could act as triggers of migraine headache in susceptible individuals. Without the PFO, these chemicals would pass first through the lungs where they could be subject to degradation or dilution. Thus elimination of right to left shunting by surgical or percutaneous techniques may ameliorate or eliminate the chemical triggers of migraine headaches without affecting the neuronal substrate. Currently, treatment for migraine cephalalgia consists only of medical management. Although the medications available may ameliorate the severity or frequency of migraine attacks, the drugs do not eliminate migraine and are less than optimal in their effectiveness.

We have been closing PFOs and ASDs with Amplatzer devices since 2001. We reported that migraine headache was present in 42% (37/89) of patients undergoing percutaneous closure of these interatrial communications. Migraine headache was present in 45% of patients with PFOs and 30% of patients with ASDs (34). At 3 months post closure of the interatrial communication, migraine disappeared completely in 22 of 37 patients (60%): in 18 of 24 patients (75%) with migraine and aura, and in 4 of 13 patients (31%) with migraine without aura. Of the remaining patients, 40% had significant improvement (≥ 2 grades by the MIDAS questionnaire). The benefit was sustained in this population over a median follow-up time of 18 months.

Table 1 summarizes the observations from six independent centers that have reported an association of PFO or ASD closure and reduction in migraine headaches. The mean incidence of resolution of migraine headaches was 55% with improvement in 42% of the residual subjects. These observational studies suggest that there may be a causal relationship between inter-atrial communications and migraine headache. This hypothesis is being tested in five different clinical trials conducted in 2005 through 2007. The information obtained by these trials should provide adequate evidence to substantiate or

Table 1 Effect of PFO closure devices on migraine headache

Authors (ref.)	*Year*	*Type of study*	*No.*	*No. (%) with migraine*	*Mean follow-up (mo)*	*% Resolved*	*Residual % improved*
Wilmshurst et al. (9)	2000	Retrospect	37	21 (57)	17	48	38
Morandi et al. (6)	2003	Prospect	17	17 (100)	12	29	59
Post et al. (7)	2004	Retrospect	66	26 (39)	6	84	N/A
Schwerzmann et al. (8)	2004	Retrospect	215	47 (22)	24	N/A	83
Azarbal, Tobis (4)	2004	Retrospect	89	37 (42)	6	60	16
Reisman et al. (5)	2004	Retrospect	162	57 (35)	12	56	14
Total			586	205 (35)		55	42

Abbreviations: N/A, not applicable; PFO, patent foramen ovale.

Source: From Tsimikas S. Transcatheter closure of patent foramen ovale: hope or hype? JACC Feb 2005; 45(6):496–498.

refute the reported association between migraine and inter-atrial shunts.

WHAT IS A MIGRAINE HEADACHE?

The etiology of migraine headache is still unclear. For many years, the mechanism of migraine headaches was explained as a vasomotor phenomenon where the cerebral arterial circulation developed intense spasm followed by dilatation. The rare occurrence of stroke associated with migraine was thought to be due to excessive vasoconstriction of a cerebral vessel. Pulsating blood through the dilated cerebral arteries was believed to be the cause of the throbbing headaches associated with migraine. More recent data using positron emission tomography (PET) imaging do not demonstrate the presence of increased blood flow in these patients during migraine headaches. PET imaging during migraine attacks with aura demonstrates decreased blood flow over the occipital visual cortex. This corresponds with animal evidence of a spreading wave of depolarization. Using transgenic mice (CK1δ-T44A) that have the human gene inserted for migraine headache with hemiplegia or familial early sleep with migraine, Charles at UCLA demonstrated that cortical spreading depression (CSD) can be reproduced and visualized in these animals (35).

TRIGEMINAL NERVE STIMULATION

One of the evolving theories of migraine headaches emphasizes the interaction between cerebral nerves and blood vessels. In this concept, migraine specific–triggers activate perivascular trigeminal nerves. The trigeminal nerve then releases vasoactive neuropeptides within the meninges, which mediate neurogenic inflammation producing vasodilation, vessel leakage, and mast cell degradation. These neuropeptides relay nociceptive impulses that produce the sensation of pain and lower the pain threshold resulting in the allodynia associated with migraine headaches. Allodynia denotes a painful response to stimuli that are usually not noxious, such as average light, sound, or touch. Of the potential culprit neuropeptides, calcitonin gene-related protein (CGRP) is elevated in the jugular vein during migraine and other forms of vascular headaches (36,37). The authors also found a transient increase in levels of IL-8 but suggest that meningeal transvascular leukocyte migration during migraine attacks may be impeded by other events, such as nitric oxide production, according to the model of sterile inflammation. In addition, infusion of CGRP induces migraine headaches in susceptible individuals. Triptans, effective agents for impeding migraine, have been shown to attach to 5-HT nerve receptors and block the release of CGRP.

Based on the association of PFO, cryptogenic stroke, and migraine headaches, there are currently two hypotheses to explain how migraine headaches might be induced in these conditions.

VENOUS EMBOLUS THEORY OF MIGRAINE

In the first theory, it is thought that the etiology of migraine headache is due to a small venous embolus that paradoxically crosses the PFO and passes to the cerebral circulation. Rather than inducing a stroke, the small embolus or platelet plug precipitates a spreading wave of depolarization, which is recognized as the neurologic phenomenon of migraine with aura. In support of this concept, a recent report from Europe has documented a higher incidence of MRI lesions in migraine patients with aura than in controls (38). In the study, there were 161 patients with migraine and aura, 134 patients with migraine without aura, and 140 controls who were case matched for age, sex, and place of residence. In the cerebellar region of the posterior circulation territory, patients with migraine had a higher incidence of MRI abnormalities than controls (5.4% vs. 0.7%; $p = 0.02$). The adjusted odds ratio was 13.7 for patients with migraine with aura compared with controls. This study suggests that patients with migraine, especially those with aura, have an increased propensity to develop brain lesions. Alternatively, they may have a significantly increased risk of having cerebral embolic events, which produce these lesions.

Although this concept is still actively debated, we suspect that paradoxical emboli are not the likely cause of migraine, although they might be the contributing factor for strokes that occur in patients who have migraine. The hypothesis that paradoxical emboli are the trigger for migraine also does not explain why migraine occurs in patients who do not have a PFO. In addition, the emboli hypothesis does not explain why migraines recur with the same neurologic pattern. Presumably emboli would distribute randomly throughout the cerebral circulation. On the other hand, a chemical trigger would distribute equally to the brain and could stimulate the same susceptible nerve receptors.

OUR HYPOTHESIS OF MIGRAINE

Our hypothesis is that some migraines are precipitated in susceptible individuals by a variety of chemical substances that are ingested or produced in the body. A PFO is not necessary for these chemical triggers to pass to the brain; however, if a PFO is also present, these chemical substances can pass directly through the atrial shunt before they can be detoxified in the first passage through the lungs. For an example of a potential chemical factor, since migraine headaches are more common in women and more prevalent around the time of menstruation, we hypothesize that one of these chemical substances may be a prostaglandin or steroid hormone that could be synthesized in the ovaries, uterus, or liver. This substance in elevated concentration could cause migraine with or without a PFO present; if a PFO is present, it could potentially shunt from the venous to the arterial system and reach the brain in a more concentrated packet than if a PFO were not present. The observation that patients who reach menopause or have a hysterectomy have a decrease in the incidence of their migraine headaches supports this hypothesis that some migraines are triggered by chemical substances. The observation that migraine headaches are significantly reduced after PFO closure leads to the hypothesis that this central shunt is an important component in the pathway to trigger migraines. We assume there are multiple chemical triggers of migraines in patients with or without a PFO. Although closing the PFO may be an effective treatment of migraine headaches by closing this short-circuit in the body, a more complete understanding of migraine may be obtained by identifying the chemical triggers that stimulate the neuronal receptors.

PFO CLOSURE AND PARADOXICAL INCREASE IN MIGRAINE HEADACHES

In contradistinction to the reports that PFO closure improves migraine headache in 60% of patients, there are reports of a small percentage of patients who experience an increase in migraine and aura for several weeks post-procedure (39,40). We addressed this apparent paradox by looking at the association of nickel allergy and post-closure adverse events in 37 patients who had ASD or PFO closure with an Amplatzer® device. These devices are composed of nitinol, which is an alloy of 55% titanium and 45% nickel.

Of 108 patients who received a PFO closure device and 42 patients who received an ASD closure device, 62 (41%) experienced chest discomfort (usually mild), palpitations (usually isolated extra beats), or increased migraine. There were seven patients (5%) who noted new-onset migraine with aura or increased frequency and severity of migraine or aura post procedure. Of the seven patients, six were tested for nickel allergy, and four of these patients (67%) had a positive nickel skin test. This finding occurred more frequently with ASD devices compared to PFO devices (12% vs. 2%, $p = 0.02$). New-onset or worsening migraine or aura (MHA/aura) was associated with nickel allergy ($p = 0.035$). When adverse events (chest discomfort, palpitations, and MHA/aura) were combined, there was a significant association with nickel allergy ($p = 0.028$). The association was strongest with the combination of chest discomfort and MHA/aura ($p = 0.005$).

The two patients who also experienced exacerbation of migraine but were not allergic to nickel had large ASD devices (38 mm). Although the sample size is small, these observations raise intriguing hypotheses. One possible mechanism to explain the new-onset or exacerbation of MHA and aura is that a local inflammatory reaction to the implanted device results in the formation of platelet adhesions. These activated platelet aggregates could then embolize to the brain causing micro-infarcts and MHA. An observation that lends support to this hypothesis is that five of the patients noted a marked increase in frequency of MHA or aura shortly after discontinuing clopidogrel, suggesting that the pharmacologic suppression of platelet aggregation on the implanted device may be preventing embolization. One other report has documented the benefit of clopidogrel in reducing MHA following nitinol device implantation (41). All five of our patients noted an improvement in MHA and aura after re-starting clopidogrel. However, there was no evidence of abnormal MRI lesions in the two cases with the most severe migraine headaches and aura. In addition, follow-up TEE did not demonstrate any thrombus on any of these Amplatzer devices. These observations are underscored by our previous work which demonstrated a 0% incidence of thrombus with the Amplatzer devices as assessed by transesophageal echocardiography at one month post implant (34). Therefore, there is no objective evidence for thrombus formation as the etiology of these neurologic symptoms.

An alternative mechanism to explain new-onset or exacerbation of MHA and aura is that a localized reaction around the device releases inflammatory mediators into the left atrium which then travel to the cerebral circulation and induce the neurologic syndrome. Presumably the inflammation is greater if the subject is sensitive to nickel, but an exaggerated response may occur without nickel allergy and produce the same symptom complex, especially if a large device is implanted. This may explain why MHA and aura are more likely to occur with ASD closure devices. This hypothesis opens research avenues to assess the effect of chemokines or other inflammatory proteins as primary triggers for migraine headaches in patients with or without implanted devices. The observation that these patients responded dramatically and rapidly to administration of clopidogrel suggests that this drug may be acting as an anti-inflammatory agent, either to decrease the release of the trigger chemicals from the inflammatory site in the left atrium, or they may be acting on nociceptive neural adenosine receptors to inhibit the cortical spreading depolarization (migraine) response to inflammatory byproducts.

CONCLUSION

This is an exciting area of medicine that combines the resources of both cardiologists and neurologists to help explain the mysterious connection between cryptogenic stroke, migraine headaches, and inter-atrial communications. We are optimistic that the randomized clinical trials will demonstrate conclusively that PFO plays an important role as a passage way for chemical triggers that stimulate susceptible neuronal receptors in the central nervous system to initiate the process of cortical spreading depolarization, which is perceived as a migraine headache. Hopefully this will lead not only to a better understanding of the mechanism of migraine headache and cryptogenic stroke, but also to improved treatment and relief for the millions of individuals who suffer from migraine.

REFERENCES

1. Wahl A, Windecker S, Meier B. Patent foramen ovale: pathophysiology and therapeutic options in symptomatic patients. Minerva Cardioangiol 2001; 49(6):403–411.
2. Hagen PT, Scholz DG, Edwards WD. Incidence and size of patent foramen ovale during the first 10 decades of life: an autopsy study of 965 normal hearts. Mayo Clin Proc 1984; 59(1):17–20.
3. Kerut EK, Norfleet WT, Plotnick GD, Giles TD. Patent foramen ovale: a review of associated conditions and the impact of physiological size. J Am Coll Cardiol. 2001; 38(3):613–623.
4. Lethen H, Flachskampf FA, Schneider R, et al. Frequency of deep vein thrombosis in patients with patent foramen ovale and ischemic stroke or transient ischemic attack. Am J Cardiol 1997; 80(8):1066–1069.
5. Cramer SC, Rordorf G, Maki JH, et al. Increased pelvic vein thrombi in cryptogenic stroke: results of the Paradoxical Emboli from Large Veins in Ischemic Stroke (PELVIS) study. Stroke 2004; 35(1):46–50.
6. Lechat P, Mas JL, Lascault G, et al. Prevalence of patent foramen ovale in patients with stroke. N Engl J Med 1988; 318(18):1148–1152.

7. Overell JR, Bone I, Lees KR. Interatrial septal abnormalities and stroke: a meta-analysis of case-control studies. Neurology 2000; 55(8):1172–1179.
8. Barratt DM, Harch PG, Van Meter K. Decompression illness in divers: a review of the literature. Neurologist 2002; 8(3):186–202.
9. Germonpre P, Dendale P, Unger P, Balestra C. Patent foramen ovale and decompression sickness in sports divers. J Appl Physiol 1998; 84(5): 1622–1626.
10. Moon RE, Camporesi EM, Kisslo JA. Patent foramen ovale and decompression sickness in divers. Lancet 1989; 1(8637):513–514.
11. Schwerzmann M, Seiler C, Lipp E, et al. Relation between directly detected patent foramen ovale and ischemic brain lesions in sport divers. Ann Intern Med 2001; 134(1):21–24.
12. Knauth M, Ries S, Pohimann S, et al. Cohort study of multiple brain lesions in sport divers: role of a patent foramen ovale. BMJ 1997; 314(7082):701–705.
13. Walsh KP, Wilmshurst PT, Morrison WL. Transcatheter closure of patent foramen ovale using the Amplatzer septal occluder to prevent recurrence of neurological decompression illness in divers. Heart 1999; 81(3):257–261.
14. Seward JB, Hayes DL, Smith HC, et al. Platypnea-orthodeoxia: clinical profile, diagnostic workup, management, and report of seven cases. Mayo Clin Proc 1984; 59(4):221–231.
15. Sorrentino M, Resnekov L. Patent foramen ovale associated with platypnea and orthodeoxia. Chest 1991; 100(4):1157–1158.
16. Rao PS, Palacios IF, Bach RG, Bitar SR, Sideris EB. Platypnea-orthodeoxia: management by transcatheter buttoned device implantation. Catheter Cardiovasc Interv 2001; 54(1):77–82.
17. Guerin P, Lambert V, Godart F, et al. Transcatheter closure of patent foramen ovale in patients with platypnea-orthodeoxia: results of a multicentric French registry. Cardiovasc Intervent Radiol 2005; 28(2):164–168.
18. Delgado G, Inglessis I, Martin-Herrero F, et al. Management of platypnea-orthodeoxia syndrome by transcatheter closure of atrial communication: hemodynamic characteristics, clinical and echocardiographic outcome. J Invasive Cardiol 2004; 16(10):578–582.
19. Belkin RN, Pollack BD, Ruggiero ML, Alas LL, Tatini U. Comparison of transesophageal and transthoracic echocardiography with contrast and color flow Doppler in the detection of patent foramen ovale. Am Heart J 1994; 128(3):520–525.
20. Chen WJ, Kuan P, Lien WP, Lin FY. Detection of patent foramen ovale by contrast transesophageal echocardiography. Chest 1992; 101(6): 1515–1520.
21. Droste DW, Silling K, Stypmann J, et al. Contrast transcranial doppler ultrasound in the detection of right-to-left shunts: time window and threshold in microbubble numbers. Stroke 2000; 31(7):1640–1645.
22. Nemec JJ, Marwick TH, Lorig RJ, et al. Comparison of transcranial Doppler ultrasound and transesophageal contrast echocardiography in the detection of interatrial right-to-left shunts. Am J Cardiol 1991; 68(15):1498–1502.
23. Windecker S, Wahl A, Chatterjee T, et al. Percutaneous closure of patent foramen ovale in patients with paradoxical embolism: long-term risk of recurrent thromboembolic events. Circulation 2000; 101(8):893–898.
24. Mathew NT. Pathophysiology, epidemiology, and impact of migraine. Clin Cornerstone 2001; 4(3):1–17.
25. Lipton RB, Scher AI, Kolodner K, Liberman J, Steiner TJ, Stewart WF. Migraine in the United States: epidemiology and patterns of health care use. Neurology 2002; 58(6):885–894.
26. Sztajzel R, Genoud D, Roth S, Mermillod B, Le Floch-Rohr J. Patent foramen ovale, a possible cause of symptomatic migraine: a study of 74 patients with acute ischemic stroke. Cerebrovasc Dis 2002; 13(2):102–106.
27. Anzola GP. Clinical impact of patent foramen ovale diagnosis with transcranial Doppler. Eur J Ultrasound 2002; 16(1–2):11–20.
28. Morandi E, Anzola GP, Angeli S, Melzi G, Onorato E. Transcatheter closure of patent foramen ovale: a new migraine treatment? J Interv Cardiol 2003; 16(1):39–42.
29. Wilmshurst PT, Nightingale S, Walsh KP, Morrison WL. Effect on migraine of closure of cardiac right-to-left shunts to prevent recurrence of decompression illness or stroke or for haemodynamic reasons. Lancet 2000; 356(9242): 1648–1651.
30. Lamy C, Giannesini C, Zuber M, et al. Clinical and imaging findings in cryptogenic stroke patients with and without patent foramen

ovale: the PFO-ASA Study. Atrial Septal Aneurysm. Stroke 2002; 33(3):706–711.

31. Li J, Zhang Z, Rosenzweig J, Wang YY, Chan DW. Proteomics and bioinformatics approaches for identification of serum biomarkers to detect breast cancer. Clin Chem 2002; 48(8): 1296–1304.
32. Lechner H, Ott E, Fazekas F, Pilger E. Evidence of enhanced platelet aggregation and platelet sensitivity in migraine patients. Cephalalgia 1985; 5(suppl 2):89–91.
33. Fragoso YD. Reduction of migraine attacks during the use of warfarin. Headache 1997; 37(10):667–668.
34. Azarbal B, Tobis J, Suh W, Chan V, Dao C, Gaster R. Association of interatrial shunts and migraine headaches: impact of transcatheter closure. J Am Coll Cardiol 2005; 45(4):489–492.
35. Charles A. Reaching out beyond the synapse: glial intercellular waves coordinate metabolism. Sci STKE 2005; 2005(270):pe6.
36. Sarchielli P, Alberti A, Vaianella L, et al. Chemokine levels in the jugular venous blood of migraine without aura patients during attacks. Headache 2004; 44(10):961–968.
37. Sarchielli P, Gallai V. Nerve growth factor and chronic daily headache: a potential implication for therapy. Expert Rev Neurother 2004; 4(1):115–127.
38. Kruit MC, van Buchem MA, Hofman PA, et al. Migraine as a risk factor for subclinical brain lesions. JAMA 2004; 291(4):427–434.
39. Yew G, Wilson NJ. Transcatheter atrial septal defect closure with the Amplatzer septal occluder: five-year follow-up. Catheter Cardiovasc Interv 2005; 64(2):193–196.
40. Wilmshurst PT, Pearson MJ, Nightingale S, Walsh KP, Morrison WL. Inheritance of persistent foramen ovale and atrial septal defects and the relation to familial migraine with aura. Heart 2004; 90(11):1315–1320.
41. Sharifi M, Burks J. Efficacy of clopidogrel in the treatment of post-ASD closure migraines. Catheter Cardiovasc Interv 2004; 63(2):255.
42. Purandare N, Burns A, Daly KJ, Hardicre J, Morris J, Macfarlane G, McCollum C. Cerebral emboli as a potential cause of Alzheimer's disease and vascular dementia: case-control study. BMJ 2006; May 13 332(7660): 1119–1124.

19

Device closure of secundum atrial septal defects

Francisco Garay, Qi-Ling Cao, and Ziyad M. Hijazi

INTRODUCTION

Secundum atrial septal defects (ASD) account for 6–10% of all congenital cardiac anomalies and are more frequent in females than in males (2:1). ASD produces a left to right shunt and consequently right cardiac chambers volume overload, increased pulmonary blood flow, and eventually pulmonary arterial hypertension and pulmonary vascular disease. King et al. demonstrated in 1976 that secundum ASD was amenable for device closure. Since that time many devices have been developed for this purpose; however, due to the low success rate and high residual shunt rates, their application was not widely accepted. In 1997, Amplatz designed a device that rendered most secundum ASDs amenable for catheter closure. His device, the Amplatzer Septal Occluder (ASO) device (AGA Medical Corporation, Golden Valley, MN), and subsequent other devices revolutionized interventional therapy for septal defects. Studies comparing closure of ASDs using the ASO with surgery have demonstrated lower complication rate, shorter length of hospital stay, and less expense than the traditional surgical treatment. Complications after device closure have been shown to occur at a rate of 2.8% for minor complications (transitory rhythm disturbances, device embolization, and bleeding) and 0.3% for major complications (cardiac tamponade, TIA or stroke, endocarditis).

Patients with ASDs are usually asymptomatic or have subtle symptoms (shortness of breath, fatigue, and palpitations). ASD closure is indicated in patients even if asymptomatic but with clinical evidence of significant hemodynamic shunt (a systolic ejection heart murmur with fixed splitting of S2, radiologic evidence of cardiomegaly and increased pulmonary blood flow). Usually transthoracic echocardiography demonstrates right heart chamber enlargement. Primum or sinus venosus types of atrial defects are not suitable for device closure. The development of non-reactive pulmonary vascular disease can occur in adults older than 40 years of age. A pulmonary vascular resistance indexed higher than 6 Woods units after a trial of vasodilators, such as oxygen and inhaled nitric oxide, is a contraindication for closure. In patients older than 65 years of age with large defects, especially if they have another form of cardiac disease (hypertensive, valvular, or coronary), it is necessary to evaluate the left ventricle compliance and determine if it will be capable of handling the volume overload produced with the ASD closure. This is achieved by measuring the left atrial pressure during balloon occlusion of the defect. We use a 27–33 mm Meditech sizing balloon (Boston Scientific, Natick, MA) advanced over the wire into the left atrium. The balloon is inflated and brought tight to the defect to close it. This is documented by echocardiography. Once cessation of shunt occurs, the wire is removed and the left atrial pressure is measured from the distal tip of the balloon. If left atrial pressure increases above 18 mmHg or by more than 5 points from baseline, the procedure is aborted and the patient is sent to the ward for left ventricle conditioning treatment using anticongestive and afterload therapy for 48–72 hours prior to attempting the closure procedure. Then the procedure is repeated and if the left atrial pressure does not exceed 18 mmHg, complete closure of the defect is attempted. However, if the left atrial pressure increases to more than 18 mmHg or more than 5 points from baseline, a fenestrated ASO device is used. Other contraindications for device closure include current systemic or local infection or sepsis within 1 month of the procedure, presence of intracardiac thrombus and bleeding disorders, or other contraindication to aspirin therapy, unless other antiplatelet agents such as clopidogrel can be used for six months.

THE DEVICE

The ASO device is a double disk device constructed from a 0.004–0.0075 in. Nitinol wire mesh (Fig. 1) with a 3–4 mm connecting waist between the two disks. The device size is determined by the diameter of its connecting waist. The device is available in sizes ranging from 4 to 40 mm (1 mm increments up to 20 mm; 2 mm increments up to 40 mm). The two flat disks extend radially beyond the connecting waist to secure the anchorage. The left atrial disk is larger than the right atrial disk. For devices ranging 4–10 mm in size, the left disk is 12 mm and the right disk is 8 mm larger than the waist. For devices ranging from 11–34 mm in size, the left disk is 14 mm and the right disk is 10 mm larger than the waist. For devices larger than 34 mm, the left disk is 16 mm and the right disk is 10 mm larger than the connecting waist. Dacron polyester patches are sewn into each disk and the connecting waist to increase thrombogenicity of the device. A stainless steel sleeve with a female thread is laser-welded to the right disk. This is used to screw the delivery cable to the device.

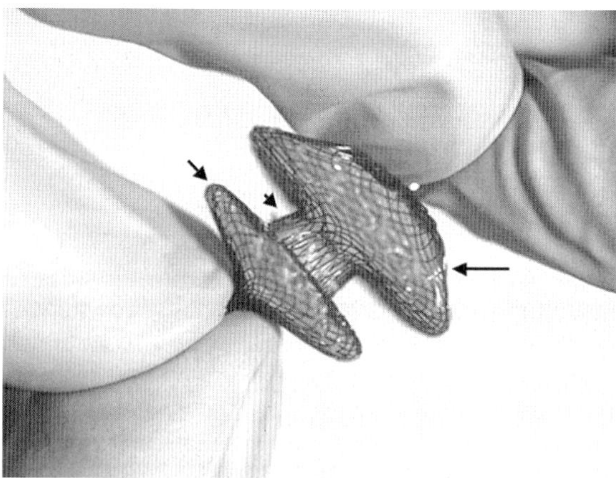

Figure 1 The Amplatzer® septal occluder. The *long arrow* denotes the left atrial disk; the *arrowhead* denotes the connecting waist; and the *short arrow* denotes the right atrial disk.

The device is implanted using the Amplatzer delivery system supplied separately from the device; it includes a 45° angled tip delivery sheath of specified French size and length, its dilator, a cable (0.081 in.), a loader to collapse the device, a side arm, and a pin vise to release the device from the cable. The 6 French sheath has a length of 60 cm; the 7 French sheath is available in lengths of 60 and 80 cm; and the 8, 9, 10, and 12 French sheaths are all 80 cm long. It is recommended to use the 6 French delivery system for devices less than 10 mm in diameter; a 7 French sheath for devices 10–15 mm; an 8 French delivery system for devices 16–19 mm; a 9 French sheath for devices 20–26 mm; a 10 French delivery system for devices 28–34 mm; and a 12 French sheath for the 36, 38, and 40 mm devices.

TECHNIQUE

Review in advance all data related to the patient and the defect to be closed need and ensure that appropriate devices, delivery systems, and exchange (rescue) system are all available in the catheterization laboratory. The exchange (rescue) system is similar to the delivery system with the exception of the dilator. The dilator inner lumen (0.088 in.) is larger than the regular dilator to allow passage of the cable inside. Aspirin 81–325 mg should be started 48 hours prior to the procedure; alternatively, clopidogrel 75 mg could be used. If the procedure is performed under transesophageal echocardiography (TEE) guidance, due to the length of the procedure and for the patient's comfort, the procedure should be done under general endotracheal anesthesia. If the procedure is performed under intra cardiac echocardiographic (ICE) guidance, mild sedation can be given. The right femoral vein is accessed with a 7 French short sheath and if ICE catheter is used, an additional 8 French short sheath is placed via a separate puncture in the same femoral vein. Arterial access could be used for monitoring, but it is not mandatory. In cases in which femoral venous access is not available it is preferable to use the trans-hepatic approach. Delivery of the device from the jugular or subclavian vein is difficult. Heparin is administered to maintain an activated clotting time (ACT) above 200 seconds at the time of device deployment. Antibiotic coverage is recommended for the procedure (cefazolin 1 g IV), the first dose at the time of the procedure and two additional doses 6–8 hours apart. Right heart catheterization is performed to measure pulmonary artery pressure and to calculate pulmonary vascular resistance and shunt (Qp:Qs) ratio. The pulmonary vascular reactivity can be evaluated if necessary. TEE or ICE images are obtained to assess the ASD location, size, additional defects and rims (Fig. 2A–D). It is important to evaluate the superior and inferior rims in the bicaval view (Fig. 2C) and the posterior and anterior rims in the short axis view (Fig. 2D). Then a 7 French multipurpose or angiographic catheter is advanced from the inferior vena cava into the left atrium and into the right upper pulmonary vein. TEE or ICE can be useful to guide the catheter across difficult defects. An angiogram in the right upper pulmonary vein in the hepatoclavicular projection (35° LAO and 35° cranial) is performed to evaluate the atrial septal length and shape (Fig. 3A) Then the multipurpose catheter is positioned in the left upper pulmonary vein and the super stiff guidewire is advanced just distal to the tip (Fig. 2E). We usually use the Amplatzer Super Stiff Exchange guidewire (0.035 in. with 1 cm floppy tip), however any extra stiff J-tipped wire could be used.

The multipurpose catheter is exchanged for an appropriate sizing balloon. We use the Amplatzer® Sizing balloon (AGA Medical Corp., Golden Valley, MN) that is a double-lumen balloon catheter with a 7 French shaft size (Fig. 2F, Fig. 3B). The balloon is made from nylon and is very compliant making it ideal for sizing ASDs by flow occlusion and preventing overstretching of the defect. We prefer to use the 34-mm balloon directly through the skin without a sheath over the wire. The balloon is placed across the defect under fluoroscopic and echocardiographic guidance and then inflated with diluted contrast until the left to right shunt ceases (stop flow technique) as observed by color flow Doppler on TEE or ICE (Fig. 2F). The indentations in the balloon made by the margins of the ASD are measured on echocardiographic (long axis view) or fluoroscopic images (beam perpendicular to the balloon)(Fig. 3B). Usually the echo measurements are more reliable than the fluoroscopic measurements. We choose a device about 1–2 mm larger than the stop flow diameter. The sizing balloon is removed and an appropriate delivery sheath for the device size is advanced over the super stiff guidewire to the left upper pulmonary vein (Fig. 2G). Extreme care must be exercised to avoid passage of air inside the delivery sheath. This can be achieved using different techniques. We have found the best technique to be advancing the sheath alone, once at the inferior vena cava-right atrial junction, over the dilator and guidewire all the way until it is in the left upper pulmonary vein. Once the sheath tip is in the left upper pulmonary vein, lower the sheath between the patient's legs (lower than the left atrium) and remove the dilator with the wire slowly out of the body allowing free back bleed.

The device is then screwed to the delivery cable and drawn into the loader under saline. A Touhy-Borst Y connector previously attached to the loader allows flushing with saline to purge any air bubble. The loader containing the device is attached to the proximal hub of the delivery sheath and the device is advanced to the distal tip of the sheath, taking care not to rotate the cable while advancing it in the long sheath to prevent premature unscrewing of the device. Then the cable and delivery sheath are pulled

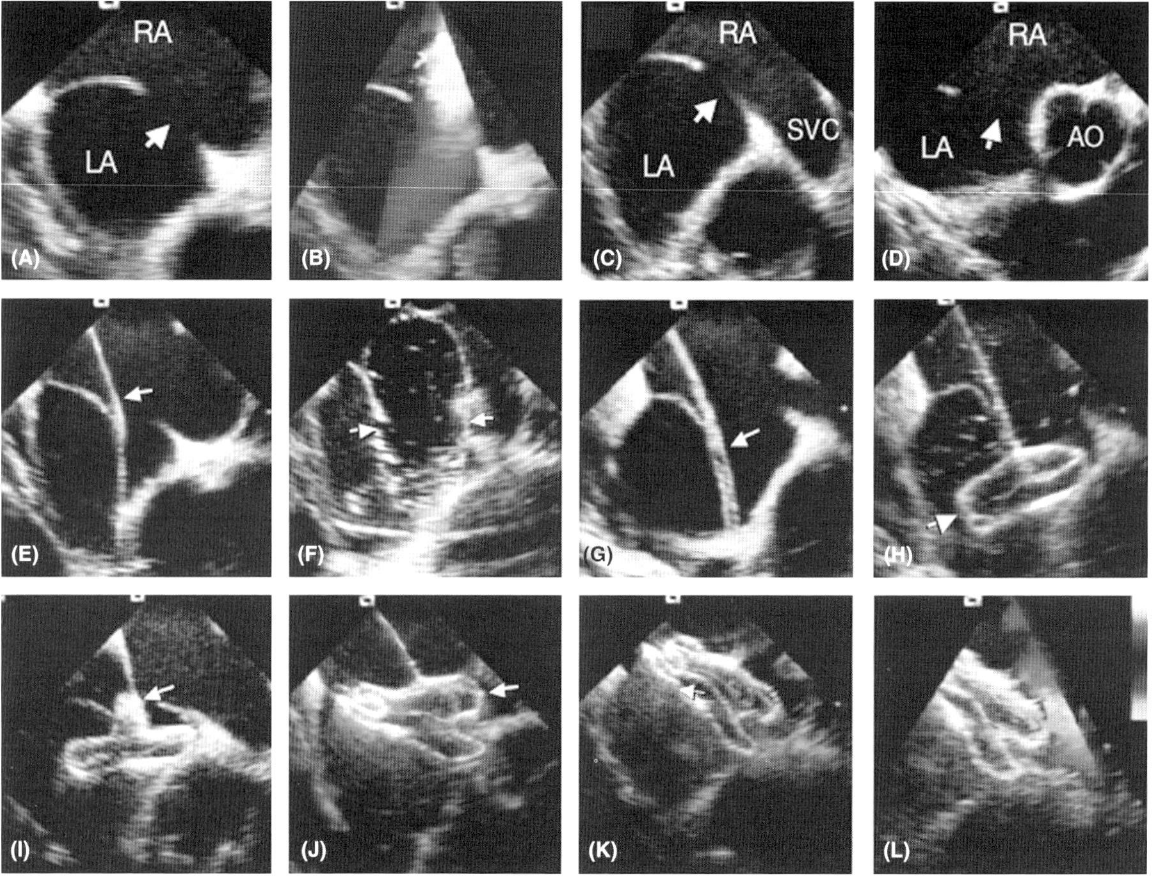

Figure 2 Intracardiac echocardiographic (ICE) images in a 42-year-old female patient with a 24 mm secundum atrial septal defect (ASD) as measured by ICE. (**A,B**) Septal view without and with color Doppler demonstrating the ASD (*arrow*) and left to right shunt. (**C**) Bicaval long axis view demonstrating the superior and inferior rims and the defect (*arrow*). (**D**) Short axis view demonstrating the absence of anterior rim, good posterior rim, and the ASD (*arrow*). (**E**) Passage of the guide wire (*arrow*) through the ASD to the left atrium to the left upper pulmonary vein. (**F**) The sizing balloon when left to right shunt ceased indicating the "stop-flow" diameter (*arrows*) of the defect. (**G**) Passage of the delivery sheath (*arrow*) through the defect to the left upper pulmonary vein. (**H**) Deployment of the left atrial disk (*arrow*) of a 30-mm Amplatzer® septal occluder in the left atrium. (**I**) Deployment of the connecting waist (*arrow*) in the defect. (**J**) Deployment of the right atrial disk (*arrow*) in the right atrium. (**K**) After the device has been released indicating good device position. (**L**) Bicaval view after the device has been released indicating good device position and no shunt. *Abbrevations*: LA, left atrium; RA, right atrium; SVC, superior vena cava; AO, aortic valve. (*See color insert.*)

back as one unit to the middle of the left atrium. This position and the next steps are verified under fluoroscopy or TEE/ICE (Figs. 2H–L) and 3C–G). The left atrial disk is deployed in mid left atrium by pulling back the sheath over the cable. Part of the connecting waist should be deployed in the left atrium very close to the atrial septum. Finally, by withdrawing the delivery sheath off the cable, the connecting waist and the right atrial disk are deployed in the ASD itself and in the right atrium respectively.

Proper device position can be assessed by fluoroscopy on hepatoclavicular projection where both disks are seen parallel to and separated from each other by the atrial septum (Fig. 3F). Gentle push forward and pull backward movement

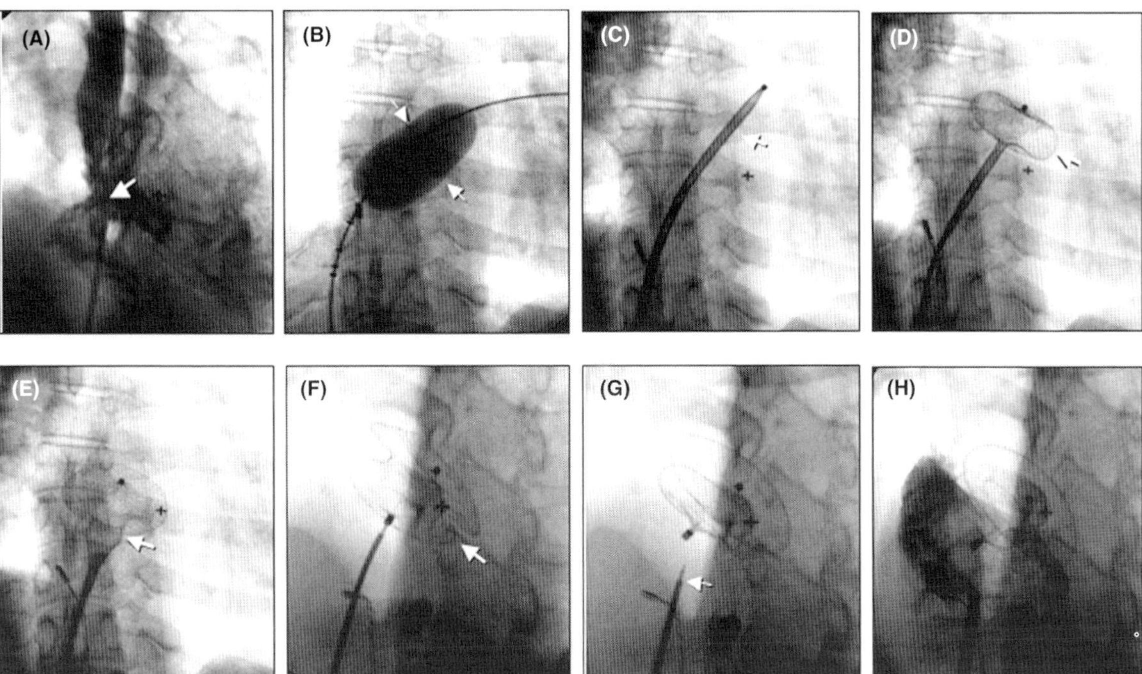

Figure 3 Cineangiographic views in the same patient during ASD closure. (**A**) Angiogram in the right upper pulmonary vein in the hepatoclavicular projection demonstrating the left to right shunt via the ASD (*arrow*). (**B**) Cine fluoroscopy in the frontal projection during sizing of the defect when color Doppler showed cessation of shunt (*arrows*). (**C**) Cine fluoroscopy in the frontal projection during passage of the device (*arrow*) inside the sheath that is positioned in the mouth of the left upper pulmonary vein. (**D**) Cine fluoroscopy in the frontal image during deployment of the left disk of a 30 mm Amplatzer® septal occluder in the left atrium. (**E**) Cine fluoroscopy in the frontal projection during deployment of the connecting waist in the defect (*arrow*). (**F**) Cine fluoroscopy in the hepatoclavicular projection just after deployment of the right disk (*arrow*) in the right atrium. (**G**) Cine fluoroscopy in the hepatoclavicular projection immediately after the device has been released from the cable (*arrow*). Note the change in position of the device that occasionally happens due to the self-centering properties of the device. (**H**) Angiogram in the right atrium in the hepatoclavicular projection using the side arm of the delivery sheath demonstrating right atrium and right disk opacification, which indicates good device position.

(Minnesota wiggle) of the cable while fixing the sheath will test stability of the device. Optional angiogram in the right atrium with pulmonary levophase using the side arm of the delivery sheath can be performed in this projection (Fig. 3H). The proper position of the device manifests by opacification of the right atrial disk alone when the contrast is in the right atrium, and the opacification of the left atrial disk alone on pulmonary levophase. In addition the echocardiogram (TEE/ICE) must demonstrate the presence of one disk in each atrial chamber (Fig. 2J–L). If the position is uncertain or questionable after all these maneuvers, the device can be recaptured and repositioned following similar steps. After the position of the device has been verified, the device is released by counterclockwise rotation of the delivery cable using the pin vise (Figs. 2K and 3G). Assessment of the final result of the closure procedure is performed immediately with TEE or ICE, and again 24 hours later with transthoracic echocardiography.

At the end of the procedure, ACT is rechecked and the sheath removed. If the ACT is higher than 250 seconds, we reverse the effects of heparin with protamine sulfate. Patients are asked to take aspirin 81–325 mg orally once daily for six months and endocarditis prophylaxis when necessary for six months after the procedure. Full activity including competitive and contact sports are allowed four weeks from implantation.

MANAGEMENT OF COMPLICATIONS

Prolapse of the left disk across the defect

This can occur during the deployment especially in patients with large defects and deficient antero/superior rims. In this situation the left atrial disk deploys perpendicular to the septum and prolapses through the anterior/superior part of the defect. There are few potential tips to prevent the prolapse: (*i*) deployment of the device in the right or left upper pulmonary veins rather than the left atrium; (*ii*) using a specially designed long sheath with a stiffer sharper posterior curve (Hausdorf sheath, Cook Inc., Bloomington, IN); (*iii*) using the long dilator of the delivery sheath from the contralateral femoral vein to hold the left atrial disk in the left atrium while deploying the waist and right atrial disk in their respective locations; and finally (*iv*) using a balloon to hold the left atrial disk during deployment of the waist and right atrial disk, in a way similar to the dilator technique.

Device embolization

If this occurs the device must be removed either surgically or by transcatheter snare techniques. Snaring is difficult and requires an experienced operator in snaring techniques. A long Mullins sheath two French sizes larger than the sheath used to deliver the device is needed. Pulling the device across valves must be avoided.

Cobra-head formation

This occurs when the left atrial disk maintains a high profile when deployed, mimicking a cobra head. This usually occurs when the left atrial disk is inadvertently opened in the pulmonary vein or left atrial appendage; when the left atrium is too small to accommodate the device; or when the device was loaded with an unusual strain. In this situation check the site of deployment or recapture the device, remove it to inspect and re-introduce it. If the same result occurs, the device should be recaptured and sent back to the manufacturer for inspection. Never release a device if the left disk has a cobra-head appearance.

Air embolism

Meticulous technique should be used to prevent air entry into the left side that may result in coronary ischemia and stroke. Free flow of blood out of the sheath when it is at the mouth of the left upper pulmonary vein must be allowed, avoiding forceful negative pressure to aspirate it. If air enters the cardiac chambers, the patient should be placed on 100% oxygen. Atropine or catecholamines are given depending on the patient condition.

Arrhythmias

An increase in atrial arrhythmias occurs following the procedure, but this is a transient phenomenon that resolves within six months. Heart block has been also rarely reported.

Device erosions

This is extremely infrequent (0.1 %). As of September 2005, a total of 36 cases of device erosions have been reported to the manufacturer. The manufacturer estimates that a total of 60,000 devices have been implanted worldwide. In the United States, a total of 17,000 devices have been implanted with a total of 18/36 erosions. Most erosions occurred in patients who received oversized devices, especially in patients with deficient anterior/superior rims. The mechanism seems to be erosion of the free atrial wall adjacent to the atrial septum by the edges of the device. To minimize this risk, one should not be oversizing the defect too much and use the stop flow technique.

CONCLUSION

In summary, the ASO device has been demonstrated to be safe and user-friendly with excellent clinical success in closing secundum ASD. The immediate success rate is greater than 97%, and our experience suggests that, with proper device selection and placement, 100% closure can be obtained.

SUGGESTED READINGS

1. Omeish A, Hijazi Z. Transcatheter closure of atrial septal defects in children and adults using the Amplatzer Septal Occluder. J Interven Cardiol 2001; 14(1):37–44.
2. Amin Z, Hijazi ZM, Bass J, et al. Erosion of Amplatzer® septal occluder device after closure of secundum atrial septal defects: Review of registry of complications and recommendations to minimize future risk. Catheter Cardiovasc Interv 2004; 63(4):496–502.
3. Schubert S, Peters B, Abdul-Khaliq H, et al. Left ventricular conditioning in the elderly patient to prevent congestive heart failure after transcatheter closure of atrial septal defect. Catheter Cardiovasc Interv 2005; (64): 333–337.
4. Harper R, Mottram P, McGaw D. Closure of secundum atrial septal defects with the Amplatzer® septal occluder device: techniques and problems. Cathet Cardiovasc Intervent 2002; 57(4):508–524.
5. Hijazi ZM, Wang Z, Cao Q, Koenig P, Waight D, Lang R. Transcatheter closure of atrial septal defects and patent foramen ovale under intracardiac echocardiographic guidance: feasibility andcomparison with transesophageal echocardiography. Cathet Cardiovasc Intervent 2000; 52(2): 194–199.
6. Du ZD, Hijazi ZM, Kleinman CS, et al. Comparison between transcatheter and surgical closure of secundum atrial septal defect in children and adults: results of a multicenter nonrandomized trial. J Am Coll Cardiol 2002; 39(11): 1836–1844.
7. Varma C, Benson LN, Silversides C, et al. Outcomes and alternative techniques for device closure of the large secundum atrial septal defect. Catheter Cardiovasc Interv 2004; 61: 131–139.
8. King TD, Thompson SL, Steiner C, Mills NL, Secundum arterial septal defeat. Nonoperative closure during cardiac catheterization, JAMA 1976; 235:2506–2509.

20

Catheter therapy of coarctation of the aorta

Francisco Garay, Qi-Ling Cao, and Ziyad M. Hijazi

INTRODUCTION

Coarctation of the aorta accounts for approximately 6–8 % of all congenital heart defects. It typically consists of a discrete stenosis or narrowing of the descending thoracic aorta immediately distal to the left subclavian artery. However, there is a wide spectrum of clinical presentations due to variable severity, anatomy, and physiology. Anatomic severity can vary from mild coarctation to complete interruption of the aorta. Hemodynamic findings can manifest as a mild pressure gradient between upper and lower extremities in asymptomatic patients or as severe hypertension with variable degrees of left ventricular hypertrophy. Some patients may complain of severe headaches or may present with signs and symptoms of subarachnoid hemorrhage due to rupture of a berry aneurysm. If coarctation is not treated, progression is complicated with stroke, premature coronary artery disease, chronic heart failure, and high mortality before 50 years of age (75% mortality by 46 years of age).

MANAGEMENT OPTIONS

Surgical therapy has resulted in significant improvement in survival, but has not corrected completely the natural history. Some patients, despite successful correction continue to have hypertension (25–75%), berry aneurysms (5–20%), coronary artery disease (5–23%), residual or recurrent coarctation (3–10%), and death (12% at 9 years). Balloon angioplasty to treat non operated (native) coarctation of the aorta or post surgical recoarctation was reported first in 1982. Results of balloon angioplasty for recoarctation of the aorta are good and it is considered the treatment of choice. However, balloon angioplasty in some centers is still considered to be controversial for the management of native coarctation.

Balloon angioplasty for recoarctation cases has produced effective and sustained reductions in arm-to-leg gradients with average immediate success (gradient <20 mmHg) in 78% to 94% of the patients. The more consistent predictor for failure is the presence of isthmus or transverse arch hypoplasia. At long-term follow-up 72% of patients remain free of reintervention. Aneurysm formation has been reported in up to 20% of the cases but they have usually been small and required no intervention. The reported mortality related to the procedure varies from none to 2.5%. Based on such data, as mentioned above, balloon angioplasty is considered the treatment of choice for recurrent coarctation of the aorta. Intervention is indicated in any patient with a gradient of 20 mmHg or more between the upper and lower extremities.

Balloon angioplasty for native coarctation of the aorta has also shown good results with acute success rate of about 73% and sustained gradient relief in adult patients. Aortic wall abnormalities have been frequently described in up to 50%, but they are usually benign and infrequently require an additional intervention.

The mechanism behind balloon angioplasty is creating a controlled tearing of the intima and part of the media. Intimal tears have been demonstrated after balloon angioplasty by intravascular ultrasound and angiography. This has been thought to be the underlying mechanism for later aneurysm formation. Advanced age and oversized balloons have also been implicated as risk factors for the development of aneurysms following aortic angioplasty. To avoid this problem it has been proposed to use stents to treat coarctation lesions, with the idea to appose any intimal flap against the aortic wall allowing healing to occur without dissection. Additionally, stents allow the treatment of long segment coarctation, and act as a rigid frame to support the aortic wall preventing the elastic recoil that may be encountered by balloon angioplasty. The stent is deployed to a chosen diameter (usually smaller than the diameter of the isthmus, especially when the narrow area is very tight!), avoiding overdilation of the adjacent normal aorta. Immediate results after stent implantation demonstrated an impressive relief of the pressure gradient usually with no or very little residual gradient. In clinical reports stenting has been associated with more predictable and uniform results that led many to consider this technique to be the preferred approach to treat native aortic coarctation in adult patients.

Despite the use of stents for aortic coarctation, aneurysm formation still occurs, albeit with a lower frequency of 7%. Anecdotal reports of aortic rupture and death still exist, raising concern about the use of bare stents that are dilated excessively as the primary treatment, and supporting either the use of covered stents or the gradual inflation (over two separate procedures) of the stent for the treatment of coarctation. Covered stents have been successfully used to treat aortic coarctation as a bail-out measure after aortic dissection or aneurysm formation after balloon angioplasty. They have also been used in severe stenotic lesions or even atretic segments protecting the vessel from dissection, aneurysm formation, or rupture. Covered stents have also been used to treat aortic coarctation associated with patent ductus arteriosus. However the use of covered stents has not been consistently evaluated and these encouraging results are based on single reports and on small non randomized retrospective series.

BALLOON CATHETERS AND STENTS

Selection of the appropriate balloon catheter to use is based on the aortic arch diameters. For native coarctation of the aorta, the area of narrowing can be safely dilated to 2–4 times the diameter of the narrowest area. However, we recommend that the diameter of the balloon does not exceed the diameter of the aorta at the isthmus or the descending aorta at the level of the diaphragm. One can be a little more aggressive in cases of recurrent coarctation and can choose a balloon diameter 3–4 times the narrowest segment or similar to the descending aorta immediately distal to the post stenotic segment.

The ideal balloon catheter to use would be a low-pressure low-profile balloon catheter. However, such balloons may rupture before an adequate result is achieved. Therefore, we often use a high-pressure balloon catheter, although currently there are few balloons that can be used for this purpose. Low-pressure balloons include TYSHAK® (NuMED Inc., Hopkinton, NY) available up to diameters of 30 mm; Proflex 5® (Mallinckrodt, Hangelwood, MO); and Accent® (Cook Inc., Bloomington, IN). High-pressure balloons include the ZMED® (NuMED Inc., Hopkinton, NY) also available up to a diameter of 20 mm; Ultrathin® (Meditech, Westwood, MA); and the XXL (Meditech).

If a stent is going to be used, the stent must have the ability to be dilated to a diameter more than 18 mm. In addition to this the stent radial strength must be high enough to avoid recoil and recoarctation. We have been using the Palmaz stents (Genesis XD, Palmaz-Schatz P308; P3110; P4010, P5010®, Johnson & Johnson, Somerville, NJ) or the Intrastent, (MAX-LD, ev3, Plymouth, MN). Outside the United States, the CP stent (NuMED Inc., Hopkinton, NY) is available as a bare or covered stent. The stent must be long enough to cover the narrowest area and the area immediately above and below this area. Balloon length must be slightly longer than the stent to avoid displacement of the stent during balloon inflation but not excessively longer to avoid the risk of balloon perforation and rupture during the inflation. A balloon length not more than 1 cm over the stent length is usually adequate. The use of the BIB balloon (NuMED Inc., Hopkinton, NY) has been particularly useful. It provides the possibility of fine positioning while the stent is partially deployed over the inner balloon and it also avoids excessive flaring of the stent ends during the inflation of the outer balloon.

TECHNIQUE FOR AORTIC ANGIOPLASTY AND STENTING

All data related to the patient and the aortic coarctation need to be reviewed prior to the procedure. All equipment necessary to perform successful intervention should be available in the laboratory. A covered stent of an appropriate size and a vascular surgeon should be readily available. A failed attempt or a complication due to lack of proper equipment is inexcusable! Additional imaging information such as magnetic resonance or computed tomography angiogram can be useful prior to the procedure to define the anatomy (Fig. 1).

The procedure is performed under general anesthesia and percutaneously through a femoral artery and vein. Heparin is administrated during the procedure to maintain an activated clotting time above 200 seconds. We only administer the heparin after we cross the area of coarctation. On rare occasions of atretic area (total interruption), one may not be able to cross in a retrograde fashion; therefore, a transseptal puncture or puncture of the brachial artery is required to delineate the exact anatomy and perhaps to cross the coarctation from above. It is good practice to do an angiogram in the descending aorta adjacent to the narrowest area to use as a roadmap for crossing from below. We usually cross the coarctation in a retrograde fashion using a Judkins right coronary diagnostic catheter with a soft tipped J-angled glide wire (Terumo medical Corp., Somerset, NJ). Routine hemodynamic evaluation is performed including measurement of the left ventricle end diastolic pressure and the pressure gradient across the coarctation site by either simultaneous recording of two catheters (one above and one below the area using the contra lateral femoral artery), by catheter pull-back, or by using the Multitrack® catheter over the wire (NuMED Inc., Hopkinton, NY). Then, the catheter is advanced to the area of the transverse arch and an angiogram is performed in biplane projection if available (Fig. 2A). If

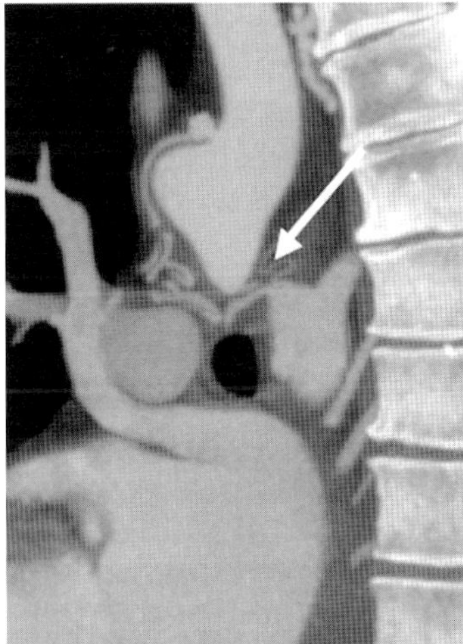

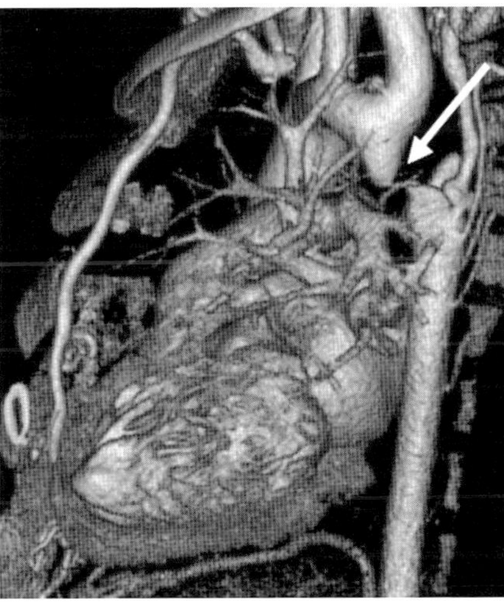

Figure 1 A multi slice CT angiogram in a 42-year-old male patient with severe coarctation of the aorta diagnosed after the patient presented with sub-arachnoid hemorrhage due to ruptured berry aneurysm. The image on the left is a two-dimensional image showing the very tight coarctation (*arrow*); the image on right is the three-dimensional reconstruction showing the coarctation (*arrow*). This patient underwent successful covered stent implantation.

biplane fluoroscopy is available, the frontal camera is angled in 30° LAO and the lateral camera is kept in straight lateral projection. The diameters of the aortic arch at the transverse arch, isthmus, narrowest diameter of the coarctation, and the descending aorta at the level of diaphragm are measured. For balloon angioplasty alone, an extra-stiff guide wire is positioned in the ascending aorta and the proper size balloon is advanced over this wire, until it reaches above the diaphragm. The size of the balloon should be 2–3 times the diameter of the narrowest area and not exceeding the diameter of the isthmus. The balloon must be purged and deaired outside the body and inflated first in the descending aorta to clear any potential air. Then the balloon is positioned across the area of coarctation (using previous landmarks from the angio) and inflated using an inflator until waisting in the balloon disappears. If the area of coarctation is not tight and to prevent the balloon from milking out the area of narrowing, we have been using right ventricle overdrive pacing to lower the cardiac output. We usually test this prior to the angioplasty. We try to achieve a blood pressure of about 40 mmHg during the pacing. Usually, this requires pacing up to 200–220 beats per minute. We usually start pacing and observe the drop in blood pressure, then we inflate the balloon until waisting disappears, then deflate the balloon, and then terminate pacing. We repeat this once to ensure that no further waisting is observed. The balloon is removed out of the body, keeping the wire across the area at all times. Repeat pressure gradient is performed as described above. Finally, repeat angiogram is performed using either the Multi-track catheter or a pigtail catheter. If the result is satisfactory, the wire is advanced inside the catheter and the catheter is removed over the wire and finally the wire is removed.

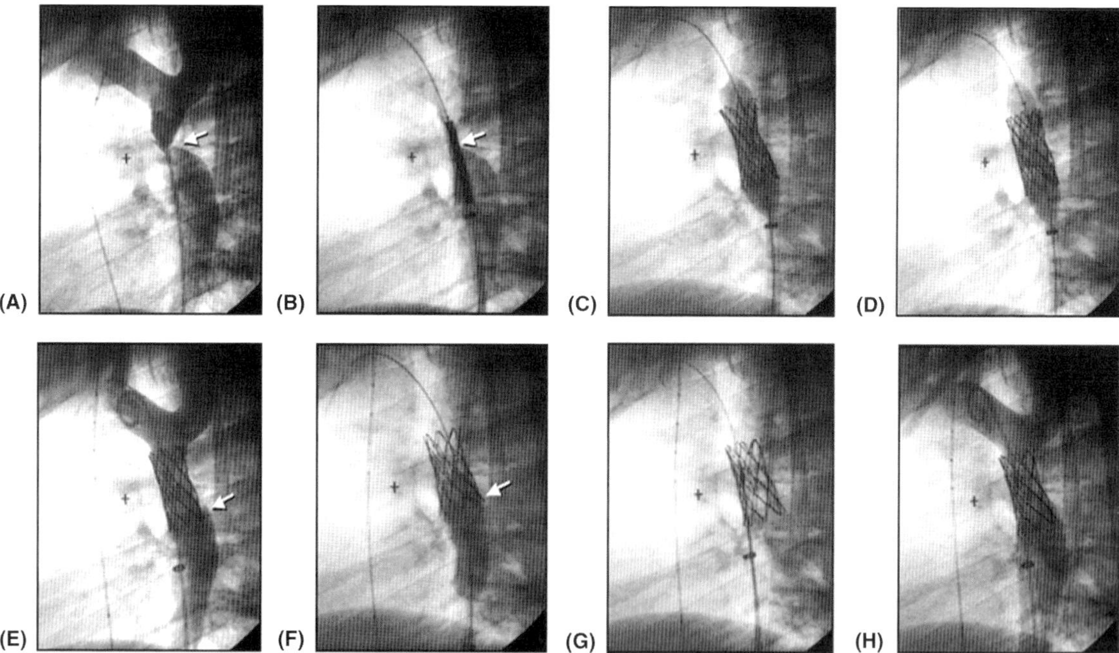

Figure 2 Cineangiograms in the lateral projection in a 30-year-old female patient with severe coarctation of the aorta with a gradient of 48 mmHg. (**A**) Angiogram demonstrating the tight coarctation measuring just about the size of a five French catheter (*arrow*). Good isthmus and descending aorta sizes. (**B**) Cine fluoroscopy during positioning of a 34-mm covered CP stent (*arrow*). (**C**) Cine fluoroscopy during inflation of the inner balloon (7mm diameter). (**D**) Cine fluoroscopy during inflation of the outer balloon (14 mm diameter). (**E**) Angiogram demonstrating good stent position. Note the distal part of the stent was not fully apposed to the wall of the aorta (*arrow*). (**F**) Cine fluoroscopy during balloon inflation using a 16 mm balloon (*arrow*). (**G,H**) Cine and angiogram of the final result demonstrating good stent position.

If the procedure is intended for stent placement, an appropriate size Mullins-type sheath is positioned over the wire above the coarctation site. If a stent is used this is mounted by hand crimping over the appropriate size balloon and introduced over the wire inside the delivery sheath until it reaches the tip of the sheath. If a stent is used, the sheath must be 1 French size larger than the recommended size for the balloon itself. Then the sheath is pulled back, trying to position the stent in the middle of the narrowest diameter of the coarctation, and finally the stent is uncovered by further pulling back of the sheath (Fig. 2). Repeated hand injections using the side arm of the sheath are performed to delineate the position of the stent and fine adjustments are done accordingly, trying not to cover the side branches of the aortic arch vessels. Once an adequate position is confirmed, the balloon is inflated until the stent is fully expanded. Again, similar to balloon angioplasty, we use right ventricle overdrive pacing to decrease the cardiac output and thus prevent movement of the stent during the inflation. After the stent has been deployed, pacing is continued until the balloon is completely deflated. The balloon is removed by advancing the sheath over the balloon inside the stent to avoid stent displacement. Our goal during the initial stenting is to deploy the stent to an acceptable diameter (usually 3–4 times the diameter of the narrowest area, not to exceed that of the isthmus). If one wishes to expand the distal part of the stent until it apposes the wall of the aorta, extreme care has to be exercised (this could result in overexpansion and results in dissection), so that the larger balloon is only in the distal part of the stent and not in the proximal portion (Fig. 2F). Some operators may elect not to expand the distal part at all during the initial procedure and bring the patient back after 6–12 months and then safely expand the distal part to appose the wall of the aorta.

Finally repeat measurement of gradient across the coarctation is performed using a Multitrack catheter (NuMED, Inc., Hopkinton, NY) or by simultaneous measurement using a pigtail catheter above the stent and the side arm of the sheath below the stent. Repeat angiography is also performed to evaluate the result (Fig. 2E, H). In adult patients, we are usually very cautious and deploy the stent to a diameter of no more than 12 mm, especially if the area is very tight. Then 6–12 months later, the patient is brought back to the catheterization laboratory for further dilatation of the stent. By that time, scar tissue has formed and it is perhaps safer to dilate the stent so that the walls of the stent are fully apposed to the wall of aorta.

At the end of the procedure, ACT is rechecked and the sheaths are removed. Antibiotic coverage is recommended for the procedure if a stent was deployed (cefazolin 1 g IV, the first dose at the time of the procedure and two additional doses 6–8 hours apart). The day following the procedure, chest radiographs and echocardiograms are performed, and non-invasive blood pressure between arm and leg is recorded. Usually patients are discharged the following day on aspirin 81 mg per day for six months and are asked to adhere to bacterial endocarditis prophylaxis when appropriate. We recommend no contact sports and no lifting of heavy objects (over 50 pounds) for the first month after the procedure. Follow-up must include clinical examination, blood pressure measurements in the arm and leg, and an echocardiogram. MRA or CT angiogram must be included in the follow-up evaluation after 6–12 months to rule out the possibility of aneurysm development.

MANAGEMENT OF COMPLICATIONS

Stent migration

If migration of a partially deployed stent occurs it can be moved into a segment of the aorta where there are no important side branches and deployed there.

Aortic aneurysm or dissection

If an angiogram shows evidence of acute aneurysm or dissection at the site of dilatation, a covered stent must be deployed as mentioned above. Usually the use of a covered stent requires a larger sheath (2 French sizes larger than recommended for the bare stent itself). If an acute aortic rupture is produced with hemodynamic instability, the balloon catheter can be inflated again trying to tamponade the bleeding site while moving with the patient to the operating room.

Balloon rupture

It can occur when a long balloon is used to flare the stent. If the rupture is circumferential, there is a chance that the distal end of the balloon may displace the stent or the distal part of the balloon may not come out the sheath. In such circumstances, one has to snare the distal tip of the balloon while it is over the wire and remove it from the contra lateral femoral artery. The availability of wide range of retrieval catheters (gooseneck or Ensnare) cannot be overemphasized.

CONCLUSION

In summary, interventional treatment of aortic coarctation has proved to be an effective alternative to surgery. The use of stents demonstrated very good results. However, extreme care should be exercised when deploying stents. Selection of the proper type stent and the proper balloon type and size is extremely important for a safe and successful procedure.

SUGGESTED READINGS

1. Cheatham J. Stenting of Coarctation of the Aorta. Cathet Cardiovasc Intervent. 2001; 54(1):112–125.
2. Ewert P, Abdul-Khaliq H, Peters B, et al. Transcatheter Therapy of Long Extreme Subatretic Aortic Coarctations with Covered Stents. Catheter Cardiovasc Interv 2004; 63(2):236–239.
3. Jenkins N, Ward C. Coarctation of the Aorta: Natural History and Outcome After Surgical Treatment. Q J Med. 1999; 92(7):365–371.
4. Johnston T, Grifka R, Jones T. Endovascular Stents for Treatment of Coarctation of the Aorta: Acute and Follow-Up Experience. Catheter Cardiovasc Interv 2004; 62(4):499–505.
5. Ovaert C, Benson L, Nykanen D, Freedom R. Transcatheter Treatment of Coarctation of the Aorta: a Review. Pediatric Cardiol. 1998; 19(1):27–44.
6. Pedra C, Fontes V, Esteves C, et al. Stenting vs. Balloon Angioplasty for Discrete Unoperated Coarctation of the Aorta in Adolescents and Adults. Catheter Cardiovasc Interv 2005; 64(4):495–506.
7. Piechaud, J. Stent Implantation for Coarctation in Adults. J Interv Cardiol. 2003; 16(5):413–418.
8. Shah L, Hijazi Z, Sandhu S, Joseph A, Cao Q. Use of Endovascular Stents for the Treatment of Coarctation of the Aorta in Children and Adults: Immediate and Midterm Results. J Invasive Cardiol In press. 2005; 17:614–618.

21

Renal stenting

Bernhard Reimers, Dimitris Nikas, and Mohamed Abdel Ghany

INTRODUCTION

Renal artery stenosis (RAS) represents the most common cause of secondary hypertension and may result in renal function deterioration as well as progressive renal atrophy (1–3). It has also been proven to be a stronger independent predictor of all-cause mortality than congestive heart failure or decreased renal function (4). Moreover, it is the presumed etiology of renal failure in 14–20% of patients over 50 years of age in hemodialysis (5,6).

Awareness of this condition is important because its prevalence is increasing and it represents a potentially treatable cause of hypertension or renal failure. Renal artery stenosis, defined as stenosis of > 60%, was present in 6.8% of 834 patients undergoing ultrasound screening (7). In a series of unselected autopsies of 221 patients older than 50 years, the prevalence of RAS (stenosis > 50%) was 27%. In the same series, the prevalence of RAS was even higher (53%) when patients had a history of diastolic hypertension (8). The prevalence of RAS is reported to range from 8.5% in patients undergoing routine cardiac catheterization for suspected coronary artery disease to 42% in patients with documented peripheral and aortoiliac disease (9–13).

Renal artery stenosis is a progressive disease. Progression of the severity of RAS has been shown in several studies despite successful control of hypertension with aggressive medical therapy (14,15). The rate of progression to occlusion is associated with the initially detected degree of stenosis. Ultrasound perspective studies proved that the higher the stenosis, the faster and more frequently it progresses to total occlusion (16–18).

PATIENT SELECTION

Surgical repair was considered the treatment of choice until the 1990s because balloon angioplasty was associated with unacceptably high restenosis rates, even though its safety has been proven from the early 1980s in selected cases (19,20). With the development of angioplasty devices and the introduction of stents, renal angioplasty became the preferred treatment of RAS. Several studies have demonstrated the benefit of renal stenting both in terms of reduction in renal insufficiency and in hypertension control (18, 21–23).

Generally, renal artery revascularization is indicated in patients with significant renal stenosis, defined as ≥ 70% angiographic stenosis or moderate angiographic stenosis (50–69%) and ≥ 20 mmHg systolic translesional pressure gradient (24), and associated with the following clinical conditions: (*i*) accelerated, malignant or resistant hypertension, hypertension with unilateral small kidney, (*ii*) renal insufficiency, (*iii*) recurrent unstable angina in association with severe renal stenosis, (*iv*) unexplained heart failure associated with renal stenosis, and (*v*) "flash" pulmonary edema (4,25,26). Contraindications for renal stenting are patients with limited life expectancy and patients with chronic dialysis depended ischemic nephropathy. It is of pivotal importance to consider the nephrotoxicity of contrast medium particularly in patients with impaired renal function. Small amounts, of contrast, hydration, N-acetyl-cystein, bicarbonates and post-procedural hemofiltration should be considered as possible means of nephro-protection. In patients with advanced renal failure, carbon dioxide can also be considered, but its use may decrease the diagnostic resolution while/whereas controversies exist regarding the protective role of gadolinium (27,28).

DIAGNOSTIC ANGIOGRAPHY

Although modern non-invasive tests such as duplex ultrasound scan, computed tomography (CT) scan, and magnetic resonance imaging (MRI) have been advanced to a degree that can accurately diagnose RAS, diagnostic angiography remains the "gold standard" in quantitative assessment of RAS before intervention (29–34). A high quality diagnostic renal angiography, performed separately or just before angioplasty procedure, is of major importance to set the appropriate revascularization strategy.

Selective angiography of renal arteries can be performed with the usage of several types of catheters according the anatomy of the origin of the renal arteries (Table 1). Special attention must be paid to avoid pitfalls by superimposed arteries originating from the aorta and not to miss possible multiple renal arteries. The origin of both renal arteries usually arises at the level of the L1–L2 vertebral interspace and can be best visualized in the LAO 20° projection (Fig. 1). Lumbar interspaces should be counted from T12, which is the vertebra giving rise to the last fluctuant rib. In the presence of a tortuous aorta, however, modified projections may be needed. Renal atherosclerotic disease usually involves the proximal one-third of the renal artery and it is rarely present without abdominal aortic plaques (35). To the contrary, renal artery fibromuscular dysplasia usually involves the body of the renal arteries but does not affect the proximal segment of the artery (36).

As an alternative to selective angiography, especially in cases of a severely diseased aorta,

Table 1 Catheters commonly used for diagnostic and angioplasty renal procedures

Judkins Right
Internal Mammary (IM)
Simmons (Type I)
Double Renal Curve (DRC)
Hockey-Stick (HS)
Right Amplatz 1
Sos-Omni
Cobra
Multi-purpose (usually in brachial approach)

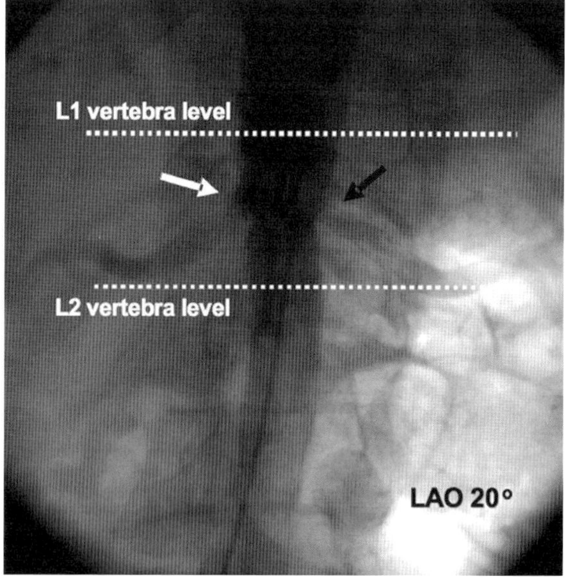

Figure 1 Non-selective angiogram in left anterior oblique (LAO) 20° projection in a patient with severe bilateral renal stenosis [de novo in the right renal artery (*white arrow*) and restenotic in the left renal artery (*black arrow*)]. Normal origin of both renal arteries is the mid-vertebra space between L1 and L2.

non-selective arteriography with a Pigtail catheter (5 or 6 French) using digital subtraction can also achieve a good visualization of the renal arteries without the risk of damaging a diseased ostium or plaque dislodgement. Moreover, less contrast medium is needed, obviating the risk of contrast-induced nephropathy. In all cases, however, maneuvers and catheter manipulation must be done with great care to avoid complications such as renal artery trauma and distal atheromatic material embolization. "Back flush" of the catheter before first selective contrast injection is also recommended to clean the catheter of debris and avoid embolization to the renal parenchyma.

RENAL ARTERY STENTING

Access sites

Since it is familiar to most interventionalists, the retrograde femoral approach is the most commonly used in renal interventions. It allows the use of guiding catheters of different types and sizes as well as application of closure devices. The femoral approach is generally preferred when the takeoff of the renal arteries is horizontal, caudal, or mildly cephalic with respect to the aorta. With the femoral approach, 6 or 7 French short sheaths (11 cm) are usually used except in the presence of tortuous iliac arteries where longer ones (23 cm) might be needed for better guidance of catheters and balloons.

The brachial approach may be used in the presence of chronic aortic occlusion or in case of infra-renal aortic wide aneurysms that do not allow cannulation of the renal arteries. An extremely cephalic origin of the renal artery may also require this approach. For the brachial approach guiding catheters or long (90 cm) preshaped sheaths can be used. For the radial approach, extra long (≥ 120 cm) guiding catheters are needed.

Cannulation of the renal artery

Guiding catheters are usually used for delivery of the balloon or stent. It reduces the time of radiation exposure and offers more comfort to the operator. Renal artery cannulation can be performed using several guiding catheters similar to those used for diagnosis (Table 21.1). Specially designed sheaths (Britetip IG™, Cordis Corp., Miami, FL) with the appropriate length (55 cm) and curve to directly engage the renal arteries are also available. In this case, a guiding catheter is not necessary and therefore sheaths of smaller diameter (usually 1 French smaller) can be used, reducing the access site complications.

In difficult anatomies a diagnostic catheter may better cannulate the renal artery than a guiding catheter. If a diagnostic catheter is employed, a 0.014 in. guidewire can be advanced in the renal artery and the guide catheter can be exchanged over the 0.014in. wire.

In order to reduce the possibility of distal aortic debris embolization during engagement of the renal artery with the guiding catheter, Feldman et al. introduced the "no-touch" technique (37). According this technique, a normal or hydrophilic 0.035 in. J-tip wire protrudes several centimeters outside the distal tip of the catheter during manipulation of the guiding itself. The wire is apposed to the vessel wall and the guiding catheter is gently maneuvered until gentle contrast injections confirm its position adjacent to the ostium of the renal artery. Once the renal artery is identified, the wire is removed and the renal ostium is cannulated in a gentle and controlled manner, reducing the risk of trauma and dissection. It is also possible to advance a 0.014 in. in the renal artery before removing the 0.035 in. wire. Using the "no-touch" technique, the contact between guiding catheter and the atheromatic aorta wall is minimized, aggressive scraping of the aorta is eliminated, and potential embolization of plaque debris is reduced. This technique is particularly *recommended in the presence of diseased atheromatic aorta or in cases of tortuous aorta* where many and probably more aggressive manipulations might be needed (Figs. 2 and 3).

Angioplasty

Once the guiding catheter is positioned a steerable 0.014 in. (more rarely a 0.018 in.) soft-tip guiding wire is used to cross the stenosis. Distal position of the wire must be meticulously avoided to prevent perforation of the renal

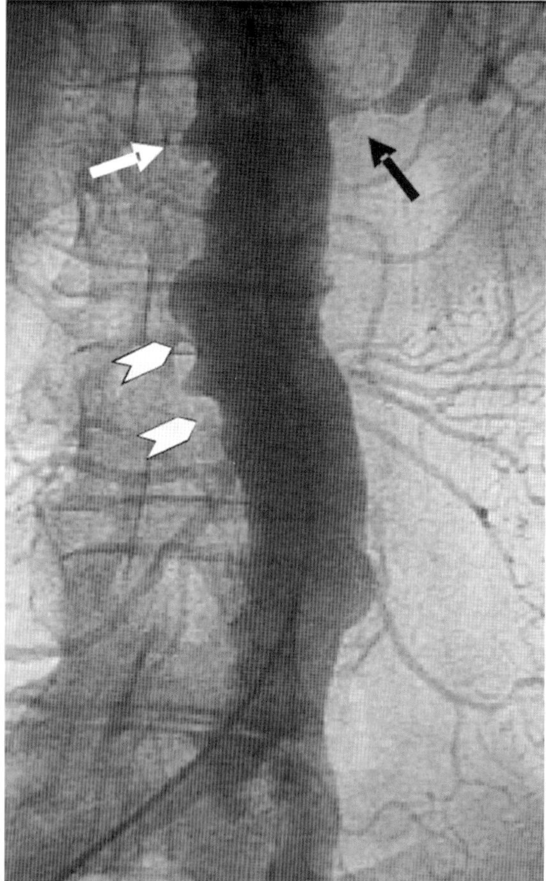

Figure 2 Severe atheromatic aorta indicated for "no touch" technique. The *white arrow* indicates occluded right renal artery; *black arrow* indicates significant stenosis of the left renal artery; *block arrows* indicate severe atheromatic plaques in the sub-renal aorta.

parenchyma. Soft-tip support wires should only be used if the position of the guiding catheter or sheath is unstable.

In severe stenosis pre-dilatation is usually recommended because it allows assessment of the actual vessel size and allows advancement of the guiding catheter into the mid renal artery over the deflated balloon for accurate stent delivery (Fig. 4). Balloons should not be oversized or inflated with very high pressures because of possible vessel rupture and elevated risk of aortic dissection in case of ostial lesions. For stenosis less than 90% (70–90%) direct stenting is preferred as it may reduce the risk of atheromatic embolization caused by the excessive manipulation of both catheters and devices at the lesion site (Figs. 5 and 6). Predilatation is recommended only in cases of calcified lesions of fibromascular dysplasia in order to evaluate whether the stenosis can be dilated before stent implantation. In cases of hard, fibrotic lesions the cutting balloons (Cutting Balloon Ultra ™, Boston Scientific International, Colombes Cedex, France) may be used. For predilatation any low-profile coronary or peripheral balloon slightly undersized compared to the vessel diameter can be used. Optimal inflation time is usually 10–20 seconds. Inflation pressure must be set not only by the lesion's characteristics (lesion calcification, balloon "waisting," degree of stenosis) but also by the patient's symptoms. Acute onset of back pain during inflation of the balloon usually means adventitia stretching, and requires prompt balloon deflation as there is an increased risk for vessel rupture or dissection.

Elective use of stents to scaffold the lesion and optimize the angiographic result is generally preferred. Balloon angioplasty has been the traditional treatment of choice for renal artery fibromuscular medial dysplastic lesions (36). However, it is not preferable in atherosclerotic renal artery stenosis as it is associated with a restenosis rate that approaches 50% mainly because of significant recoil (19,38–40). Stents demonstrated both a superior hemodynamic result compared with balloons in atherosclerotic RAS (41) and had a more favorable long-term outcome (23,39,42–45). For renal arteries, balloon-expandable stents are strongly recommended because they offer more precise positioning, stronger radial forces, and reduce the incidence of early vessel recoiling (Fig. 7). Dedicated renal stents are deployed with gradual inflation of the balloon so that the ends of the balloon, which are not covered by the stent, expand first giving a "dumbbell" appearance to the balloon. This could prevent stent dislodgement in cases of asymmetric balloon inflation. In some cases, when a higher stability of the guiding wire is needed, the catheter can be advanced into the renal artery. Once the stent is correctly positioned the guiding catheter or the guiding sheath is withdrawn, uncovering the stent that is now ready for implantation.

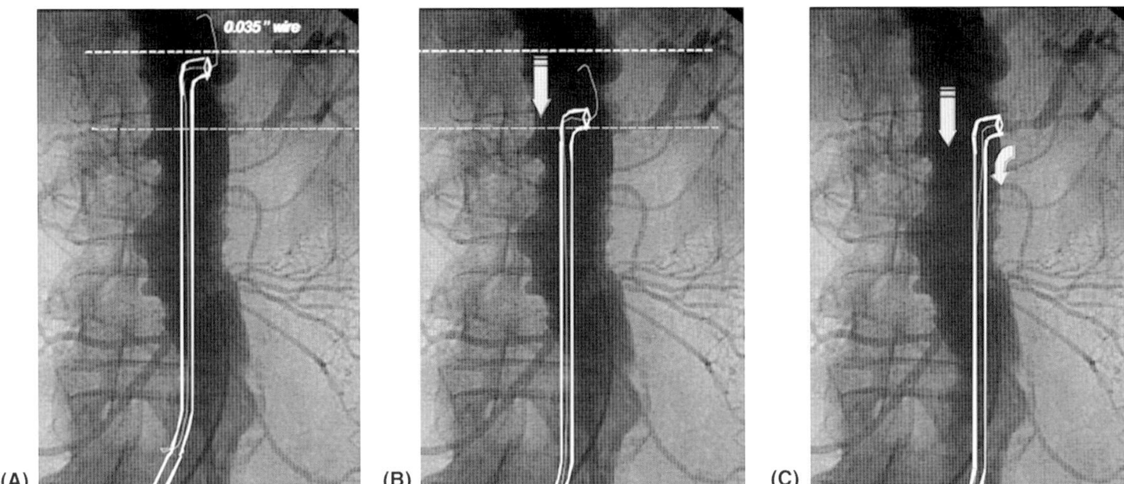

Figure 3 Schematic representation of the left renal artery cannulation in a very atheromatic aorta using the "no touch" technique. The catheter is first placed in the aorta over a J-tip 0.035 in. wire sitting against the aorta wall (**A**). The catheter then is pulled back near the ostium of the renal artery with the wire in place (**B**). With a gentle manipulation the catheter is engaged into the renal artery ostium while the wire is simultaneously retrieved into the catheter (**C**).

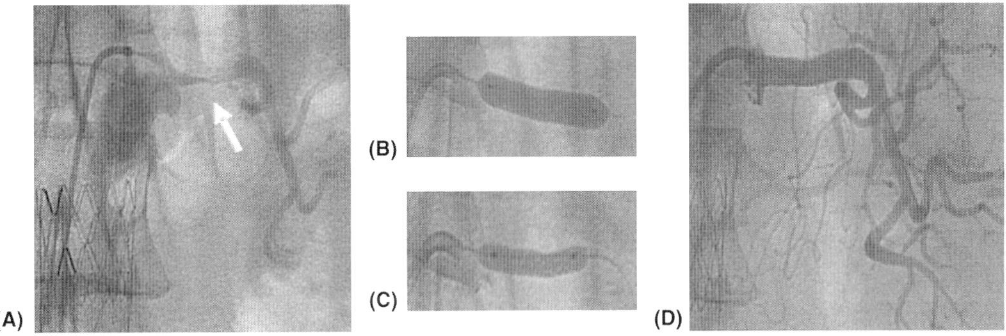

Figure 4 Renal stenting in a patient with previous aortic endoprosthesis. (**A**) Tight stenosis of the right renal artery (*arrow*); (**B**) predilatation with 3.0 × 20 mm balloon; (**C**) 5 × 28 mm stent implantation; and (**D**) good angiographic result.

Special care must be taken when treating ostial lesions; the stent should protrude approximately 1 or 2 mm into the aorta to ensure complete ostium coverage. Contrast injection in different angiographic projections may be necessary to ensure precise positioning just outside the ostium. A minimum shortening of the stent needs to be taken into account (Fig. 4).

The use of drug-eluting stents (DES) is questionable. Currently the only possible application of DES in renal artery stenting is the presence of unilateral kidney (anatomical or functional) or bilateral renal artery stenosis. At present the only DES which may reach a 5 mm diameter suitable for some renal arteries is the Taxus stent (Boston Scientific, Natick, MA). In the only available randomized trial (Palmaz Genesis peripheral stainless steel balloon expandable stent, comparing the sirolimus-coated vs. bare stent in *RE*nal *A*rtery *T*reatment, or the *GREAT* trial), DES reduced the restenosis rate by 50% (from 14% to 7%) compared to bare metal stenting (46). Because only stents of 5 or 6 mm in diameter were used in that study, it is recommended to use DES in renal arteries equal or less than 6 mm. Given the lower stenosis rate in big vessels, bare metal stents may be used in larger

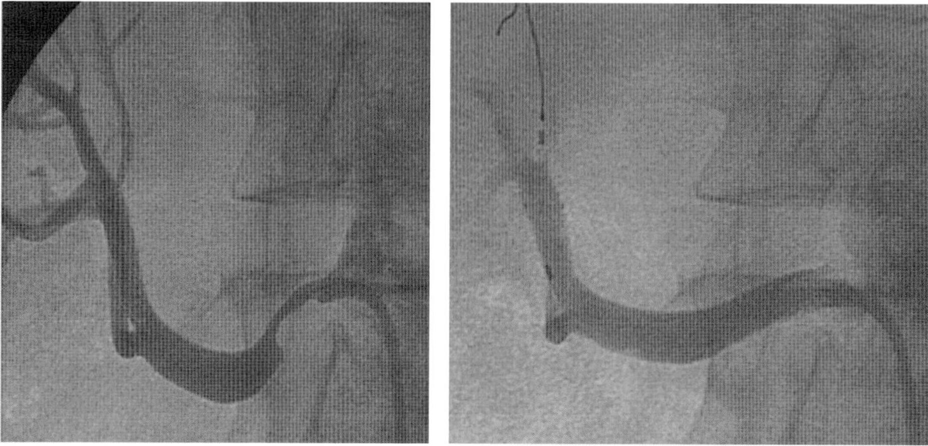

Figure 5 Good result after successful direct stenting of ostial renal stenosis (bulky lesion) under protection of Angioguard™ Emboli Capture Guidewire System (Cordis Europa NV, Roden, The Netherlands).

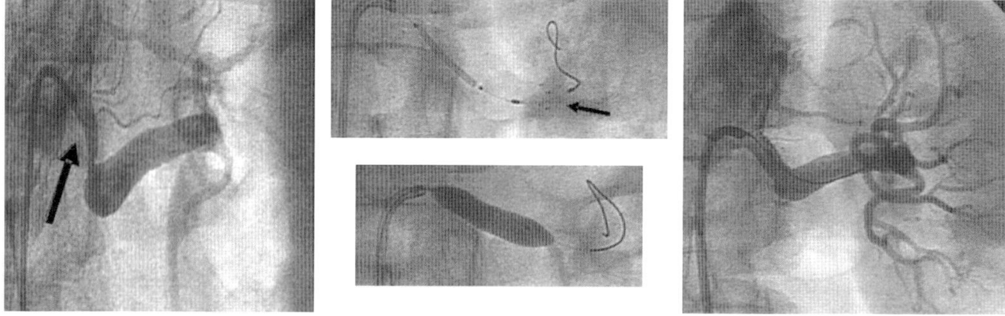

Figure 6 Severe ostial stenosis of the left renal artery in a downward origin (*large arrow*). Utilization of the IM (7 French) guiding catheter and direct stenting with a 5 × 18 mm stent. Protection with Angioguard™ (8 mm) Emboli Capture Guidewire System (Cordis Europa NV, Roden, The Netherlands) (*small arrow*). Post-dilatation with 7 × 20 mm balloon with good final angiographic result.

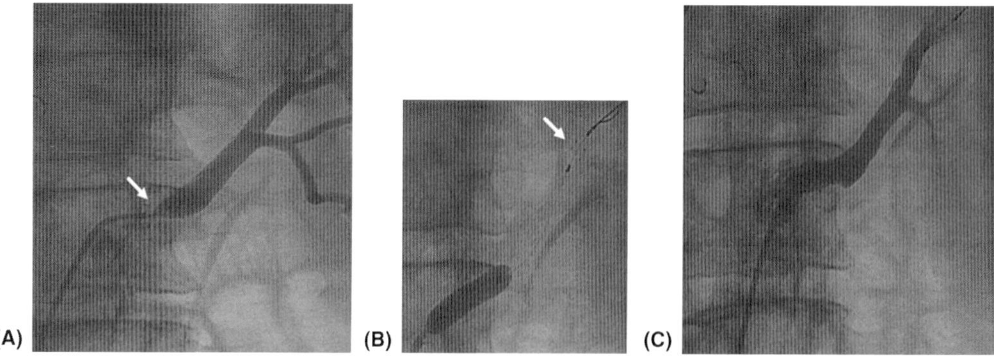

Figure 7 (**A**) Severe ostial stenosis of the left renal artery. (**B**) Cannulation with a 7 French JR4 guiding catheter. Direct stenting with a 6 × 18 mm stent under protection of the Angioguard™ (6 mm) Emboli Capture Guidewire System (Cordis Europa NV, Roden, The Netherlands) (*arrow*). (**C**) Final result.

renal arteries. Another potential indication for DES is to treat restenotic lesions.

DISTAL PROTECTION

Up until now, many different types of protection devices have been tested in several trials, both occlusive balloon and filter-based types (47–49) (Figs. 5 to 7). The benefit, however the routine usage of protection devices in renal intervention has not yet proven. Even though visible debris from the protection device has been retrieved in most cases (47,48), the number of patients included in these trials and their retrospective features does not justify the routine use of protection devices in renal stenting. A large randomized trial comparing the renal stenting with vs. without protection devices is ongoing (50).

At the present, no protection device specifically designed for renal stenting is available. The majority of those devices were designed either for coronary or for carotid interventions; this sets an important limitation to their effectiveness. Particularly in large vessels, filter-based devices may be too small, leaving enough free space for debris passage. Moreover, in cases of proximal renal artery bifurcation (<20 mm from the ostium), only one branch is protected with the usage of protection device. Additionally, protection devices may prolong the procedure and increase its cost.

Complications regarding the use of protection devices have been reported but are generally rare (47,49).

PHARMACOLOGIC PROTOCOL

Before the procedure all patients must be pretreated with double antiplatelet therapy; that is, aspirin 75–150 mg once daily and clopidogrel 75 mg once daily, or ticlopidine 250 mg twice daily. Clopidogrel or ticlopidine should have been started at least three days prior to the procedure. Otherwise, a loading dose of clopidogrel (300 mg) is administered just before the procedure.

During the procedure heparin 100 IU/kg of body weight is given intra-arterially through the arterial sheath in order to achieve an ACT of 250–350 seconds. Additional antiplatelet drug administration, such as IIb/IIIa, is under investigation and is not as yet recommended in routine renal stenting. Fluids should be administered liberally prior to, during, and following the procedure.

After the procedure, patients are prescribed aspirin (75–150 mg/day) indefinitely and 1 month of clopidogel (75 mg/day) or ticlopidine (250 mg twice a day).

PATIENT FOLLOW-UP

All patients should undergo periodical duplex ultrasound evaluation of the renal artery 3 and 6 months after the procedure in order to detect possible restenosis. Furthermore, renal function must be carefully monitored with repeated measurements of the serum creatinine during the 2–3 days post-procedure and monthly afterwards for the first 6 months. Continuous comparison of these values during follow-up is of major importance in order to promptly detect any renal function deterioration. Effects on arterial blood pressure also need careful monitoring.

RESTENOSIS

Restenosis rates after successful renal stent placement vary from 6% to 20% and increased rates have been correlated to smaller vessel diameters. Treatment of in-stent restenosis includes mainly balloon dilation or re-stenting (Fig. 8). Other methods like cutting balloons or brachytherapy have been also reported but their value has not been tested in any cohort series of patients (51–53). Both balloon restenosis and in-stent restenosis can be treated with balloon-only angioplasty; however, the recurrence of restenosis in cases of in-stent restenosis is significantly lower than in case of balloon-restenosis (54).

COMPLICATIONS

A number of published series report a complication rate associated with renal angioplasty and/or stenting ranging from 5–20%, mostly involving the access site (55,56). In general, major complications such as myocardial infarction,

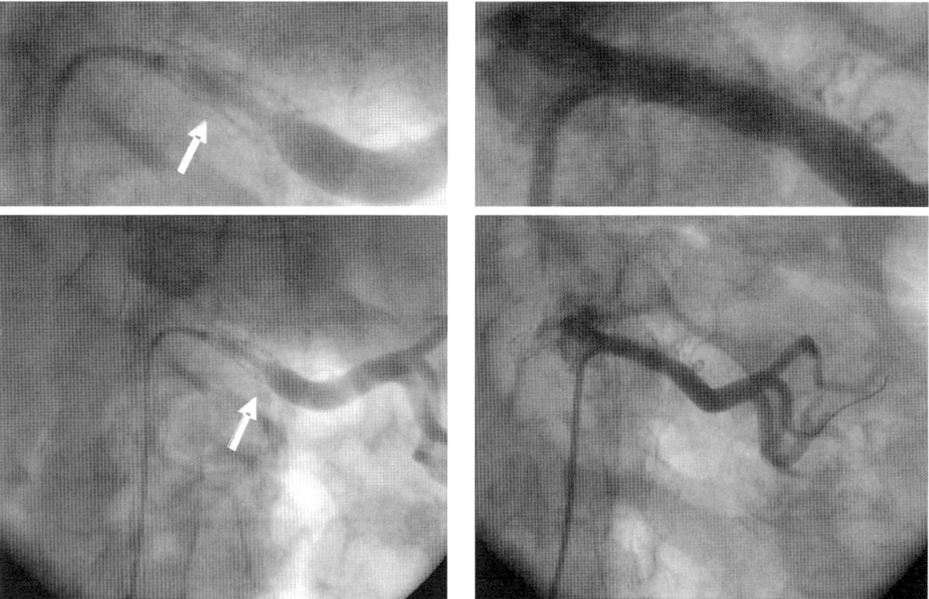

Figure 8 Severe intrastent restenosis. IM 6 French guiding catheter. Good angiographic result after treatment with balloon only angioplasty.

emergency dialysis, or need for emergency surgery are infrequent (23, 57, 58) and it has been shown that some of these complications correlate to the operator's experience level, degree or type of stenosis, and patient comorbidities (59).

The most dangerous complications are dye nephropathy and atheroembolism either in the renal or peripheral vascular bed during the stent procedure. Other complications include dissection of the renal artery or the aorta, acute or delayed thrombosis, infection, rupture of the artery, or renal perforation with guidewires (60–62) (Fig. 9). Technical advancements in material manufacturing—such as softer guiding catheters, more flexible and lower-profile balloons, and stents specifically dedicated for renal arteries—may further decrease the incidence of complications during renal stenting (63,64).

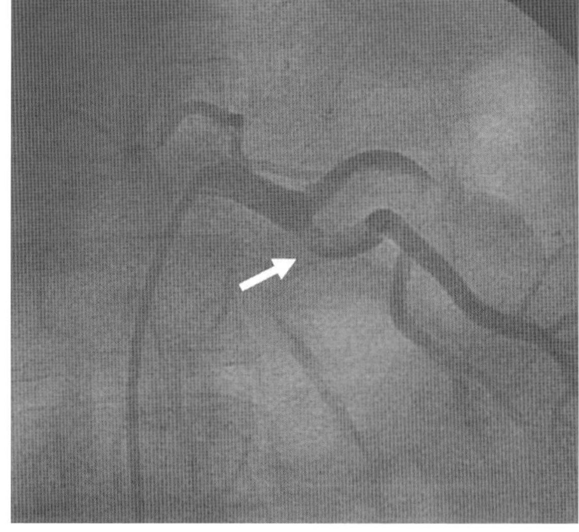

Figure 9 Acute stent thrombosis. The *arrow* indicates angiographically visible thrombus at the distal part of the stent.

CLINICAL OUTCOME

Renal stenting has become the preferable treatment in patients with symptomatic RAS, targeting mainly those with hypertension who are not or are responding poorly to drug treatment for preservation of renal function. The effectiveness of renal angioplasty for blood pressure control was tested in three randomized studies in which relatively small numbers of patients were randomized to receive optimal medical treatment or angioplasty. In all these trials, renal angioplasty did not offer any significant benefit compared to patients who were treated conservatively

(18,21,22). However, all these trials had several important limitations, such as the small number of patients, the high rate of "crossover" between treatment arms, and the fact that most patients were treated with balloon angioplasty only, resulting in a high rate of restenosis. Contrarily, several studies in which patients were treated with stenting reported favorable outcomes of those patients (39,61–63,65).

Contradictory data have also been published regarding the impact of renal stenting in renal function. A meta-analysis that included all renal stenting studies published until 1999 concluded that renal function was improved in 26% of patients with some degree of renal impairment deteriorated in 26% of them and remain unchanged in 48% of them (66). Given the progressive nature of RAS in terms of renal dysfunction, these results might indicate that renal stenting can possibly halt the progression of the disease. In the literature several studies report improvement or at least stabilization of renal function (23,67–71), while others report impairment of renal function especially in patients with stable renal function prior to intervention(72). Severe atheroembolization during renal stenting could be an important reason for the deterioration of renal function in those patients (73,74).

To clearly identify the true benefits of renal stenting, large-scale, prospective and better-controlled trials to determine the thresholds for renal impairment and renal stenosis, with or without protection devices, are clearly needed. Until then, renal stenting remains a catheter-based procedure with high technical success and a relatively low procedural complication rate that is suitable for patients with fibromuscular dysplasia or atherosclerotic RAS. Careful patient selection with appropriate indications is mandatory for the long-term success of the procedure.

REFERENCES

1. Caps MT, Zierler RE, Polissar NL, et al. Risk of atrophy in kidneys with atherosclerotic renal artery stenosis. Kidney Int 1998; 53(3):735–742.
2. Kothari SS. ACE inhibitors and unilateral renal artery stenosis—what price? Int J Cardiol 1996; 53(3):199–201.
3. Woolfson RG. Renal failure in atherosclerotic renovascular disease: pathogenesis, diagnosis, and intervention. Postgrad Med J Feb 2001; 77(904): 68–74.
4. Safian RD, Textor SC. Renal–artery stenosis. N Engl J Med 2001; 344(6):431–442.
5. van Ampting JM, Penne EL, Beek FJ, et al. Prevalence of atherosclerotic renal artery stenosis in patients starting dialysis. Nephrol Dial Transplant 2003; 18(6):1147–1151.
6. Coen G, Calabria S, Lai S, et al. Atherosclerotic ischemic renal disease. Diagnosis and prevalence in an hypertensive and/or uremic elderly population. BMC Nephrol 2003; 4:2.
7. Hansen KJ, Edwards MS, Craven TE, et al. Prevalence of renovascular disease in the elderly: a population-based study. J Vasc Surg 2002; 36(3): 443–451.
8. Holley KE, Hunt JC, Brown AL, Jr., et al. Renal Artery Stenosis. A Clinical-Pathologic Study In Normotensive And Hypertensive Patients. Am J Med 1964; 37:14–22.
9. Cohen MG, Pascua JA, Garcia-Ben M, et al. A simple prediction rule for significant renal artery stenosis in patients undergoing cardiac catheterization. Am Heart J 2005; 150(6):1204–1211.
10. Harding MB, Smith LR, Himmelstein SI, et al. Renal artery stenosis: prevalence and associated risk factors in patients undergoing routine cardiac catheterization. J Am Soc Nephrol 1992; 2(11):1608–1616.
11. Siogas C, Goudevenos J, Pappas S, et al. Usefulness of Renal Arteriography Following Coronary Angiography. J Invasive Cardiol 1996; 8(5):223–227.
12. Aqel RA, Zoghbi GJ, Baldwin SA, et al. Prevalence of renal artery stenosis in high–risk veterans referred to cardiac catheterization. J Hypertens 2003; 21(6):1157–1162.
13. Weber-Mzell D, Kotanko P, Schumacher M, et al. Coronary anatomy predicts presence or absence of renal artery stenosis. A prospective study in patients undergoing cardiac catheterization for suspected coronary artery disease. Eur Heart J 2002; 23(21):1684–1691.
14. Schreiber MJ, Pohl MA, Novick AC. The natural history of atherosclerotic and fibrous renal artery disease. Urol Clin North Am 1984; 11(3): 383–392.
15. Crowley JJ, Santos RM, Peter RH, et al. Progression of renal artery stenosis in patients undergoing

cardiac catheterization. Am Heart J 1998; 136(5): 913–918.

16. Caps MT, Perissinotto C, Zierler RE, et al. Prospective study of atherosclerotic disease progression in the renal artery. Circulation 1998; 98(25):2866–2872.
17. Zierler RE, Bergelin RO, Isaacson JA, et al. Natural history of atherosclerotic renal artery stenosis: a prospective study with duplex ultrasonography. J Vasc Surg 1994; 19(2):250–257; discussion 257–258.
18. van Jaarsveld BC, Krijnen P, Pieterman H, et al. The effect of balloon angioplasty on hypertension in atherosclerotic renal-artery stenosis. Dutch Renal Artery Stenosis Intervention Cooperative Study Group. N Engl J Med 2000; 342(14):1007–1014.
19. Sos TA, Pickering TG, Sniderman K, et al. Percutaneous transluminal renal angioplasty in renovascular hypertension due to atheroma or fibromuscular dysplasia. N Engl J Med 1983; 309(5):274–279.
20. Surowiec SM, Sivamurthy N, Rhodes JM, et al. Percutaneous therapy for renal artery fibromuscular dysplasia. Ann Vasc Surg 2003; 17(6):650–655.
21. Plouin PF, Chatellier G, Darne B, et al. Blood pressure outcome of angioplasty in atherosclerotic renal artery stenosis: a randomized trial. Essai Multicentrique Medicaments vs Angioplastie (EMMA) Study Group. Hypertension 1998; 31(3): 823–829.
22. Webster J, Marshall F, Abdalla M, et al. Randomised comparison of percutaneous angioplasty vs continued medical therapy for hypertensive patients with atheromatous renal artery stenosis. Scottish and Newcastle Renal Artery Stenosis Collaborative Group. J Hum Hypertens1998; 12(5):329–335.
23. Dorros G, Jaff M, Mathiak L, et al. Four-year follow-up of Palmaz-Schatz stent revascularization as treatment for atherosclerotic renal artery stenosis. Circulation1998; 98(7):642–647.
24. Rundback JH, Sacks D, Kent KC, et al. Guidelines for the reporting of renal artery revascularization in clinical trials. American Heart Association. Circulation 2002; 106(12):1572–1585.
25. White CJ. Catheter-based therapy for atherosclerotic renal artery stenosis. Circulation 2006; 113(11):1464–1473.
26. Hirsch AT, Haskal ZJ, Hertzer NR, et al. ACC/AHA 2005 guidelines for the management of patients with peripheral arterial disease (lower extremity, renal, mesenteric, and abdominal aortic): executive summary a collaborative report from the American Association for Vascular Surgery/Society for Vascular Surgery, Society for Cardiovascular Angiography and Interventions, Society for Vascular Medicine and Biology, Society of Interventional Radiology, and the ACC/AHA Task Force on Practice Guidelines (Writing Committee to Develop Guidelines for the Management of Patients With Peripheral Arterial Disease) endorsed by the American Association of Cardiovascular and Pulmonary Rehabilitation; National Heart, Lung, and Blood Institute; Society for Vascular Nursing; TransAtlantic Inter-Society Consensus; and Vascular Disease Foundation. J Am Coll Cardiol 2006; 47(6):1239–1312.
27. Ailawadi G, Stanley JC, Williams DM, et al. Gadolinium as a nonnephrotoxic contrast agent for catheter-based arteriographic evaluation of renal arteries in patients with azotemia. J Vasc Surg 2003; 37(2):346–352.
28. Kaufman JA, Geller SC, Waltman AC. Renal insufficiency: gadopentetate dimeglumine as a radiographic contrast agent during peripheral vascular interventional procedures. Radiology 1996; 198(2):579–581.
29. Blebea J, Zickler R, Volteas N, et al. Duplex imaging of the renal arteries with contrast enhancement. Vasc Endovascular Surg 2003; 37(6):429–436.
30. Olin JW, Piedmonte MR, Young JR, et al. The utility of duplex ultrasound scanning of the renal arteries for diagnosing significant renal artery stenosis. Ann Intern Med 1995; 122(11):833–838.
31. Manganaro A, Ando G, Salvo A, et al. A comparison of Power Doppler with conventional sonographic imaging for the evaluation of renal artery stenosis. Cardiovasc Ultrasound 2004; 2(1):1.
32. Kaatee R, Beek FJ, de Lange EE, et al. Renal artery stenosis: detection and quantification with spiral CT angiography versus optimized digital subtraction angiography. Radiology 1997; 205(1): 121–127.
33. Attallah N, Yee J, Gutierrez A, et al. Likelihood ratios in the diagnosis of renal artery stenosis by magnetic resonance angiography compared with renal angiography. Am J Hypertens 2003; 16(12):987–992.

34. Leung DA, Hoffmann U, Pfammatter T, et al. Magnetic resonance angiography versus duplex sonography for diagnosing renovascular disease. Hypertension 1999; 33(2):726–731.
35. Kaatee R, Beek FJ, Verschuyl EJ, et al. Atherosclerotic renal artery stenosis: ostial or truncal? Radiology 1996; 199(3):637–640.
36. Slovut DP, Olin JW. Fibromuscular dysplasia. N Engl J Med 2004; 350(18):1862–1871.
37. Feldman RL, Wargovich TJ, Bittl JA. No-touch technique for reducing aortic wall trauma during renal artery stenting. Catheter Cardiovasc Interv 1999; 46(2):245–248.
38. Boisclair C, Therasse E, Oliva VL, et al. Treatment of renal angioplasty failure by percutaneous renal artery stenting with Palmaz stents: midterm technical and clinical results. AJR Am J Roentgenol 1997; 168(1):245–251.
39. Blum U, Krumme B, Flugel P, et al. Treatment of ostial renal-artery stenoses with vascular endoprostheses after unsuccessful balloon angioplasty. N Engl J Med 1997; 336(7):459–465.
40. Plouin PF, Darne B, Chatellier G, et al. Restenosis after a first percutaneous transluminal renal angioplasty. Hypertension 1993; 21(1):89–96.
41. Dorros G, Prince C, Mathiak L. Stenting of a renal artery stenosis achieves better relief of the obstructive lesion than balloon angioplasty. Cathet Cardiovasc Diagn 1993; 29(3):191–198.
42. Dorros G. Long-Term Effects of Stent Revascularization Upon Blood Pressure Management Renal Function and Patient Survival. J Invasive Cardiol 1998; 10(1):51–52.
43. Lederman RJ, Mendelsohn FO, Santos R, et al. Primary renal artery stenting: characteristics and outcomes after 363 procedures. Am Heart J 2001; 142(2):314–323.
44. Leertouwer TC, Gussenhoven EJ, Bosch JL, et al. Stent placement for renal arterial stenosis: where do we stand? A meta-analysis. Radiology 2000; 216(1):78–85.
45. van de Ven PJ, Kaatee R, Beutler JJ, et al. Arterial stenting and balloon angioplasty in ostial atherosclerotic renovascular disease: a randomised trial. Lancet 1999; 353(9149):282–286.
46. Zeller T, Rastan A, Rothenpieler U, Muller C. Restenosis after stenting of atherosclerotic renal artery stenosis: Is there a rationale for the use of drug-eluting stents? Cathet Cardiovasc Interv 2006; 68(1):125–130.
47. Henry M, Henry I, Klonaris C, et al. Renal angioplasty and stenting under protection: the way for the future? Catheter Cardiovasc Interv 2003; 60(3):299–312.
48. Holden A, Hill A. Renal angioplasty and stenting with distal protection of the main renal artery in ischemic nephropathy: early experience. J Vasc Surg 2003; 38(5):962–968.
49. Hagspiel KD, Stone JR, Leung DA. Renal angioplasty and stent placement with distal protection: preliminary experience with the FilterWire EX. J Vasc Interv Radiol 2005; 16(1):125–131.
50. RESIST Trial www.clinicaltrials.org, accessed at Jun 17,2006.
51. Munneke GJ, Engelke C, Morgan RA, et al. Cutting balloon angioplasty for resistant renal artery in-stent restenosis. J Vasc Interv Radiol 2002; 13(3):327–331.
52. Ellis K, Murtagh B, Loghin C, et al. The use of brachytherapy to treat renal artery in-stent restenosis. J Interv Cardiol 2005; 18(1):49–54.
53. Spratt JC, Leslie SJ, Verin V. A case of renal artery brachytherapy for in-stent restenosis: four-year follow-up. J Invasive Cardiol 2004; 16(5): 287–288.
54. Wohrle J, Kochs M, Vollmer C, et al. Re-angioplasty of in-stent restenosis versus balloon restenoses—a matched pair comparison. Int J Cardiol 2004; 93(2-3):257–262.
55. Guerrero M, Syed A, Khosla S. Survival following renal artery stent revascularization: four-year follow-up. J Invasive Cardiol 2004; 16(7):368–371.
56. Sivamurthy N, Surowiec SM, Culakova E, et al. Divergent outcomes after percutaneous therapy for symptomatic renal artery stenosis. J Vasc Surg 2004; 39(3):565–574.
57. White CJ, Ramee SR, Collins TJ, et al. Renal artery stent placement: utility in lesions difficult to treat with balloon angioplasty. J Am Coll Cardiol 1997; 30(6):1445–1450.
58. Burket MW, Cooper CJ, Kennedy DJ, et al. Renal artery angioplasty and stent placement: predictors of a favorable outcome. Am Heart J 2000; 139(1 Pt 1):64–71.
59. Ivanovic V, McKusick MA, Johnson CM, 3rd, et al. Renal artery stent placement: complications at a single tertiary care center. J Vasc Interv Radiol 2003; 14(2 Pt 1):217–225.
60. Bloch MJ, Trost DW, Sos TA. Type B aortic dissection complicating renal artery angioplasty and

stent placement. J Vasc Interv Radiol 2001; 12(4):517–520.

61. Henry M, Amor M, Henry I, et al. Stents in the treatment of renal artery stenosis: long-term follow-up. J Endovasc Surg 1999; 6(1):42–51.
62. Iannone LA, Underwood PL, Nath A, et al. Effect of primary balloon expandable renal artery stents on long-term patency, renal function, and blood pressure in hypertensive and renal insufficient patients with renal artery stenosis. Cathet Cardiovasc Diagn 1996; 37(3):243–250.
63. Nolan BW, Schermerhorn ML, Rowell E, et al. Outcomes of renal artery angioplasty and stenting using low-profile systems. J Vasc Surg 2005; 41(1):46–52.
64. Zeller T, Frank U, Muller C, et al. Technological advances in the design of catheters and devices used in renal artery interventions: impact on complications. J Endovasc Ther 2003; 10(5): 1006–1014.
65. Zeller T, Frank U, Muller C, et al. Stent-supported angioplasty of severe atherosclerotic renal artery stenosis preserves renal function and improves blood pressure control: long-term results from a prospective registry of 456 lesions. J Endovasc Ther 2004; 11(2):95–106.
66. Isles CG, Robertson S, Hill D. Management of renovascular disease: a review of renal artery stenting in ten studies. Qjm 1999; 92(3):159–167.
67. Leertouwer TC, Derkx FH, Pattynama PM, et al. Functional effects of renal artery stent placement on treated and contralateral kidneys. Kidney Int 2002; 62(2):574–579.
68. Airoldi F, Palatresi S, Marana I, et al. Angioplasty of atherosclerotic and fibromuscular renal artery stenosis: time course and predicting factors of the effects on renal function. Am J Hypertens. 2000; 13(11):1210–1217.
69. Geroulakos G, Abel P. Effect of renal-artery stenting on progression of renovascular renal failure. Lancet 1997; 349(9068):1840.
70. Harden PN, MacLeod MJ, Rodger RS, et al. Effect of renal-artery stenting on progression of renovascular renal failure. Lancet 1997; 349(9059): 1133–1136.
71. Rocha-Singh KJ, Ahuja RK, Sung CH, et al. Long-term renal function preservation after renal artery stenting in patients with progressive ischemic nephropathy. Catheter Cardiovasc Interv 2002; 57(2):135–141.
72. Muray S, Martin M, Amoedo ML, et al. Rapid decline in renal function reflects reversibility and predicts the outcome after angioplasty in renal artery stenosis. Am J Kidney Dis 2002; 39(1):60–66.
73. Krishnamurthi V, Novick AC, Myles JL. Atheroembolic renal disease: effect on morbidity and survival after revascularization for atherosclerotic renal artery stenosis. J Urol 1999; 161(4): 1093–1096.
74. Scolari F, Tardanico R, Zani R, et al. Cholesterol crystal embolism: A recognizable cause of renal disease. Am J Kidney Dis 2000; 36(6):1089–1109.

22

Endovascular repair of abdominal and thoracic aneurysms

Alexandra A. MacLean and Barry T. Katzen

ENDOVASCULAR REPAIR OF ABDOMINAL AORTIC ANEURYSMS

The endovascular approach to repair of abdominal aortic aneurysms (AAA) is a particularly attractive alternative to open surgical repair, especially for high-risk patients with comorbidities like respiratory insufficiency. Endovascular repair (EVAR) is minimally invasive, requires a shorter operative time, and incurs less blood loss. Both asymptomatic and symptomatic aneurysms can be repaired using this approach. This chapter describes how to select patients for the procedure, carry out the operation including choosing the best device for the patient and aneurysm, manage complications, and follow the patients after the procedure.

Patient selection

The appropriate selection of patients for this procedure is the most important factor leading to successful EVAR. Patients who are older and have substantial comorbidities (renal, respiratory, and cardiac dysfunction) are more likely to benefit from this procedure than those who are young and, apart from the presence of an abdominal aortic aneurysm, otherwise healthy (1). The patient with few risk factors should be counseled to the proven durability of open surgical repair (transabdominal or retroperitoneal approach). The sex of the patient is important because female patients and those with a smaller body habitus have a higher EVAR procedure abortion rate due to the presence of smaller access arteries (2,3). In addition, patients must be able to undergo close follow-up for many years with annual computed tomography (CT) scans, as EVAR has complications that occur many years after the procedure.

The clinical recommendation remains to offer treatment for aneurysms between 5 and 5.5 cm dependent on clinical trials (4). An exception to this guideline is that intervention should be offered despite the size of the aneurysm if symptoms develop or the aneurysm increases in size by 1 cm per year (5). In addition, if the patient is female with smaller native vessels the relative size that represents aneurysmal disease may be less than the conventional 5 to 5.5 cm range.

Preoperative assessment and imaging

The devices currently used for EVAR of AAAs are designed for aneurysms with particular features and are contraindicated in a host of others (Table 1). The aneurysm is evaluated using a three-dimensional reconstruction from CT

Table 1 EVAR eligibility and contraindications

CT scan assessment for EVAR eligibility:
- *Proximal neck*: Diameter, length, angle, presence or absence of thrombus
- *Distal landing zone*: Diameter and length
- *Iliac arteries*: Presence of aneurysms and occlusive disease
- *Access arteries*: Diameter, presence of occlusive disease

Contraindications for EVAR:
- Short proximal neck (less than 15 mm)
- Thrombus presence in proximal landing zone
- Conical proximal neck
- Greater than 120° angulation of the proximal neck
- Critical inferior mesenteric artery
- Significant iliac occlusive disease
- Tortuosity of iliac vessels

angiography or aortography with a calibrated catheter. The access arteries are measured; femoral arteries measuring less than 8 mm in diameter are viewed as a contraindication to femoral access and therefore retroperitoneal access to the iliac arteries or aorta must be entertained. The iliac arteries are assessed for tortuosity and presence of calcification (Fig. 1). Extensive mural thrombus in the proximal neck is not a favorable situation for endography fixation (Fig. 2). The length of the neck is measured from the lowest renal artery to the beginning of the aneurysmal dilatation. The neck should be greater than or equal to 15 mm in length in order to provide an adequate seal of the proximal portion of the device. The ability to achieve good fixation and seal has a direct impact on the endoleak rate. In addition, significant angulation of the neck can make this an unfavorable approach to aneurysm repair (Fig. 3). The aneurysm sac cannot involve visceral vessels (Fig. 4). Extensive calcification in the delivery route can make passage of the device challenging, and this requires careful and continual assessment of the ease of passing wires. The presence of significant stenosis in the celiac and superior mesenteric arteries is examined because in this procedure, the inferior mesenteric artery is always covered and there is no opportunity to reimplant it. If significant stensoses are seen, the patient may have ischemic issues with bowel perfusion after EVAR since there is a greater reliance on blood flow from the inferior mesenteric artery (IMA). The fitness of the distal seal zone in the common iliac arteries is assessed. If the common iliac artery is aneurysmal, then the device will have to land in the external iliac artery, thereby covering the

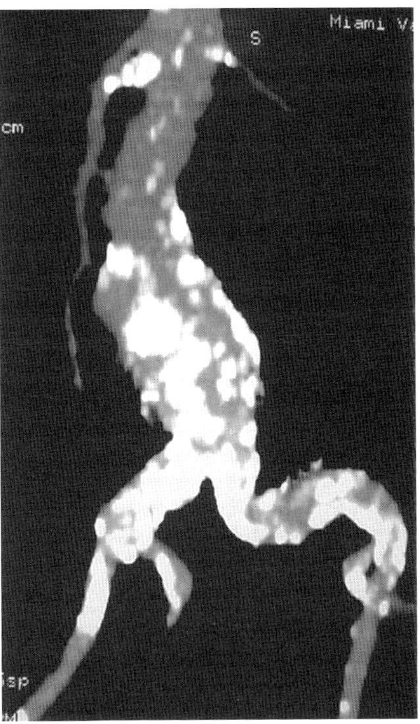

Figure 1 Extensive calcification.

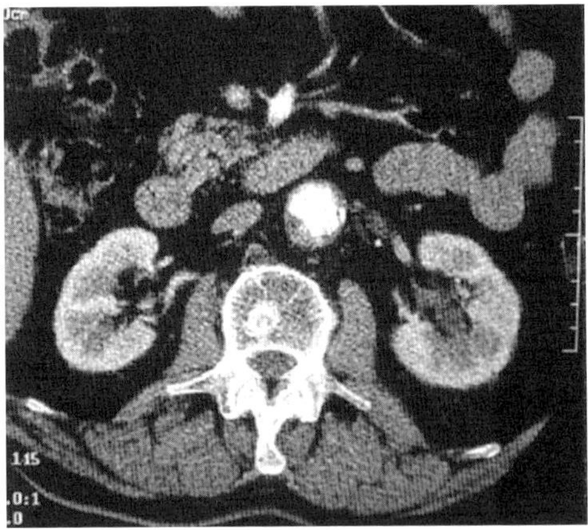

Figure 2 Mural thrombus in proximal neck.

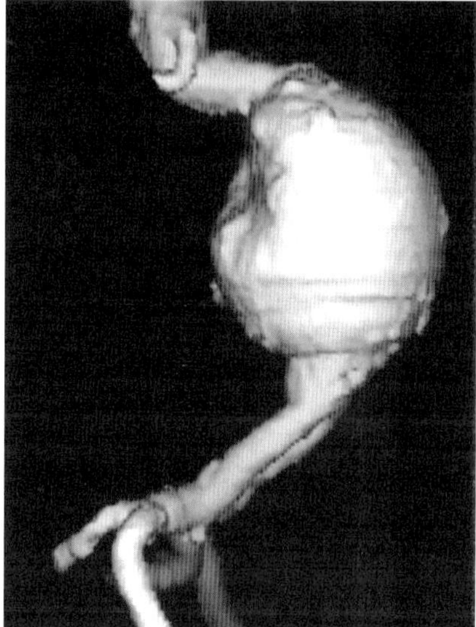

Figure 3 Neck angulation.

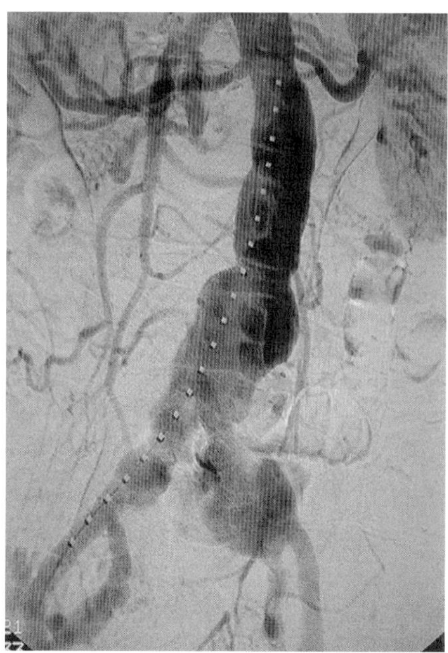

Figure 5 Iliac aneurysms.

internal iliac artery (Fig. 5). Persistent backflow from the internal iliac artery would lead to a type IB endoleak and, to prevent this from happening, the internal iliac artery is therefore embolized preoperatively (Fig. 6). There are risks to this procedure including buttock claudication. Internal iliac embolization is usually carried out as a separate procedure before aneurysm repair but it can be performed concurrently. If this is performed at the same time as EVAR, the fluoroscopic time is inevitably increased. Therefore, for the less experienced endovascular physician, the procedures should be performed separately. The distal aorta must be able to accommodate the expanded device; if it is too narrow, this is not possible (Fig. 7).

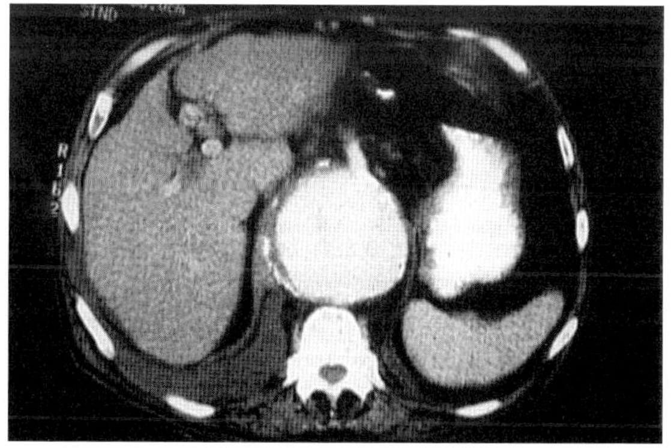

Figure 4 Visceral vessel involvement.

Choosing the device

The devices have many different features that must be understood to match the device to the aneurysm. This is less important in patients with "ideal" anatomic features, but as features such as neck angulation, calcification, and access tortuosity develop, challenges may be better addressed with one device than another. Most devices are bifurcated with a supported structure throughout the endograft (Fig. 8). The device is characterized by the location of the fixation: suprarenal or infrarenal. Most devices are infrarenal and therefore require the 15 mm sealing zone distal to the lowest renal artery. On some occasions suprarenal attachment may be necessary and desirable; in others infrarenal fixation may be sufficient. Also, the devices have different profiles with smaller ones permitting access through smaller vessels. Four devices are currently FDA-approved for commercial use in the United States (AneuRx®, Excluder®, Zenith®, and PowerLink®); the other devices are in clinical trials or are in use only in Europe. (See Table 2 for product specifications.)

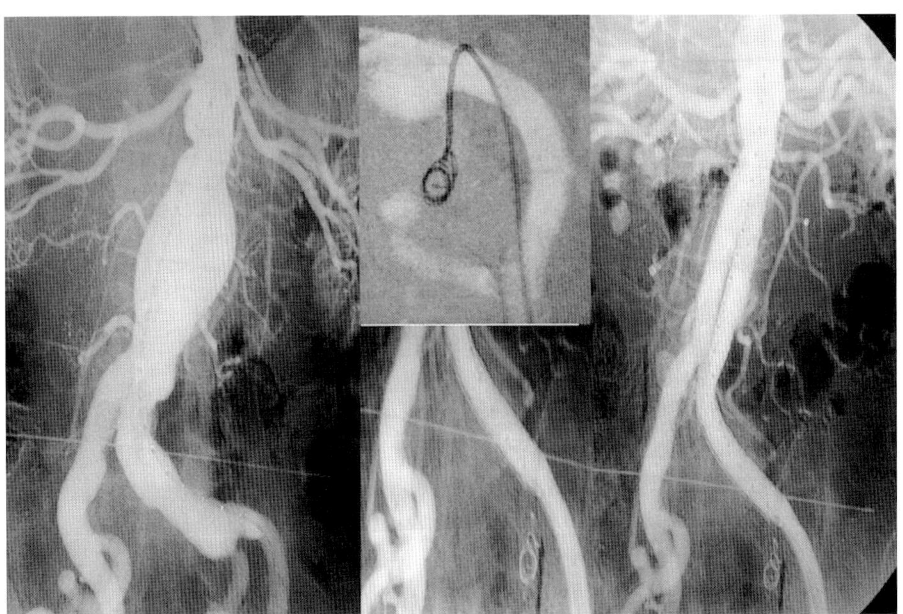

Figure 6 Internal iliac embolization.

Table 2 Endograft devices

Device (company)/ market	*Date of FDA approval*	*Main body diameter (mm)*	*Fixation*	*Profile*
Ancure (Guidant) Off the market in 2003	Sep–99	20–26	Infrarenal	21 French
AneuRx® (Medtronic, Bloomington, IN) Worldwide	Sep–99	22–28	Infrarenal	21 French
Excluder (W.L. Gore & Assoc., Phoenix, AZ) Worldwide	Nov–99	23–31	Infrarenal	18 French
Fortron (Cordis) Europe	No	26–34	Suprarenal	N/A
Lifepath (Edwards) Europe, Australia	No	21–29	Infrarenal	21 French
Powerlink (Endologix) Europe	No	25–34	Infrarenal Suprarenal	21 French
Stentor/Vanguard (Boston Scientific, Natick, MA) Off the market in 1999	No	22–26	Infrarenal	21 French
Talent (Medtronic, Bloomington, IN) Europe, Australia, Asia	No	24–34	Suprarenal	22/24 French
Trivascular (Boston Scientific, Natick, MA) In research	No	16–26	Infrarenal	16 French
Zenith (Cook Medical Inc., Bloomington, IN) Worldwide	May–03	22–32	Suprarenal	18/20 French

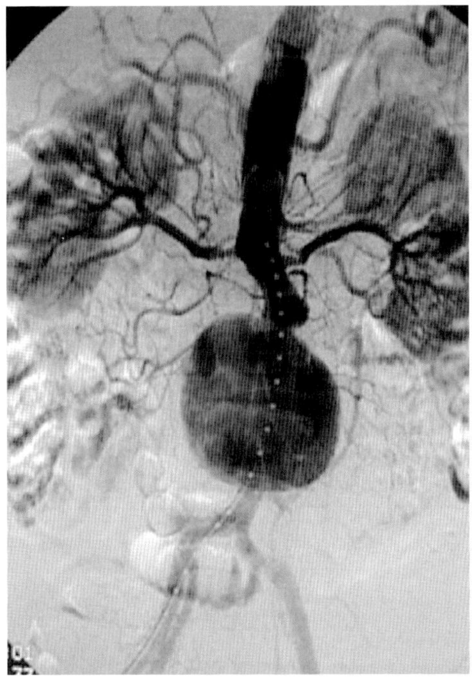

Figure 7 Narrow distal aorta.

The procedure

Preoperative preparation

The patient should have a peripheral pulse examination that is documented in the chart so comparison postoperatively is facilitated. In addition, the glomerular filtration rate is noted by looking at the BUN and creatinine as this will help the physician choose the appropriate contrast agent for the procedure and again allows for easy postoperative assessment. An appropriate antibiotic is given just prior to the procedure. The procedure can also be performed on patients who are on dialysis; in these cases, the physician must assess if the patient still has some spontaneous diuresis, as do most patients who are on peritoneal dialysis. In this case, care must be taken to preserve the integrity and flow of the renal arteries in order not to eliminate the spontaneous diuresis of the patient, which will help avoid any condition associated with fluid overload.

Anesthesia

The procedure can be performed under local, epidural, or general anesthesia. Local anesthesia is chosen for patients who are able to lie still for a couple of hours and have favorable anatomy rendering EVAR straightforward. Epidural anesthesia is appropriate for patients with significant respiratory and cardiac issues that make general anesthesia more risky. Of course, the experience of the team of endovascular physicians and anesthesiologists also plays an important role in determining the mode of anesthesia used for the procedure. General anesthesia provides the physician with a patient who is perfectly still and a mode where the ventilator can be held during crucial pictures as respiratory variation leads to inaccurate images.

Percutaneous versus open access

This choice is usually determined by the type of device, the size of the sheath required for introduction of the endograft, and the presence of significant plaque in the access arteries. The Excluder® endograft (W. L. Gore & Assoc., Phoenix, AZ) permits percutaneous access. The

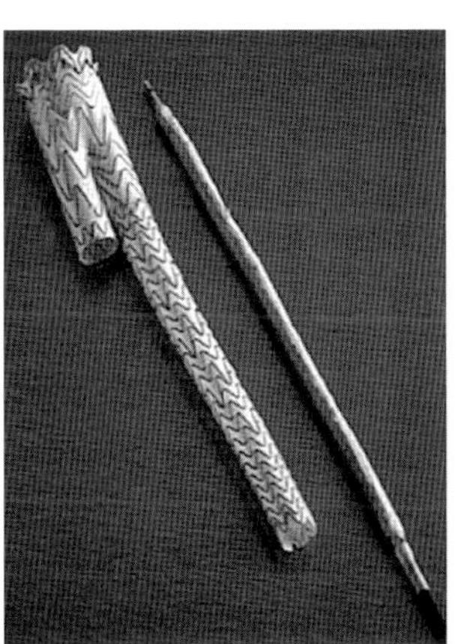

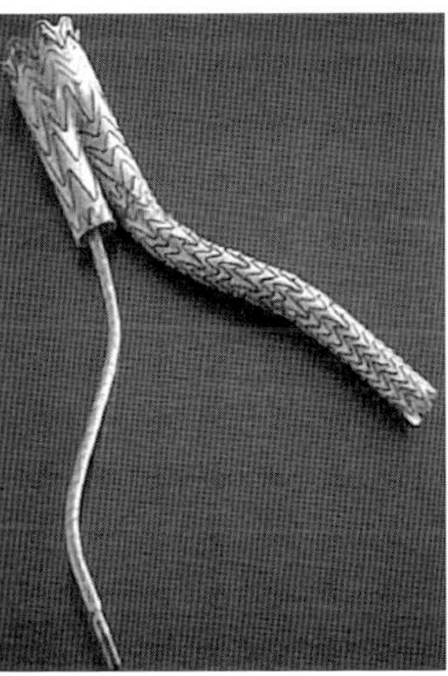

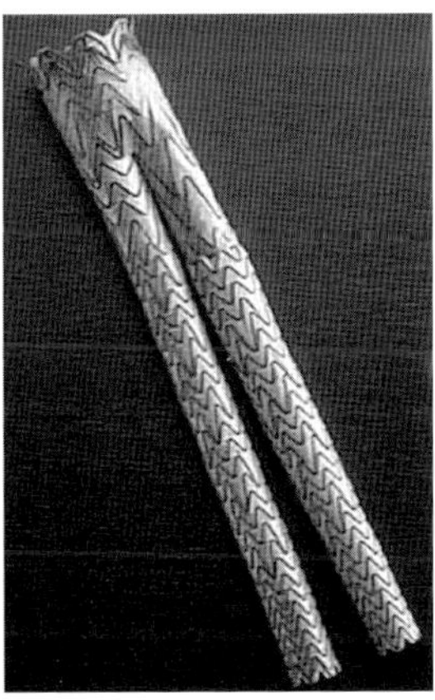

Figure 8 Bifurcated supported endograft.

use of the percutaneous access route mandates the employment of a closure device at the end of the procedure. Patients who have plaque in the femoral arteries or who have undergone previous groin explorations are likely to benefit from open access so the soft portion of the artery can be accurately accessed thereby limiting arterial dissections.

Femoral versus retroperitoneal access

The measurement of the femoral artery diameter is an important determinant of whether to insert the device into this artery as opposed to the retroperitoneal iliac arteries or aorta. Femoral arteries smaller than 8 mm force the physician to think about using the larger iliac artery or aorta for device insertion. In addition, the presence of substantial plaque in the femoral arteries also makes the larger arteries more favorable for device sheath placement.

Procedure overview

Once the patient is selected and the appropriate device is in hand to deal with the particular aneurysm morphology, the patient is brought into the interventional or operating room suite for the procedure. The procedure is now performed by interventional radiologists, cardiologists, and vascular surgeons with the patient under general, regional, or local anesthesia (6). The access arteries are chosen and an aortogram is performed to locate the renal and internal iliac arteries. The main body of the device is then inserted through either arteriotomy but the largest and most disease free artery is preferred. The patient is anticoagulated as at this point in the procedure, blood flow to the legs is interrupted by the size of the sheath and in addition, anticoagulation helps prevent embolization. Heparin or a direct thrombin inhibitor (e.g., bivalirudin) may be used (7). The location of the renal arteries with respect to the top of the endograft is reassessed and the endograft is then deployed. Next, the limbs of the device are inserted through each groin into the respective leg of the endograft. Once again the location of the internal iliac arteries are verified before the limbs are landed just proximal to their orifices or distally if the internal iliac artery was embolized preoperatively.

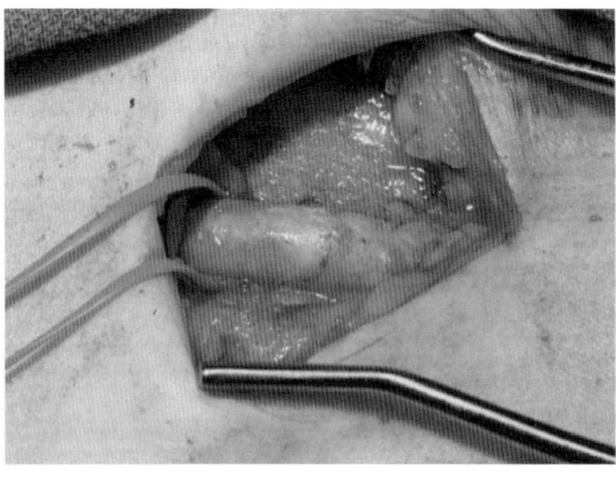

Figure 9 Femoral arteriotomy.

Closure

Percutaneous closure devices can be used to close the arteriotomy but if there is a problem such as bleeding or loss of distal pulses, the artery should be evaluated by an open approach.

Postoperative care

The patient is monitored for distal pulses, renal function, and abdominal pain. Any significant change in these should lead to an imaging study to evaluate the femoral artery, renal arteries, and endograft seal of aneurysm sac flow that can result in sac expansion and possible rupture.

Procedural challenges and solutions

Difficult iliacs

If the iliac artery has substantial plaque and stenosis, an iliac angioplasty can be performed prior to inserting the large sheath. In the case of a tortuous ileofemoral system, a second stiff buddy wire can be passed through the arteriotomy to facilitate straightening of the ileofemoral system and permit easier delivery of the device along its wire. In addition, if one iliac cannot be negotiated then an aortouniiliac device may be inserted with occlusion of the tortuous/calcified iliac with a plug. Then, a femoral–femoral bypass is performed to provide flow to the leg.

Difficult neck

The difficult neck comes in a variety of types: angulated, conical, and stenotic. The angulated neck makes wire passage challenging, but this can be overcome with the use of flexible sheaths and if necessary brachial artery insertion of the initial wire for retrieval from the femoral artery. In addition, the angulation often straightens during endograft placement and therefore the ability to judge the exact post-procedure location of the graft is difficult, especially with respect to the renal arteries. The conical neck increases in diameter from the renals to the aneurysm sac. This neck is a challenge for endograft sizing and achievement of graft seal. The former is often dealt with by decreasing the amount of usual graft oversizing to 10–15%; this reduces stretching the narrower portion of the conical neck. Endografts that require balloon expansion as opposed to radial force may facilitate graft seal when dealing with the conical neck. The third type of challenging neck is the stenotic neck. Once again, the issue centers on the importance of sizing the graft correctly. If the graft is oversized for the stenotic portion, graft infolding may occur. On the other hand, if the graft is undersized, then the neck may seal but the remainder of the repair does not fit properly, leading to endoleak and possible graft migration.

Large aneurysm

A large aneurysm sac can render contralateral limb cannulation challenging. There are methods to help with this situation: use of a stabilizing sheath close to the limb; snaring a wire that was inserted through the ipsilateral limb and placed up and over the bifurcation into the contralateral limb; or snaring a wire that has been inserted through the brachial artery down into the contralateral limb.

Ruptured AAA

In case of ruptured AAA, mortality reaches 90%; as many as 50% of patients who make it to the operating room for open repair die (8). Emergency repair of the ruptured AAA using the endovascular approach shows great promise. The Montefiore Endovascular Graft (MEG) device uses placement of a proximal occlusion balloon through the brachial artery to lodge in the descending thoracic artery. This device permits intraoperative adjustments for proximal neck diameter and distal limb length. Some of the key maneuvers include permissive hypotension, placement of the brachial wire under local anesthesia, performance of a diagnostic angiogram, and of course, readiness for conversion to an open procedure if necessary. This endovascular approach to ruptured AAAs has been used in an increasing number of patients and there are some small studies that show it has some real benefits in these critically ill patients, including decreased mortality and complication rates (9,10).

Complications

As with any procedure, there is an important list of complications that the practitioner of EVAR for AAA must keep in mind during the procedure and of course during the surveillance period. A fair number of these complications are minor and can simply be watched carefully, whereas a smaller number require reintervention in the form of either surgery or other catheter based procedures (11). Table 3 displays one way of categorizing the complications.

Access-related complications

As with any procedure that accesses the femoral arteries, distal embolization of plaque or thrombus may occur. This may be treated by embolectomy and heparinization. In addition, dissection of the iliac, profunda, and/or superficial femoral artery may lead to an ischemic limb. Dissection of the iliac artery is often treated with stenting, whereas problems with the profunda and/or superficial femoral artery may require stenting, endarterectomy, or bypass.

Deployment-related complications

Failed deployment of the device is often treated by surgical conversion, whereas iliac artery

Table 3 EVAR Complications

Access-related
Hematoma
Lymphocele
Infection
Embolization
Ischemic limb
Deployment-related
Failed deployment
Arterial rupture
Dissection
Device-related
Structural failure
Implant-related
Endoleaks
Limb occlusion
Stent graft kink
Sac enlargement
Proximal neck dilatation
Stent migration
AAA rupture
Infection
Buttock/leg claudication
Systemic
Cardiac
Pulmonary
Renal insufficiency
Cerebrovascular
Deep vein thrombosis
Pulmonary embolism
Coagulopathy
Bowel ischemia
Spinal cord ischemia
Erectile dysfunction

rupture and dissection can be dealt with by stenting or conversion.

Device-related complications

Structural failure is usually noted during the follow-up period and was more common with earlier devices where there were breaks in the struts. This is less of a problem today.

Implant-related endoleaks

Endoleaks are the complication that is unique to EVAR. Endoleak describes the continuation of blood flow into the extragraft portion of the aneurysm (12). It is either graft-related or non-graft-related; a classification system has been developed (Table. 4) (13). These are diagnosed by a variety of techniques: arteriography, pressure monitoring during the procedure, CT scan, abdominal X-ray, and duplex scanning. The preferred method for detecting endoleaks is by CT scanning.

Treatment of Endoleaks

The methods employed to treat endoleaks include coil embolization, placement of stent-graft cuffs and extensions, laparoscopic ligation of inferior mesenteric and lumbar arteries, open surgical repair, and EVAR redo procedures. Type I and III endoleaks require fairly urgent intervention because blood flow and sac pressure will continue to increase and lead to rupture. Type IV endoleaks usually resolve on their own.

The management of Type II endoleaks is more controversial because some of them will thrombose on their own while others will lead to sac enlargement. The challenge with Type II endoleaks is determining when to intervene (14). One approach is to monitor with a 6-month post-procedure CT scan. If the aneurysm has increased in size then a plan for intervention is formulated.

Table 4 Classification of endoleaks

I	Attachment site leaks
	• Proximal end of endograft
	• Distal end of endograft
	• Iliac occluder (plug)
II	Branch leaks (without attachment site connection
	• Simple or to-and-fro (from only 1 patent branch)
	• Complex or flow-through (with 2 or more patent branches)
III	Graft defect
	• Junctional leak or modular disconnect
	• Fabric disruption (midgraft hole)
	• Minor (<2 mm; e.g., suture holes)
	• Major (≥ to 2 mm)
	• Graft wall (fabric) porosity (<30 days after graft placement)

There are at least 3 approaches to manage Type II endoleaks: transarterial, translumbar embolization, and laparoscopic ligation (15).

Limb occlusion

Limb occlusion is an infrequently encountered problem, occurring in less than 5% of patients, but its morbidity is serious as it may lead to limb loss (16). Small limb diameter and graft extension to the external iliac artery, as opposed to the common iliac, is a risk factor for the development of limb occlusion. The majority of limb occlusions will require intervention: surgical (femoro-femoral, axillary-femoral, axillary-bifemoral bypasses) and/or endoluminal techniques (rheolytic and pharmacologic thrombolysis).

Stent graft kinks

Stent graft kinks are more often seen when unsupported endografts are used (17). This finding is associated with Types I and III endoleaks, graft stenosis, graft limb thrombosis, graft migration, and conversion to open repair (18). In addition, women with angulated AAA necks are at most risk for stent graft kink. This problem is usually managed with stenting of the kink.

Sac enlargement

Sac enlargement is usually attributed to the presence of an endoleak. Once this is located, then it should be treated to prevent sac rupture.

Proximal neck dilatation

This problem is found during the surveillance period and is associated with proximal stent migration, a wide preoperative neck, large aneurysm diameter, short necks, proximal endoleak, and absence of suprarenal fixation. If a proximal endoleak is noted it should be fixed expediently, otherwise this finding can be followed closely.

Stent migration

The risk factors for this complication include low initial deployment, below the renals, and short proximal fixation length. The majority of patients will require no treatment and others will require placement of extender modules or surgical conversion. Devices with an active fixation design (e.g., Zenith™, Cook Medical, Inc., Bloomington, IN) may be protective against migration.

Ischemia

Ischemia to the viscera and extremities can also occur and can present with subtle signs like decreased pulses, mild abdominal pain, buttock claudication, or with more obvious problems such as lower extremity mottling, severe abdominal pain, elevated creatinine phosphokinase levels, or gastrointestinal bleeding. Lower extremity ischemia can result from problems at the femoral access site (dissection, atheroembolization) or from issues with the endograft (limb occlusion, kinking). The former often requires surgical intervention whereas the latter can be managed by interventional techniques like placing additional stents. The endograft covers the inferior mesenteric artery and if the remainder of the visceral and hypogastric circulation is poor or compromised, this can lead to colonic ischemia. In addition, spinal cord ischemia can manifest in paresis or paralysis due to the coverage of intercostal arteries; this complication is rare but serious.

Rupture

Rupture is fortunately a rare event; if it occurs in a stable patient, it is usually treated with surgical conversion or the placement of an occluding balloon followed by a covered stent. The presence of a Type I or III endoleak indicates a risk of aneurysm rupture.

Follow-up

Endograft surveillance is important to document normal and abnormal morphological changes in the repair and the involved vessels. This process is vital for the detection of endoleaks, increased aneurysm diameter, and possible device migration (19). Perigraft air, accompanied by leukocytosis and fever, can be

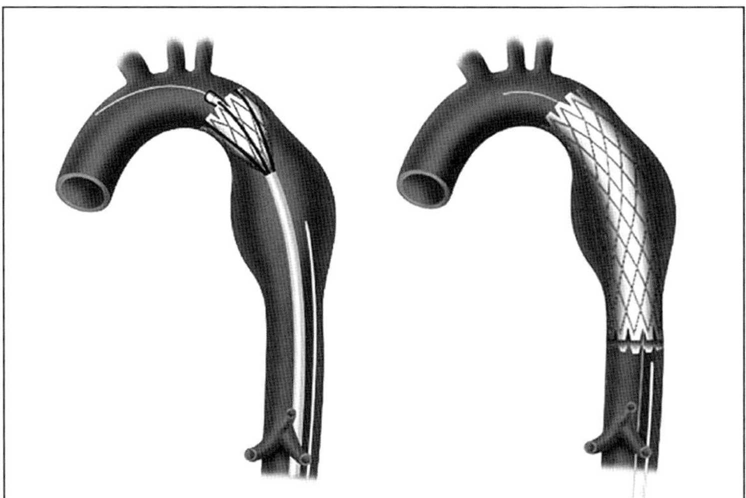

Figure 10 Endovascular repair of thoracic aneurysms.

detected following repair and has been shown to be nonspecific and not indicative of graft infection (20).

The recommended surveillance routine is for a CT scan at 1, 6, and 12 months and annually thereafter. If an endoleak is detected, the frequency of the scans increases to every 6 months until resolution of the endoleak is detected. CT scan is superior to duplex or magnetic resonance imaging (MRI) for endoleak detection (21). MRI can also be used for graft surveillance especially in older patients with decreased renal function (22). A recent development for endograft surveillance is the monitoring of sac pressure within treated aneurysms through an implanted sensor device (23, 24). Trials with this implanted sensor are currently being conducted.

ENDOVASCULAR REPAIR OF THORACIC ANEURYSMS

Endovascular repair of thoracic aneurysms caused by degenerative or traumatic diseases has had a major impact on the treatment of these difficult lesions. This approach is minimally invasive and involves the placement of one or more covered stents across the aneurysm sac to exclude it from high pressure aortic blood flow (Fig. 10). This results in eventual thrombosis of the aneurysm sac. Open surgical repair of this lesion involves thoracotomy, aortic cross-clamping, ligation of intercostal arteries, and suturing the graft proximally and distally to often poor-quality aortic tissue. Many surgeons routinely place the patient on partial or full cardiopulmonary bypass to permit visceral perfusion during the procedure. EVAR of thoracic aneurysms is particularly attractive because the morbidity and mortality of open repair is high and much greater than that for open repair of AAAs. The indications for treating thoracic aneurysms are detailed in Table.5.

Patient selection

Endografts are considered to be part of the algorithm for thoracic aneurysm repair in patients who are at high risk for open repair and who have favorable anatomy for this approach. Without the longterm data on how this approach fares, many physicians advise young and medically fit patients to undergo open surgical repair.

Table 5 Indications for TAA Repair
1. $\geq$ 60 mm diameter or $>$2 $\times$ transverse diameter of an adjacent normal aortic segment
2. Symptomatic regardless of size
3. Growth rate of aneurysm to $>$3 mm/yr

Table 6 Anatomic requirements for endovascular repair of thoracic aortic aneurysm

1. A proximal neck at least 15 to 25 mm from the origin of the left subclavian artery
2. A distal neck at least 15 to 25 mm proximal to the origin of the celiac artery
3. Adequate vascular access—absence of severe tortuosity, calcification, or atherosclerotic plaque burden involving the aortic or pelvic vasculature
4. The transverse diameter of the proximal and distal neck should be within the range that available devices can appropriately accommodate

Preoperative assessment and imaging

The aneurysm and access vessels are evaluated with detailed preoperative imaging using spiral CT, MRI, or angiography with a calibrated catheter. Sometimes additional studies using transesophageal echocardiography or intravenous ultrasound can help delineate the anatomy (Table 6). The distance of normal aorta between the aneurysm neck and the left subclavian artery take-off is an important measurement. Ideally the first stent is landed between 1.5 and 2.5 cm distal to this vessel. It is paramount that an adequate seal with normal aortic wall is obtained with the endograft to prevent the development of Type I endoleaks. The device is oversized by 10–20% to obtain sufficient radial force for fixation and seal. In some situations the diameter of the normal aortic landing zone is too large for current devices. If an adequate landing zone would involve coverage of one or more of the great vessels, then debranching of these vessels can be achieved through a carotid–subclavian bypass or more extensive operative procedures using a partial median sternotomy. The angulation of the descending aorta must be noted because sometimes the delivery system is not able to navigate this angle into the arch.

The size, tortuosity, and calcification of the femoral and iliac arteries must be visualized adequately with these preoperative images. Since thoracic endografts are large and therefore require larger sheaths for insertion, small femoral and/or iliac arteries can pose a problem that is usually overcome by sewing a conduit (Dacron or PTFE) onto the aorta or iliac artery through a retroperitoneal incision.

Choosing the device

Two devices are currently approved by the FDA for treatment of thoracic aneurysms in the United States (TAG®, W.L. Gore and Associates, Inc., Phoenix, AZ and TX2®, Cook Medical Inc., Bloomington, IN), and one other is undergoing clinical trials for FDA approval (Talent™, Medtronic, Inc., Minneapolis, MN) (Table 7). Each has its advantages and disadvantages.

TAG®

The TAG® endograft is made of a self-expanding nitinol stent lined with polytetrafluoroethylene (PTFE) graft material. The device is very flexible and this helps when the device is delivered into the aortic arch with its natural angulation. The device is covered at the proximal end.

TX2®

The TX2® thoracic endograft is a two-component device made with stainless steel Gianturco Z-stents and polyester fabric. The distal end of the distal component is uncovered and both ends have barbs to facilitate fixation to the aortic wall.

Talent™

The Talent™ stent-graft is stiffer than the aforementioned devices because it has longitudinal bars that provide support. This device is composed of sinusoidal nitinol stent elements with polyester graft material. It has an uncovered proximal end thereby permitting fixation across the left subclavian artery origin without preventing flow.

Table 7 Available devices for thoracic gneanrysm repair

Device (company)	*Stent/graft material*	*Delivery profile*	*Unique properties*
TAG (W. L. Gore, & assoc., Phoenix, AZ)	Nitinol/PTFE	20–24 Fr	Flexible
Talent (Medtronic, Bloomington, IN)	Nitinol/polyester	22–27 Fr	Uncovered proximally
TX2 (Cook Medical, Inc., Bloomington, IN)	Stainless steel/ polyester	20–22 Fr	Fixation barbs

Abbreviation: PTFE, Polytetrafluoroethylene.

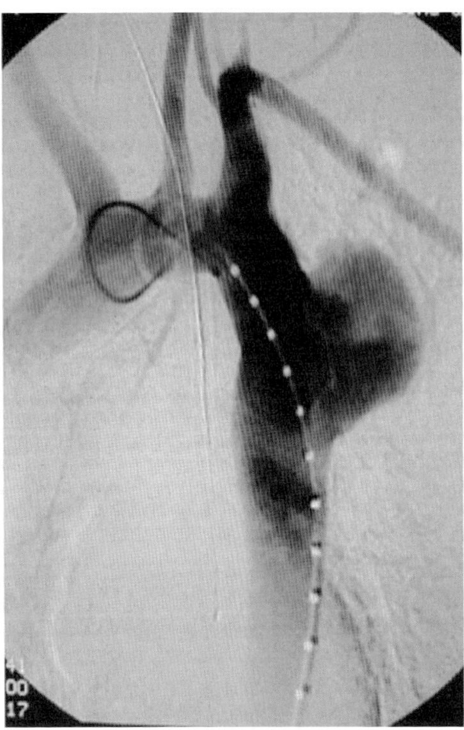

Figure 11 Arch aortogram.

The procedure

Preoperative preparation, anesthesia, and access route

The same factors as mentioned in the endovascular treatment of AAAs also apply to this scenario. The vascular access route, however, is a particularly important consideration in the endovascular treatment of thoracic aneurysms. Due to the large delivery system, access is obtained by an open surgical approach in the groin. This facilitates accurate closure of the arteriotomy at the completion of the procedure. Also, the left and right arm pressures are noted as these are monitored postoperatively.

Procedure overview

The device is chosen after assessment of preoperative imaging. The patient is brought into the operating room or interventional suite. The groins are prepped and the procedure is performed under general, regional, or local anesthesia. Usually one groin is accessed percutaneously and a short sheath is inserted. This is followed by insertion of a long wire (Bentson, for example) and a diagnostic catheter that will reach up into the aortic arch. At this point, some physicians image the left subclavian and aneurysm neck whereas others wait until the device is inserted.

The other groin and common femoral artery is accessed by open surgical technique to provide passage for the endograft and its large sheath. Generally the less tortuous and atherosclerotic artery is chosen for this portion of the procedure. An 18-gauge baseplate needle punctures the common femoral artery that is controlled with vessel loops. Next a floppy wire (Bentson) is placed through this access and placed up in the aortic arch. A Kumpe catheter (or its equivalent) helps negotiate this wire up into the arch and serves for the next exchange. Then, the floppy wire is exchanged for a stiff wire (Lunderquist® Cook Medical Inc., Bloomington, IN, or Amplatz™, Boston Scientific, Natick, MA; often a particular type is recommended by the device manufacturer). The patient is then systemically heparinized to an ACT of 250.

The device is prepped according to the manufacturer's instructions. The device is now inserted through its large sheath. Some devices are packaged within the sheath, whereas others require a separate sheath and device. The device is delivered just distal to the left subclavian artery essentially to the landing zone. Attention is paid to negotiation of the sheath and device through the iliac artery. At this point, an arch aortogram is performed using the diagnostic catheter that was inserted through the short sheath in the other groin (Fig. 11). Preoperative measurements are confirmed. The blood pressure is dropped to a systolic of about 100 mmHg and the diagnostic catheter is withdrawn just distal to the device. Sometimes, adenosine is used to temporarily stop the heart while the device is deployed. Once delivery is achieved, another arch aortogram is performed with the diagnostic catheter now placed through the device up into the arch. A balloon is now inserted through the device sheath to secure the proximal and distal device landing zones. Once again, an arch aortogram is performed to assess device placement and look for endoleaks. If another endograft is needed distally, this is now inserted. Once the aneurysm is excluded by one or more stents, the procedure is completed and the sheath is removed under direct vision. We prefer to leave the wire in place while the sheath is removed in case there is evidence of an iliac artery rupture. This allows us to insert a balloon and or covered stent to treat this problem. The arteriotomy is closed in the usual fashion and distal pulses are assessed. The diagnostic catheter and short sheath are removed and manual pressure is applied. If the distal pulses are intact, we give protamine to reverse heparinization. Attention is paid to the secure closure of the open groin to prevent development of a hematoma or lymphocele.

Closure

This is performed in the usual surgical fashion with attention to post closure Doppler signals and postoperative distal pulses.

Postoperative care

The patient is monitored for distal pulses, renal function, and chest/abdominal pain. Any significant change in these should be evaluated by an imaging study to assess the femoral and iliac arteries, aorta, and endograft seal of aneurysm sac flow leading to expansion and possible rupture. In addition, the arm pressures are examined and any ischemic symptoms in the left arm are noted and diagnosed.

Procedural challenges and solutions

Large sheath insertion

If the artery is too small or calcified, the iliac artery or distal aorta should be evaluated for possible retroperitoneal exposure with the anastomosis of a conduit or direct access at this level. Stenosis in the iliac artery can be treated with balloon angioplasty to facilitate large sheath insertion.

Difficult iliacs

If the iliac artery has substantial plaque and stenosis, an iliac angioplasty can be performed prior to inserting the large sheath. A second stiff buddy wire can be passed through the arteriotomy to facilitate straightening of the iliofemoral system and permit easier delivery of the device along its wire.

Aorta or arch tortuosity

A wire advanced through the right brachial artery through the arch and down to the femoral artery can be used to deliver the device through a tortuous aorta and/or arch.

Landing

If the landing zone distal to the left subclavian artery is inadequate, then the arch can be debranched with a prior left carotid–left subclavian bypass or transposition procedure. Also, many patients will tolerate intentional coverage of the left subclavian artery. If the left common carotid artery orifice must also be covered, then an additional right carotid-left carotid bypass can be performed.

Inadvertent coverage of the left subclavian artery or left common carotid artery

Most patients will tolerate coverage of the left subclavian artery with the device. If the brachial artery pulse is lost following this maneuver or the patient is symptomatic, then a left carotid–left subclavian bypass or transposition can be performed. If the left common carotid artery is inadvertently covered, then a balloon can be placed up into the orifice and inflated to permit perfusion into the left common carotid system. If this fails, then a carotid–carotid bypass is performed. Patients in whom the left internal mammary artery was used for coronary artery bypass grafting will likely not tolerate left subclavian artery coverage.

Complications

Most of the complications detailed in Table 3 for endovascular AAA repair also apply to repair of thoracic aneurysms with stents.

Access and deployment-related complications

Hematomas, lymphoceles, and wound infection can occur if either the groin or retroperitoneum is accessed directly. Proper anticoagulation with heparin or a direct thrombin inhibitor can help prevent distal embolization and ischemia especially given the large occlusive size of most thoracic endograft sheaths. The key maneuver to avoid arterial rupture and dissection is to properly judge the diameter and calcification severity of the access arteries prior to the procedure. If the femoral arteries are not of an appropriate size or are too calcified, then the retroperitoneal vessels should be evaluated for direct access.

Device-related complications

Metal fracture, fabric erosion, and suture breakage are rare but reported complications are seen during the surveillance period.

Implant-related complications

As with EVAR for AAAs, endoleaks are a prominent complication of thoracic stenting but the incidence is smaller in this group (25). However, the majority of the endoleaks occur at the proximal or distal fixation sites (Type I) (26). These require immediate attention and formulation of a treatment plan, as it is well known that type I endoleaks can lead to aneurysm sac growth and increased risk of rupture. The modalities used to treat these include endovascular graft extensions or cuffs, balloon angioplasty, coil/glue embolization, and open repair (27,28).

If the proximal fixation and seal are not adequate, device collapse can occur as the high blood flow in the aorta pushes one stent wall onto the other. This can occur when device sizing is not accurate. Another consequence of poor proximal fixation and seal is device migration and kinking, but this tends to occur more often with unsupported early grafts.

Systemic complications

A particular risk with thoracic aneurysm repair either by endovascular or open technique is paraplegia that thought to result from exclusion of blood flow into the spinal artery (29–32). The incidence of this complication is lower with endovascular repair (0–5% vs. 5–25%) since the added insult of hypotension and aortic cross-clamping is eliminated. Adjunctive methods are commonly employed in open surgical repair of thoracic aneurysms (spinal cord drainage, epidural cooling, etc.) and these are also being investigated in endovascular repair (51).

Follow-up

The protocol for surveillance post thoracic stenting is similar to what is used for endovascular AAA repair. The main purpose is to detect problems that lead to increased risk of aneurysm rupture. Follow-up surveillance with serial CT scans at 1, 6, and 12 months and annually thereafter is recommended to monitor changes in aneurysm morphology, identify device failures, and detect endoleaks.

FUTURE OF ENDOVASCULAR TREATMENT OF AAA AND THORACIC ANEURYSMS

The future of endovascular treatment of AAAs and thoracic aneurysms rests in the ability to design and deploy devices that can deal with visceral and arch branches emanating from the aneurysm sac. This advance will bring this low morbidity and mortality procedure to a greater number of patients who now can only be repaired by open surgical techniques. In addition, work is being undertaken in new implantable sac pressure monitoring devices that may lead to less reliance on CT scanning for follow-up. And finally, the results of trials to assess durability of endovascular repair will become available for analysis.

REFERENCES

1. Huber TS, Wang JG, Derrow AE, et al. Experience in the United States with intact abdominal aortic aneurysm repair. J Vasc Surg 2001; 33(2):304–310; discussion 10–11.
2. Mathison M, Becker GJ, Katzen BT, et al. The influence of female gender on the outcome of endovascular abdominal aortic aneurysm repair. J Vasc Interv Radiol 2001; 12(9):1047–1051.
3. Mathison MN, Becker GJ, Katzen BT, et al. Implications of problematic access in transluminal endografting of abdominal aortic aneurysm. J Vasc Interv Radiol 2003; 14(1):33–39.
4. Powell JT, Greenhalgh RM. Clinical practice. Small abdominal aortic aneurysms. N Engl J Med 2003; 348(19):1895–1901.
5. Scott RA, Tisi PV, Ashton HA, Allen DR. Abdominal aortic aneurysm rupture rates: a 7-year follow-up of the entire abdominal aortic aneurysm population detected by screening. J Vasc Surg 1998; 28(1):124–128.
6. Parra JR, Crabtree T, McLafferty RB, et al. Anesthesia technique and outcomes of endovascular aneurysm repair. Ann Vasc Surg 2005; 19(1): 123–129.
7. Katzen BT, Ardid MI, MacLean AA, et al. Bivalirudin as an anticoagulation agent: safety and efficacy in peripheral interventions. J Vasc Interv Radiol 2005; 16(9):1183–1187; quiz 7.
8. Bown MJ, Sutton AJ, Bell PR, Sayers RD. A meta-analysis of 50 years of ruptured abdominal aortic aneurysm repair. Br J Surg 2002; 89(6):714–730.
9. Lee WA, Hirneise CM, Tayyarah M, Huber TS, Seeger JM. Impact of endovascular repair on early outcomes of ruptured abdominal aortic aneurysms. J Vasc Surg 2004; 40(2):211–215.
10. Ohki T, Veith FJ. Endovascular therapy for ruptured abdominal aortic aneurysms. Adv Surg 2001; 35:131–151.
11. Elkouri S, Gloviczki P, McKusick MA, et al. Perioperative complications and early outcome after endovascular and open surgical repair of abdominal aortic aneurysms. J Vasc Surg 2004; 39(3):497–505.
12. White GH, Yu W, May J. Endoleak—a proposed new terminology to describe incomplete aneurysm exclusion by an endoluminal graft. J Endovasc Surg 1996; 3(1):124–125.
13. Veith FJ, Baum RA, Ohki T, et al. Nature and significance of endoleaks and endotension: summary of opinions expressed at an international conference. J Vasc Surg 2002; 35(5): 1029–1035.
14. Maldonado TS, Gagne PJ. Controversies in the management of type II "branch" endoleaks following endovascular abdominal aortic aneurysm repair. Vasc Endovascular Surg 2003; 37(1):1–12.
15. Hinchliffe RJ, Singh-Ranger R, Whitaker SC, Hopkinson BR. Type II endoleak: transperitoneal sacotomy and ligation of side branch endoleaks responsible for aneurysm sac expansion. J Endovasc Ther 2002; 9(4):539–542.
16. Carroccio A, Faries PL, Morrissey NJ, et al. Predicting iliac limb occlusions after bifurcated aortic stent grafting: anatomic and device-related causes. J Vasc Surg 2002; 36(4):679–684.
17. Carpenter JP, Neschis DG, Fairman RM, et al. Failure of endovascular abdominal aortic aneurysm graft limbs. J Vasc Surg 2001; 33(2):296–302; discussion 3.
18. Fransen GA, Desgranges P, Laheij RJ, Harris PL, Becquemin JP. Frequency, predictive factors, and

consequences of stent-graft kink following endovascular AAA repair. J Endovasc Ther 2003; 10(5):913–918.
19. Corriere MA, Feurer ID, Becker SY, et al. Endoleak following endovascular abdominal aortic aneurysm repair: implications for duration of screening. Ann Surg 2004; 239(6):800–805; discussion 5–7.
20. Velazquez OC, Carpenter JP, Baum RA, et al. Perigraft air, fever, and leukocytosis after endovascular repair of abdominal aortic aneurysms. Am J Surg 1999; 178(3):185–189.
21. Raman KG, Missig-Carroll N, Richardson T, Muluk SC, Makaroun MS. Color-flow duplex ultrasound scan versus computed tomographic scan in the surveillance of endovascular aneurysm repair. J Vasc Surg 2003; 38(4):645–651.
22. Engellau L, Albrechtsson U, Hojgard S, Norgren L, Larsson EM. Costs in follow-up of endovascularly repaired abdominal aortic aneurysms. Magnetic resonance imaging with MR angiography versus EUROSTAR protocols. Int Angiol 2003; 22(1):36–42.
23. Baum RA, Carpenter JP, Cope C, et al. Aneurysm sac pressure measurements after endovascular repair of abdominal aortic aneurysms. J Vasc Surg 2001; 33(1):32–41.
24. Ellozy SH, Carroccio A, Lookstein RA, et al. First experience in human beings with a permanently implantable intrasac pressure transducer for monitoring endovascular repair of abdominal aortic aneurysms. J Vasc Surg 2004; 40(3):405–412.
25. Thurnher SA, Grabenwoger M. Endovascular treatment of thoracic aortic aneurysms: a review. Eur Radiol 2002; 12(6):1370–1387.
26. Resch T, Koul B, Dias NV, Lindblad B, Ivancev K. Changes in aneurysm morphology and stent-graft configuration after endovascular repair of aneurysms of the descending thoracic aorta. J Thorac Cardiovasc Surg 2001; 122(1):47–52.
27. Chuter TA, Faruqi RM, Sawhney R, et al. Endoleak after endovascular repair of abdominal aortic aneurysm. J Vasc Surg 2001; 34(1): 98–105.
28. Kato N, Semba CP, Dake MD. Embolization of perigraft leaks after endovascular stent-graft treatment of aortic aneurysms. J Vasc Interv Radiol 1996; 7(6):805–811.
29. DeBakey ME, McCollum CH, Graham JM. Surgical treatment of aneurysms of the descending thoracic aorta: long-term results in 500 patients. J Cardiovasc Surg (Torino) 1978; 19:571–576.
30. Moreno-Cabral CE, Miller DC, Mitchell RS, et al. Degenerative and atherosclerotic aneurysms of the thoracic aorta. Determinants of early and late surgical outcome. J Thorac Cardiovasc Surg 1984; 88(6):1020–1032.
31. Svensson LG, Crawford ES, Hess KR, Coselli JS, Safi HJ. Experience with 1509 patients undergoing thoracoabdominal aortic operations. J Vasc Surg 1993; 17(2):357–368; discussion 68–70.
32. Livesay JJ, Cooley DA, Ventemiglia RA, et al. Surgical experience in descending thoracic aneurysmectomy with and without adjuncts to avoid ischemia. Ann Thorac Surg 1985; 39(1):37–46.
33. Dake MD, Miller DC, Mitchell RS, Semba CP, Moore KA, Sakai T. The "first generation" of endovascular stent-grafts for patients with aneurysms of the descending thoracic aorta. J Thorac Cardiovasc Surg 1998; 116(5):689–703; discussion 4.
34. Bergeron P, De Chaumaray T, Gay J, Douillez V. Endovascular treatment of thoracic aortic aneurysms. J Cardiovasc Surg (Torino) 2003; 44(3): 349–361.
35. Cartes-Zumelzu F, Lammer J, Kretschmer G, Hoelzenbein T, Grabenwoger M, Thurnher S. Endovascular repair of thoracic aortic aneurysms. Semin Interv Cardiol 2000; 5(1): 53–57.
36. Czerny M, Cejna M, Hutschala D, et al. Stent-graft placement in atherosclerotic descending thoracic aortic aneurysms: midterm results. J Endovasc Ther 2004; 11(1):26–32.
37. Ehrlich M, Grabenwoeger M, Cartes-Zumelzu F, et al. Endovascular stent graft repair for aneurysms on the descending thoracic aorta. Ann Thorac Surg 1998; 66(1):19–24; discussion 5.
38. Grabenwoger M, Hutschala D, Ehrlich MP, et al. Thoracic aortic aneurysms: treatment with endovascular self-expandable stent grafts. Ann Thorac Surg 2000; 69(2):441–445.
39. Greenberg R, Resch T, Nyman U, et al. Endovascular repair of descending thoracic aortic aneurysms: an early experience with intermediate-term follow-up. J Vasc Surg 2000; 31(1 Pt 1): 147–156.
40. Heijmen RH, Deblier IG, Moll FL, et al. Endovascular stent-grafting for descending thoracic aortic aneurysms. Eur J Cardiothorac Surg 2002; 21(1): 5–9.

41. Lepore V, Lonn L, Delle M, Mellander S, Radberg G, Risberg B. Treatment of descending thoracic aneurysms by endovascular stent grafting. J Card Surg 2003; 18(5):436–443.
42. Marin ML, Hollier LH, Ellozy SH, et al. Endovascular stent graft repair of abdominal and thoracic aortic aneurysms: a ten-year experience with 817 patients. Ann Surg 2003; 238(4):586-593; discussion 93–95.
43. Najibi S, Terramani TT, Weiss VJ, et al. Endoluminal versus open treatment of descending thoracic aortic aneurysms. J Vasc Surg 2002; 36(4): 732–737.
44. Ouriel K, Greenberg RK. Endovascular treatment of thoracic aortic aneurysms. J Card Surg 2003; 18(5):455–463.
45. Schoder M, Cartes-Zumelzu F, Grabenwoger M, et al. Elective endovascular stent-graft repair of atherosclerotic thoracic aortic aneurysms: clinical results and midterm follow-up. AJR Am J Roentgenol 2003; 180(3):709–715.
46. Sunder-Plassmann L, Scharrer-Pamler R, Liewald F, Kapfer X, Gorich J, Orend KH. Endovascular exclusion of thoracic aortic aneurysms: midterm results of elective treatment and in contained rupture. J Card Surg 2003; 18(4): 367–374.
47. Temudom T, D'Ayala M, Marin ML, et al. Endovascular grafts in the treatment of thoracic aortic aneurysms and pseudoaneurysms. Ann Vasc Surg 2000; 14(3):230–238.
48. Leurs LJ, Bell R, Degrieck Y, Thomas S, Hobo R, Lundbom J. Endovascular treatment of thoracic aortic diseases: combined experience from the EUROSTAR and United Kingdom Thoracic Endograft registries. J Vasc Surg 2004; 40(4): 670–679; discussion 9–80.
49. Makaroun MS, Dillavou ED, Kee ST, et al. Endovascular treatment of thoracic aortic aneurysms: Results of the Phase II multicenter trial of the GORE TAG thoracic endoprosthesis. The Society for Vascular Surgery Annual Meeting 2004, Anaheim, CA, USA, 2004.
50. Mitchell RS, Miller DC, Dake MD. Stent-graft repair of thoracic aortic aneurysms. Semin Vasc Surg 1997; 10(4):257–271.
51. Carroccio A, Marin ML, Ellozy S, Hollier LH. Pathophysiology of paraplegia following endovascular thoracic aortic aneurysm repair. J Card Surg 2003; 18(4):359–366.
52. Dake MD. Endovascular stent-graft management of thoracic aortic diseases. Eur J Radiol 2001; 39(1):42–49.
53. Hausegger KA, Oberwalder P, Tiesenhausen K, et al. Intentional left subclavian artery occlusion by thoracic aortic stent-grafts without surgical transposition. J Endovasc Ther 2001; 8(5): 472–476.
54. Burks JA Jr, Faries PL, Gravereaux EC, Hollier LH, Marin ML. Endovascular repair of thoracic aortic aneurysms: stent-graft fixation across the aortic arch vessels. Ann Vasc Surg 2002; 16(1): 24–28.
55. Gorich J, Asquan Y, Seifarth H, et al. Initial experience with intentional stent-graft coverage of the subclavian artery during endovascular thoracic aortic repairs. J Endovasc Ther 2002; 9(suppl 2): II39–II43.
56. Tiesenhausen K, Hausegger KA, Oberwalder P, et al. Left subclavian artery management in endovascular repair of thoracic aortic aneurysms and aortic dissections. J Card Surg 2003; 18(5): 429–435.
57. Stanley BM, Semmens JB, Lawrence-Brown MM, Goodman MA, Hartley DE. Fenestration in endovascular grafts for aortic aneurysm repair: new horizons for preserving blood flow in branch vessels. J Endovasc Ther 2001; 8(1): 16–24.
58. Inoue K, Hosokawa H, Iwase T, et al. Aortic arch reconstruction by transluminally placed endovascular branched stent graft. Circulation 1999; 100(19 suppl):II316–II321.
59. McWilliams RG, Murphy M, Hartley D, Lawrence-Brown MM, Harris PL. In situ stent-graft fenestration to preserve the left subclavian artery. J Endovasc Ther 2004; 11(2):170–174.
60. Heinemann MK, Buehner B, Jurmann MJ, Borst HG. Use of the "elephant trunk technique" in aortic surgery. Ann Thorac Surg 1995; 60(1):2–6; discussion 7.
61. Fann JI, Dake MD, Semba CP, Liddell RP, Pfeffer TA, Miller DC. Endovascular stent-grafting after arch aneurysm repair using the "elephant trunk." Ann Thorac Surg 1995; 60(4):1102–1105.
62. Dake MD, Kato N, Mitchell RS, et al. Endovascular stent-graft placement for the treatment of acute aortic dissection. N Engl J Med 1999; 340(20):1546–1552.
63. Kato N, Dake MD, Miller DC, et al. Traumatic thoracic aortic aneurysm: treatment with endovascular stent-grafts. Radiology 1997; 205(3): 657–662.

64. Eggebrecht H, Baumgart D, Schmermund A, et al. Penetrating atherosclerotic ulcer of the aorta: treatment by endovascular stent-graft placement. Curr Opin Cardiol 2003; 18(6):431–435.
65. Eggebrecht H, Baumgart D, Schmermund A, et al. Endovascular stent-graft repair for penetrating atherosclerotic ulcer of the descending aorta. Am J Cardiol 2003 1; 91(9):1150–1153.
66. Kato N, Hirano T, Ishida M, et al. Acute and contained rupture of the descending thoracic aorta: treatment with endovascular stent grafts. J Vasc Surg 2003; 37(1):100–105.

Index